How To Get
Your Kid To Eat...
But Not Too Much

Ellyn Satter, R.D., A.C.S.W.

Bull Publishing Company
Boulder, Co.

Bull Publishing Company
P.O. Box 1377
Boulder, Co. 80306
(800) 676-2855

ISBN 0-915950-83-9
www.bullpub.com

Distributed in the U.S. by:
Publishers Group West
1700 Fourth Street
Berkeley, CA 94710

Library of Congress Cataloging-in-Publication Data

Satter, Ellyn.
How to get your kid to eat—but not too much.

Bibliography: p.
Includes index.
1. Children—Nutrition. 2. Child rearing.
I. Title.

RJ206.S243 1987	*649'.3*	*87-25620*

ISBN 0-915950-83-9

Cover Design: Robb Pawlak
Cover Illustration: Kit C. King
Interior Design: Detta Penna
Text Illustrator: Ken Miller
Chapter Opening Art: Karen Foget
Production Manager: Helen O'Donnell
Compositor: Frank's Type, Mountain View, CA
Text Face: Aster
Display Face: Gill Sans Italic
Printer: Malloy Lithographing, Inc.

To
Donald Williams,
who knows children,
and David Bull,
who knows books.

Acknowledgements

This book did not come from me alone. My family, friends and colleagues gave generously of their time, expertise and encouragement, and I thank them.

For professional contributions and evaluation of the manuscript: Jack Bailey, Ph.D.; Melinda Bailey, Ph.D.; Bonnie Broderick, R.N.; Crista Dean, R.D.; Richard Guthrie, M.D.; Thomas Linscheid, Ph.D.; Deb McMillan, M.S.; Susan Nitzke, Ph.D.; Karen Ostrov, Ph.D.; Gail Price, Ph.D.; Deborah Roussos, M.S., R.D.; Erica Serlin, Ph.D.; Leona Shapiro, Ph.D.; Tom Tatum, M.A., CCC-SP; and Donald Williams, M.S.S.W., A.C.S.W.

For expert and resilient collaboration in putting together our mutual endeavor: Pat Anderson, David Bull, and Helen O'Donnell.

For love, encouragement, tolerance, distraction, humor, family maintenance and *even* word processing: Larry Satter, Kjerstin Satter, Lucas Satter, and Curtis Satter.

For her exquisite drawings: Karen Foget.

Table of Contents

Basic Principles of Feeding

Feeding As Your Child Grows

Figures

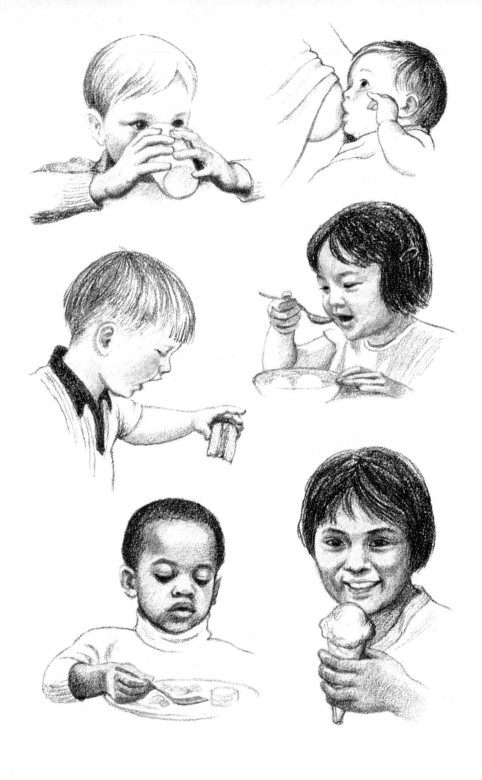

1

All About Eating

Eating well is one of life's great pleasures. If a child is to be
healthy and strong, and fit well into the world, she has to be
able to eat the food. At the same time, if she is to keep eating in
its proper place as only one of life's issues, she has to be able to
take care of it in a matter-of-fact way.

Too many people today are unsuccessful with eating, and
unsuccessful with feeding their children*. Parents worry about
their children's eating habits, their growth and weight, their
nutrition and their manners. Adults are anxious and ambivalent
about their own eating, and those feelings rub off on their parenting with food. They get into struggles with feeding their children, struggles that seemingly have no satisfactory resolution:

---

*The incidence of significant childhood eating problems is estimated
at 25 to 30%—and those are only situations that parents consider
problematic and are brought to professional attention. Problem eating behaviors include poor food acceptance, eating "too much" or
"too little," delay or difficulty in learning the mechanics of eating or
progressing to appropriately-mature eating styles, objectionable
mealtime behaviors and bizarre food habits.

1

"Jason hardly eats anything—at least compared with the other babies I know. He only takes three or four ounces at a time. He's growing all right, but it worries me. I try to get him to take more, but it just makes him mad—he cries and yells and arches his back and throws his body around."

"Eric won't eat his vegetables. In fact, there are just a lot of foods he won't eat. I put peas on his plate and he has a fit until I take them back off again. I have tried serving vegetables cooked and raw and dressed up in a sauce and even let him help prepare them. But he still won't eat. If I try making him stay at the table until he eats some, he sits there for an hour, until I finally break down and let him go."

"Mary eats so much I am afraid she will get fat. I give her as much as I think she should have, but she just wolfs it down and cries for more. She can never wait four hours until the next feeding and sometimes she cries an hour before it is time to feed her."

"I am so sick of cooking for my children, I could just scream. I end up making two or three meals. They say, 'what's that' and I tell them and then they say 'ack, I won't eat that.' And so I say, 'all right, what will you eat?' I feel like a short-order cook. Sometimes I feel like saying, 'that's your dinner, like it or lump it, and better luck next time.'"

"It's gotten to the point where I positively dread dinner time. My husband is on the kids all the time about their eating. 'Eat this, eat that, use your fork, don't use your fingers. You can't leave until you eat all of that.' One of the kids will do it, but the other one won't eat a thing. I think he would sit there for the rest of his life before he gave into his father."

"I don't eat until the kids are in bed. The way they behave at the table really gets on my nerves. They hurry up and eat some, and make a mess, or whine about what's there. Then they get down and run off and then come back and eat a little more. And they hound me for things when I am trying to eat."

We are talking about the feeding relationship: an interactive process in which both parent and child participate. Parents offer food, the child eats it—or fails to eat it. The child gives information about what she wants or doesn't want, and demonstrates her ability to eat, or lack of it. And parents give information about what's available and in what setting and what kind of eating is acceptable to them.

Eating times can be happy times, when children and parents feel they are getting along well enough with each other, and getting the job done in a satisfactory way. Or they can be painful times, when both are anxious and frustrated.

Early problems with feeding can persist, and can get even worse, and can distort lifelong eating and weight management attitudes and behaviors. Most, if not all, adolescent and adult eating disorders, obsessive (and often failed) weight management efforts, and neurotic attitudes and behaviors about eating have their roots in early childhood feeding interactions.

What It's Like For The Child

Painful as feeding problems are for *parents*, think what they must be like for *children*.

Learning about eating starts at birth. The way a child eats and accepts food and *feels* about eating is determined to a large extent by her early experiences with eating. But it goes farther than that. The way eating is managed can have an enormous impact on the way a child feels about herself and about the world.

Especially for the very young child, eating and feeding is central to her relationship with the world. If she is hungry, she is miserable and feels alone. Hunger is, after all, a very powerful and potentially painful drive. Whether a child learns to fear or accommodate hunger depends on her early experience with eating.

If she cries to be fed, and someone shows up promptly and feeds with some sensitivity to her abilities and preferences, she associates hunger with pleasure and it makes her look forward to what happens next. And she thinks, on whatever level babies think, that she must be a very important and fine person and that people must like her to go to such trouble on her behalf.

But feeding can be handled in other ways, ways that make her feel anxious and desperate when she gets hungry. Her caretakers can be slow or inconsistent about responding to her hunger signals. They can force her to eat more than she wants or insist that she eat food that revolts her. They can let her just get started eating well and then take it away.

Very few adults would be willing to deliberately do something that would hurt a child's feelings or lower her self esteem. But that happens all the time in feeding. It happens because adults have their own hangups about eating and play them out in the way they feed their children.

Why This Book?

Most struggles over feeding grow out of genuine concern for the child, and bad advice. Parents are regularly encouraged to overrule information coming from their children, and impose certain foods, or amounts of food, or feeding schedules. Whenever you impose rigid expectations, feeding will be distorted.

In *How to Get Your Kid to Eat*, I'm going to give you some good advice. The advice is about the feeding relationship. I'll tell you how to work it out with your child with eating. I'll talk about parenting in general, and parenting as it applies to eating. I'll emphasize doing your part, but also depending on your child to share responsibility with you for her eating. I'll emphasize what you should do so your child *can* eat and regulate her food intake to the best of her abilities. And, most of all, I'll detail how to make feeding a cooperative process, not just one of outsmarting or controlling your child.

How to Get Your Kid to Eat grows out of my concern about children and their eating. It also grows out of my concern for their parents, and *their* eating.

I have worked with eating for most of my professional life, first as a clinical dietitian in a medical group practice, doing outpatient nutrition counseling for adults and children. I am now a clinical social worker/dietitian in a private mental health clinic, doing family therapy and individual counseling with people who are immobilized by their concerns about eating.

In the over twenty years I have spent working with people of all ages*, I have seen a lot of misery. People can feel upset and immobilized and absolutely terrible about themselves because

---

*I will describe many of my patients, but to protect their privacy, I have changed the non-essential details.

of their inability to manage their eating. Many times they have carried these struggles with them from childhood.

I have worked with families of young children, and have observed what happens in childhood feeding interactions that distorts the way children eat—and the way they feel about eating. My adult patients remember experiencing these distortions as children, and they tell how painful it was to be over-managed or ignored with eating. Eventually, they have grown up to over-manage and ignore themselves—and they continue to experience the same conflict and anxiety about their eating.

And the cycle repeats. Unless adults are able to correct their own distorted eating attitudes and behaviors, they are likely to parent their children with feeding the way *they* were parented.

It doesn't have to be that way. There is a healthy and positive way to manage feeding, and I'll tell you about it.

It's a way that grows out of trust: trust in your child to eat in a way that's right for her and to find the body that's right for her. It's the opposite of being managing and controlling. It's a process that depends on the child's internal cues of hunger, appetite and satiety to guide the feeding process.

You'll be amazed at how being positive and trusting about feeding frees you. It makes an enormous difference in feeding if you don't have to worry about getting your child to eat. You can pay attention, instead, to doing a good job with parenting, to sharing her delight in learning to eat, and to watching her growth unfold.

A New Look At Feeding

Maintaining a positive feeding relationship demands a division of responsibility. The parent is responsible for what the child is offered to eat, the child is responsible for how much, and even whether, she eats.

That basic principle both charges you with what you must do, and lets you off the hook when you have done it. You must get good food into the house, you must get a meal on the table and provide satisfying snacks, and you must do it all in a pleasant and supportive fashion.

But once you have done all that, you simply have to let go of it, turn the rest over to your child, and trust her to do her part.

She will. Based on research and experience, here are the facts about children's eating:

Children will eat.
They are capable of regulating their food intake.
They generally react negatively to new foods but will usually accept them with time and experience.
Parents can either support or disrupt children's food acceptance and food regulation.

Children are interested in eating and capable of doing it. Research, and the survival of the species have shown this to be true. Children, like other people, are endowed with an insistent hunger and appetite. They are invested in their own survival. But they can't get food for themselves—they can only appeal to their adults.

Even as newborns, children know how much they need to eat and are capable of taking the lead with feeding. To function effectively, however, they need a supportive parent who is willing and able to be sensitive and responsive to their messages about feeding. Parents who, for whatever reason, are unable to be attentive to infant eating cues make their children feel afraid that they won't be provided for, and that distorts the feeding process.

If children seemingly have no interest in eating and in food, the problem is NOT that they lack a basic desire to eat. There is something else going on. A child's negative experiences with eating can make her behave in contradictory ways. If parents are remote, a child might give up. If parents force, a child might lose interest.

In most cases, when you try to overrule a child's natural eating cues, her eating ends up getting worse, not better. Children who are forced, cajoled, enticed or even tricked to eat, end up revolted by food and prone to avoid eating if they get a chance. Children who are deprived of food in an attempt to keep them thin become preoccupied with food, afraid they won't get enough to eat, and prone to overeat when they get a chance.

6

Problems With Feeding

The feeding interaction should always be examined when a child's growth is puzzling or when she is doing poorly with eating. If parents and children get into struggles about eating, it can interfere with the child's ability to accept a variety of food or eat the right amount of food. Too often, health workers trying to resolve feeding problems look only at the foods that are being offered and at the child's medical history. While those issues are important, they deal with only part of the story.

If a child is too fat or too thin, if she eats too much or too little, the problem could be the feeding interaction. Prevention of obesity can be started at birth by establishing a positive and supportive feeding relationship, one that allows the infant to accurately regulate her own food intake. It can be continued throughout the growing-up years by maintaining a division of responsibility in feeding.

If a distorted feeding relationship is not the cause of poor growth, it is almost certain to be the effect. People try too hard to feed children who grow poorly, and children end up eating less, not more, when feeders are over active.

If children are picky about eating, the problem is either too much pressure or too little support. Children eat best when parents follow their lead, set appropriate limits, and feed in a smooth, comfortable, and emotionally satisfying fashion. Children eat worst when parents are either domineering or neglectful in feeding.

Adolescent and adult eating disorders can have their antecedents in early childhood feeding interactions. Parents may be insensitive about feeding, and children can grow up feeling confused and anxious about their eating. The best way to prevent eating disorders is to have a positive feeding relationship throughout the growing-up years.

If a child is sick, it is especially difficult, and especially important, to maintain a positive feeding relationship. Illness often requires special feeding regimens which, in turn, puts pressure on parents to take over with feeding. It doesn't work any better to be over-managing with a sick child than with a well child.

Advances in modern medicine are presenting a whole set

7

of feeding problems that no one has had to deal with before. Babies survive who haven't previously, and the methods used to insure their survival deprive them of the opportunity to learn to eat. (They are fed through the veins, or by tubes, for the first year, or even first several years, of life.) They can learn, but they—and their parents—need special help to do it—and special sensitivity to the feeding relationship.

Summary Of The Book

In the early chapters, in the BASIC PRINCIPLES OF FEEDING section, I have laid out what works and what doesn't with feeding. Much is known. I have based my recommendations on my own experience, on extensive reading (I'll share references with you as I go along) and on much consultation with parents and professionals

In the middle section of the book, FEEDING AS YOUR CHILD GROWS, I talk in concrete detail about how to feed children from infancy through adolescence. This middle section is about parenting—and parenting-through-feeding.

I think you will find, as I have, that applying parenting principles to feeding will allow you to understand some things about raising children that you've not understood before. I also think you will find it helpful to follow child—and feeding—development in an orderly fashion from one stage to the next. Each stage builds on and reflects the achievements of the one before—or exposes limitations resulting from earlier failure to achieve.

The final section of the book, SPECIAL FEEDING PROBLEMS, deals with children and their specific needs. I have referred to the problems earlier. Here, I will simply underscore what it takes to work with special-needs children—or, if at all possible, to prevent their becoming special needs children in the first place. The key is normal feeding.

To prevent feeding problems, or to confine them to the lowest possible level, you have to maintain a healthy feeding relationship throughout the growing-up years. Preventing obesity, eating disorders, aversion to food and objectionable eating behaviors starts at birth—with sympathetic and supportive nipple feeding. It continues throughout childhood, with appropriate management of feeding based on the child's emotional and developmental needs.

Throughout, the emphasis is on parenting. The best parenting provides both love and limits. These themes play themselves out in feeding, the same that they do in every other aspect of a child's life. Feeding is a metaphor for the parent/child relationship overall. Appropriate feeding and healthy feeding relationships are part and parcel of appropriate parenting and healthy family relationships.

The best parenting grows out of a healthy marriage. Parents who get along well with each other, and support each other, do the best job with parenting—and feeding. Many times distortions in the feeding relationship can be traced back to distorted interactions between the adults in the family.

Feeding doesn't just happen. What you do with feeding can make a difference. I'll give you lots of information that is helpful, and methods that WORK. Children will eat, and they can be positive and joyful about it. And you can help them eat, and, with any luck, discover some of those positive and joyful feelings yourself.

Some day I will write a book about adults' eating and tell you how you can learn to eat in a way that is fun and intelligent. For now, you will have to let your children lead you. And you will. If you go through the motions (that I will tell you about) and keep your mouth shut and fingers crossed and the look of incredulity off your face, they will show you what healthy and normal eating is all about. They will, that is, unless your eating is too distorted.

I'll be talking in the following pages about approaches and tactics that enhance feeding and the feeding relationship. This book is about real life feeding situations and the things that go wrong. And what it takes to fix them. And the things that go right. And how they got that way. Maybe you'll find your situation here. If you do, I hope you can fix it. If you can't fix it, I hope you will get help. It's that important.

There is only so much that a book on feeding, or a book on parenting, can do to help. You can improve basically good parenting with a book like this. You can correct a lot of the conflict and misgivings that you feel about managing eating. But you can't fix poor parenting by reading, and you can't correct seriously distorted eating attitudes and behaviors. You need more help than that. If you find this book does more to expose your limitations than to enable you to improve, you would benefit from getting professional help.

The issue at hand is how to work it out with your child with feeding. So, if you have ever had a toddler who came to the table and crossed his arms and said, "I won't eat," read on.

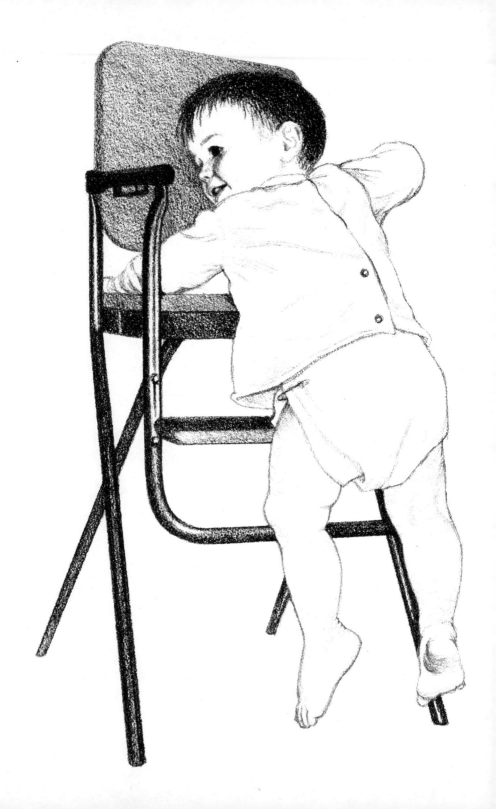

2

Quit When The Job Is Done

Helping your child to eat as well as possible requires that you do your own job with feeding but not your child's job, and that you know the difference. Parenting well with food demands that you find that gray area somewhere between the extremes of being neglectful (and not trying to help at all) and being domineering (and helping so much that it's harmful rather than helpful). It's very tricky business.

You find out what works by starting out with your intuition and some observations of your child, then using trial and error until you come up with something that is effective. It doesn't pay to be rigid and opinionated, because you could be wrong. But it also doesn't pay to do nothing at all because kids *do* need *some* help.

It's much worse to be rigid and wrong (or even right) than to be flexible and wrong. Families that get into trouble are not the ones who try and fail. They are the ones who try and fail and try the same thing again and again even though it is not working. Families that get into trouble are also the ones who don't even try at all[1].

The Division of Responsibility In Feeding

To find the middle ground in feeding between rigidity and uninvolvement, I have found it enormously helpful to think in terms of a division of responsibility. Here, suitable for framing, is the golden rule for parenting with food:

> *Parents are responsible for* **what** *is* **presented to eat and the** *manner in* **which it is presented.**
>
> *Children are responsible for* **how much and even** *whether* **they eat.**

Blow it up, and post it on a placard in the middle of your table. Mail it to your Aunt Fanny, the one who is always bugging your kids to eat "one more bite," and telling them they "have to eat. . .I made it especially for you." You know, she's the one who takes you to one side and tells you that in her day, kids weren't allowed to leave food on their plates. Kids in her day also were undoubtedly not as picky as kids are nowadays. (It's apparent, she will go on to tell you, that the problem is mothers working outside the home, or all those fast food franchises, or whatever happens to be your particular tender spot.)

Other than twitting Aunt Fanny, however, what does that golden rule really mean?

How The "Division" Applies

In the first place, the division of responsibility in feeding means that parents have a very real responsibility for choosing food for the family. They are the ones who have to know enough about nutrition and about children's abilities to ingest and digest food to select healthful food that is appropriate for them. They have to see to it that food gets bought and cooked, and that meals are on the table.

It all begins with choosing the milk feeding for a baby. Then moves up through choosing the right solid foods and knowing when to offer them, the transition to table food, eating for little children, helping school-age children be successful with their eating, giving teenagers enough (but not too much) help— all these ages and topics demand that parents know enough about food and nutrition, and about their child's characteristics and abilities, to present appropriate food in a helpful way.

The division of responsibility assumes that parents will present food to children in a positive and supportive fashion. I will be using a lot of print in this book talking about the intricacies of *that*, so I will pretty much let it go for now. I *will* point out to you here, however, that to present food well to a child you have to feel good about it yourself. If you are really anxious about eating or finicky or have some real negative feelings, you had better get them resolved. Those feelings can permeate *everything* about your child's eating.

The division of responsibility in feeding also means that parents have to *agree* on food. I know a couple (in fact, several couples) who are both so opinionated about food that neither will accept what the other cooks. In those situations I can absolutely guarantee you finicky children who will use their own likes and dislikes to manipulate their parents at mealtime. There are ways of working these situations out, but you have to *want* to, and have to like each other well enough to make the effort. Kids don't do well with eating (or with anything else) when their parents don't reach agreements with each other.

You can cause just as much havoc by doing too much as you can by doing too little. Maybe more. Once you have chosen food and presented it in a positive fashion, your job is done. You don't have to get food into your child. That's his job. The great majority of babies have the ability to suck and swallow, know how much they need to eat in order to grow properly, and can communicate that to you. The older children get, the more autonomy they have in managing their food intake. But the basic division of responsibility still holds—**Parent:what/ Child:how much.**

How The "Division" Helps

Parents of sick children and children who are growing poorly feel very relieved when they begin to share responsibility

15

for feeding with their child. All parents, but these parents in particular, need to know when they have done enough. Knowing they have done all they can frees them to respect their child and to maintain their relationship, rather than getting caught up in struggles and anxiety over eating. And it saves their child, with his poor appetite, from becoming even more repulsed by food that is not only unappealing but is being forced on him. It also prevents the child from figuring out that he can blackmail his parents into almost anything by holding out the promise that he will eat. Even sick children don't feel any happier when they are allowed to be tyrants.

There's a lot of power in eating or not eating. If parents are over concerned about food acceptance, they are likely to let children get by with unacceptable behavior just to keep them around their food, hoping they will eat it. It follows from a child's reasoning that if he has to be indulged to keep him at the table, it must not be such a special place to be. It is so much better to expect and enforce good behavior at mealtimes. THAT gives the message that the table is a special place to be, and if the child is going to be there, he needs to be pleasant.

Limiting Your Efforts

Not every problem feeding situation involves power struggles and manipulation. In most cases, in fact, children are simply communicating what they want and parents can hear it and respect it or not. Sometimes it takes real courage for parents to limit their efforts.

I'm remembering Alice Black. She was referred to me several years ago by a pediatrician asking me what I would recommend to increase the growth rate in little Alice. She was six months old, a beautiful, alert little child. However, she had gained only three pounds and five inches since birth. Alice's parents had taken her for a chromosomal examination and for endocrine tests but no one could find anything wrong with her. Actually, other than her size, nothing WAS wrong with Alice. She was just tiny.

Her parents, of course, were concerned. They wanted to be sure that they were doing everything they could to encourage Alice to grow. But they said that she was very emphatic about how much she wanted to eat, and cried and fussed when they

16

tried to encourage her to take more food. We decided we would try concentrating her formula.

We knew we would have to be careful in doing this, because if we concentrated it too much we might dehydrate her. So we carefully figured it all out, and added enough sugar to her formula so it was about 7% higher in calories than it had been before. But Alice was a good little regulator, and rather than overeating a bit on the more-concentrated formula, she simply cut back the volume of her intake by 7%. No more, no less.

Undaunted, we decided that, rather than adding extra sugar to the formula we would add extra fat. Maybe, we reasoned, it was too sweet for her. So again we figured it all out and added enough fat to increase the calories by 7% from the regular formula. But, again, Alice was ahead of us and again she cut back her intake by 7%.

Again, we put her back on regular formula while we reconnoitered (whereupon she again increased the volume of her intake to the usual amount). Finally, we simply decreased the water to concentrate the formula, and down went her intake. At that point, we gave up. Our only other option would have been to tube feed her, and none of us wanted to do that. (Tube feeding *is* an appropriate option for some kids who have real problems with the mechanics of eating or who simply don't have the strength to eat enough. We'll talk more about this in The Child Who Grows Poorly (Chapter 13).

The parents decided they simply had to support the growth pattern that was normal for Alice. They moved away, and I did not see them until Alice was nine months old and weighed nine pounds. She was feeding herself tiny amounts of food from the table. She was pulling herself up and walking around things and startling everyone because she looked like a newborn.

Hard as it was, Alice's parents did what they could and then let go of it. The outcome wasn't ideal, but at least the parents weren't making it harder for themselves and for her by struggling with her about her food intake.

It could have turned out like the little Louisiana boy I heard about when I was there doing a workshop. His parents were feeding him in the bathtub because they forced so hard and he fought back so hard, that together they made a terrible mess. He, too, was growing really poorly and his parents and doctor were pretty desperate to do something about it. So they

17

tried to force the food in, and life became one long sequence of trying to feed him, dreading meals or recovering from them, and feeling terrible about the situation.

If you try too hard to help, you can destroy the very thing you are trying to save. You can get so fixated about a certain outcome you lose all perspective on the people involved.

Dividing Responsibility As Children Grow Up

The basic division of responsibility holds true throughout the growing-up years. It is based on respect for your child as an individual and on your taking appropriate responsibility to help out with the child's growing up. The way the division of responsibility is applied, however, shifts as children grow.

Babies

With babies, it is relatively easy. You give them their milk feeding and they let you know when they are full or hungry. You try to please them and make them comfortable, because during the early months they are learning trust. You can't spoil them, except by not giving them what they need. Babies whose needs are met become easier babies to take care of, not harder, because they learn that they are not going to have to put up such a fuss to get your attention. Babies whose parents respond promptly to their crying cry less, not more[2].

To help your baby with the emotional task of becoming aware of and trusting both self and the world around, you need to be accepting, curious, and sporting about going along with what he seems to want and need. Your task is to look for and accept information coming from him. Generally, you try to figure out the small infant, find out what he wants, what works with him, and how to make him comfortable.

Nipple feeding

You have to present breastmilk or a proper formula. As I pointed out in detail in *Child of Mine*, the young infant has special food needs, and you have to respect those if he is to grow well. Only breastmilk or a specially-constituted baby formula will work during most of the first year, when a child is at first only on a milk feeding, and then making the transition to table foods. Pasteurized milk doesn't work because it's not digestible enough and doesn't have the right nutrients in the right proportions. There are other reasons, too, that I won't go into here. Trust me.

Every baby is the same with respect to needing appropriate food, but each one is different with respect to schedule and the way they regulate their food intake. You should feed based on *your* baby's times and let him eat as much as he is hungry for.

The amount children eat varies from one feeding to another and one day to another. Overall, they know how much they need to eat in order to grow properly. One child eats more than another child, and you can't tell by looking, or even weighing and measuring, how much they will need to eat. The only way you can know how much a child *should* be eating is by observing how much he *is* eating. You won't need charts to figure it out ahead of time; your most important tools are trust, patience, perseverance, and a willingness to develop ways that work.

Figure 7-1, "Division of Responsibility in Nipple Feeding," expands on feeding during the earliest months of your child's life. It says to trust your child's information about amounts, tempo, and frequency, and work to comfort him so he can eat in a smooth and continuous fashion. The Newborn (Chapter 7) talks in more detail about feeding little babies.

Spoon Feeding

Somewhere between five and twelve months your baby will make a transition in feeding from all breast milk or formula to modified adult food. What you feed him during the transition period must provide for nutritional needs and also teach feeding skills. He will start between five and seven months by learning to get semi-solid food from a spoon and swallow it. Later he will learn to manipulate and gum thicker, lumpier food, and finally to pick up and chew pieces of soft, cooked food.

The child around age six months who is ready to start solid foods is still an infant. You can continue to trust what he wants and to go along with his needs. Your job of *food selection,* however, becomes more complicated because you have much to choose from and because your baby's eating skills will be changing all the time.

We are feeding babies a lot different than we did ten or fifteen years ago. Years ago, some babies were started on solids at one month of age, or even at birth. We kept them on pureed baby food for a long time, because that was all they could get down. Now we start them on solids at around age six months, and progress them rapidly to thick, lumpy food and finally to table food.

There weren't any real good reasons for the earlier pattern. Babies tolerated it, they did OK on it, but they didn't really NEED it. The solid foods weren't even as good for them as the breastmilk or formula they replaced. If we had really paid attention to what babies were *doing*, we wouldn't have fed them solids at all. We would have seen that those little babies were most comfortable and ate best when they were cuddled and nursed. We would have realized the stupidity of the instructions we got for getting food down their throats when they couldn't swallow properly. (For what it's worth, you put them in a reclining position and put the food way back on their tongue.) Now we *are* paying attention, and the introducing-solids phase has changed a lot. Babies (and parents) are better off for it.

Children go through lots of changes in their feeding capabilities and nutritional needs during the first year. Figure 8-2 in Chapter 8, "Introducing Solid Foods," summarizes when to add solid foods and why. I will very briefly describe the process here, and discuss it in more length in The Older Baby (Chapter 8).

Babies start by learning to get semi-solid food from a spoon and swallow it. They learn to manipulate and gum thicker, lumpier food, and finally to pick up and chew pieces of soft, cooked food.

During the transition period from milk feeding to table food, most people add foods in this order:

• **Starting:** Iron fortified infant cereal mixed with the milk feeding.

• **Progressing:** Pureed, fork-mashed or milled fruits and vegetables. "Finger" breads and cereals.

• **Beginning table food:** Soft or cooked table food. Finely-divided meats.

20

This whole process usually starts around age six months, and finishes at around 10 to 12 months.

How quickly you progress from one food to the next, and from pureed to mashed to chopped food, depends on whether your baby is cautious, and needs time to get used to new things, or adventurous, and dives right in. It depends on a lot of other things, too, that only your baby can teach you about. That's the fun of having a baby.

All of this is new and strange to a child. It can also be frightening, if parents expect him to do more than he is really ready to do. Children sometimes gag, and that can put them off on spoon feeding, especially if it happens too often. Kids get *really* turned off if a parent acts frightened by that, or pushes too hard so it happens repeatedly. Some kids have a special problem with gagging and choking. I will talk about them more in Feeding the Child With Special Needs (Chapter 16).

Children do best at this and every other stage of feeding if: 1) There is an adult standing by who is available to act as a backup, and (2) They are allowed to retain as much control as possible. I can talk most effectively about these two important factors by discussing something else entirely.

Like most parents, I have spent many hours lifeguarding. I have perched on beaches or at the side of pools, watching my offspring with an eagle eye to keep them from drowning themselves. The major form of entertainment in that occupation is watching other children and other families. But since my own children never fail to interest me the most, I will tell you about them first.

When they were little we went to the beach. (We do have beaches in Wisconsin. We haul in the sand from a nearby quarry.) My daughter Kjerstin loved to play in the sand. At first, when she could sit up, she just sat and played. When she started to crawl, she gradually worked herself down from the beach to sit in the very edge of the water. She crawled around, getting out farther and farther, until she got her face wet. She jerked it up out of the water and immediately checked me to make sure I was still on the job and to find out how I felt about it. I just looked at her.

She sat and thought about the situation for a while and watched the older children going out farther. Then she went back to playing, only this time when she got her face wet she

21

wasn't as startled. Eventually she was going in very comfortably, not worrying about getting under water. The first time we went to a swimming pool, she went under water very enthusiastically and was entirely willing to jump off the side of the pool and into my arms.

As I said, I did at times tear myself from my own offspring and observed those of other people. I noticed that the children who did best with this process were the ones who did it more or less on their own. The parents helped by being there, and like all children the little ones would check back every now and again to make sure the parents were still paying attention. But the children did less well if the parents helped too much or too little.

If the parents were clearly ignoring them, the children didn't go very far; they stuck close by and kept trying to keep their parents' attention. If the parents got involved in the exploration and tried to help too much, it frightened the children. A father was entirely too ready to rescue, and ran and grabbed his child the first time she came up sputtering. That scared her, and gave her the idea that there was something *to* be scared of.

Another carried his child out and lowered her in the water until she was in over her head. A mother simply put her child's face in the water, even though it was apparent he didn't want her to. Both of the children looked frightened and screamed and fought. It seemed to me that those pressure tactics made the process harder, not easier.

I hope you have learned from this swimming lesson that children do best when parents are appropriately supportive and allow children as much control as they can handle. Now let's go back to talking about introducing solid foods.

Figure 8-1, "Division of Responsibility in Early Spoon Feeding," repeats and breaks down the division of responsibility for your infant during the first half of the second year. Essentially, it says what we said earlier: Challenge your child in a way that he can handle, give appropriate support, work with him to figure out what he is capable of doing and what he is telling you, and give him as much control over the process as possible.

The Toddler

Compared to the baby, the toddler is a whole different breed of cat—compared to almost anyone else, in fact, except maybe the adolescent. If things have gone well for him and for his parents when he was a baby, he has learned trust. Now, as a toddler, he begins to assert himself. He begins to suspect that he is a person separate from those who take care of him the most.

His job as a toddler is to confirm that. And he takes the job very seriously. The toddler learns about his separateness by exploring and asserting himself. He becomes oppositional, because by saying "no" to other people he proves he is separate from them.

The healthy toddler is engaging, curious, energetic and recalcitrant. If you treat him like you did when he was an infant, and simply accept and support his desires, you will fail him utterly. He needs reasonable and firm limits in order to feel secure.

You don't have to make up the limits. The toddler is generally an aggressive little explorer who needs a lot of room to find out about the world. But he will go too far and he will get on your nerves and he will violate your civil rights and endanger himself and property. You will recognize it when you see it.

To help you distinguish reasonable limits from harsh intrusions, it helps to elaborate on the division of responsibility we talked about earlier. Figure 9-1 "Division of Responsibility in Feeding the Toddler," summarizes tasks in feeding.

The division of responsibility still holds true: You are responsible for what your child is offered to eat, he is responsible for how much he eats. In the toddler period, you add on the responsibilities of timing and location. You no longer feed the toddler on demand—you ask him to come to the table with the rest of the family. And you time his snacks so he can last until mealtime. You also have to decide if you want eating done at the table or will allow eating elsewhere.

It is important to your child's eating that you see that he has regular and pleasant meals and snacks. (Food and mealtime climate are important features to check out in the day care setting.) It is equally important not to get *so* concerned that you take responsibility for getting food IN to your child. Getting meals on the table regularly is difficult enough without also devoting yourself to getting people to eat them.

If you try to do that with a toddler, you will *really* have your work cut out for you. The toddler, in his struggle for autonomy, is capable of making you do a shocking array of things in

23

order to make him eat: Order, scream, be unkind, beg, play silly games.

You must also remember that during the toddler period, neophobia is at its worst. The toddler's neophobia is his fear of anything new, which translates in feeding to his aversion to any new food. This natural (and largely self-protective) suspicion of new foods will be glaringly apparent at around ages two and three.

Your reassurance will not make it go away. He is not being suspicious of you and contrary in clinging to his neophobia. He is simply behaving in a very normal way for a child that age. If a child is exposed to the same foods over and over he will get to the point where he tastes, then likes the food. But you can't rush it. Only his own time and experience will make neophobia go away. You can help only by continuing to cook a variety of food, by eating and enjoying your own food, and by leaving him alone to work it out with his food in his own way.

It's the old water-wearing-away stone approach to child feeding. If you approach it right, it won't wear *you* away.

We'll talk more about feeding tactics with toddlers in Is Your Toddler Jerking You Around At the Table? (Chapter 9).

The Preschooler

Individuating was the toddler's task. Integrating is the preschooler's task. By the preschool period, a child knows who he is, he is just getting better at it. After the toddler period, the preschool period is EASY.

The division of responsibility from the toddler period works as a guide throughout the growing up years. Preschoolers, like older children, still need a certain amount of structure, but they need autonomy within those limits.

The preschooler's eating skills continue to develop and improve. Neophobia diminishes as he gains experience with food, and he can talk well enough to talk about his fears about food, rather than just acting them out. He gets better at chewing and swallowing. He gets neater and more consistent at using utensils to eat and at drinking from a cup without spilling. He takes pride in his eating abilities and likes eating with the rest of the family.

24

Remember that. Almost everyone knows that children like to gain skills and feel pride in mastering their world. But when it comes to eating, grownups forget that important fact. For some reason we regard eating as different– that unless we make it happen, the child will never really grow up with his eating. It's not true. At least, not to start with. You can make it true by putting a lot of pressure on eating, but without pressure it really isn't so.

Children can recognize pressure on feeding even in its most cleverly disguised forms. Leanne Birch, a child development researcher in Illinois, rewarded one group of preschoolers for trying new food[3]. Another group of preschoolers was simply introduced to the foods with no comments or encouragement of any kind. A few days later, they again presented the new food to the two groups of children. The rewarded preschoolers were LESS likely to go back to the new food than the ones who had been allowed to approach the food in their own way. It appears that children recognize even the most positive enticement as pressure and are put off by it.

We'll talk more about preschoolers in The Popular Preschooler (Chapter 10).

The School-age Child

School-age children are busy finding out about the world, and they need both challenges and support. Children at this stage develop a view of themselves as good workers or failures. They become more independent of their parents, and they work at whatever tasks their world provides. They get better at self control and at understanding the point of view of other people. Children this age need adults to provide them with tasks that are equal to their abilities and with recognition when they achieve those tasks. Not TOO much recognition, however, or that will interfere with the pride they take in themselves.

Friends become very important at this stage, and children put in a lot of effort learning ways of behaving and even talking that help them fit in with other kids. You may have heard recently on the playground some of the chants you used has a child. Do you recognize "Eenie, meenie, minie, moe..."?

Their concerns and interests separate them from adults. That's the point. Most of us have had the experience of having

25

our child cringe and the other children look at him with pity when we kissed him in public. He was letting us know that he was moving from the parent-centeredness of the preschooler to the friend-centeredness of the school-age child.

To live comfortably with this child, you can begin by stopping kissing him in public. That doesn't mean you have to stop being his parent. You just do it differently. You work behind the scenes. You do the same with eating.

The division of responsibility in feeding works the same for the school-age child as it did for younger children. You have to let go a little. You are still primarily responsible for what, when and where, when your child is around home. He continues to be responsible for how much and whether. But now you are going to depend on the larger community to provide your child with some of the what, when and where. He'll have the opportunity to eat school lunch and to be exposed to new foods there. He'll eat at friends' houses. And he and his friends will save their money and stop at the candy store when they go to the shopping center or to the movies.

At home, it's important to continue offering meals and snacks and to keep good food around. It's all right to say "don't eat now, dinner is in an hour," and, "get out of the refrigerator— you've had your snack." Scheduled eating times are still important. It's good to eat, and then forget about it. When you can eat any old time, food becomes an issue *all* the time.

For eating away from home, you can only offer advice, backup and support. Encourage him to try new foods at school lunch or at friends' homes. If he won't try them, teach him at least to be civilized about it so other people can enjoy their food. Tell him you don't want him to spoil his appetite for dinner by late snacking at friends' houses. Tell him if you think he's eating too many candy bars, and encourage him to choose something more nutritious for snacks. There are suggestions for snacks in *Tools and Strategies,* in the Appendix.

But don't have showdowns over his eating. The really important thing he is learning at this stage is to make it in the outside world, and that is something he has to learn on his own. If you get hard-nosed and domineering, he'll depend too much on you to tell him what to do and he won't develop his own judgment. Or he'll get contrary and do the opposite of what you want, and he STILL won't develop his own judgment.

We'll talk more about his age group in The Industrious Schoolager (Chapter 11).

Teenagers

Not too long ago I gave a talk at the high school about eating in the teen years. As part of my research for the talk I interviewed Kris, then 15, while he rode home from school with me. I found Kris at the bus stop; he had missed the bus after football practice when he ran over to The Little Store (every high school has one) to get himself a quart of pop and some potato chips. He was grateful for the ride home because he didn't want to be late for dinner.

I asked Kris about his nutritional concerns, and he said he felt his mom didn't let him eat enough junk food. I happen to know his mom is a dietitian and that she makes a real effort to see that her family gets good food. I also happen to know that she is not overly rigid about it—she gave us the recipe for best chocolate chip cookies I have ever eaten.

Actually, Kris and his mom have worked it out quite well. Kris is big and active and he needs a lot of calories. He can eat everything he needs and still have room for some nutritionally marginal food. So his mom provides the basic nutrition and Kris provides the extra calories. They don't fight about it—she just lets him spend his money the way he wants to for snacks.

During the teen years, boys get into eating and girls get into dieting. The latter is more of a concern. I'll deal with the dieting topic in Helping All You Can to Keep Your Child From Being Fat (Chapter 14), and with teens in general in The Individualistic Teenager (Chapter 12).

Parents of teens worry about control just the same as parents of younger children. And it is an appropriate worry. Or concern, maybe. The division of responsibility still holds true.

Parents continue to be the ones who have to see that there is a meal on the table. The teen can help shop for it, and cook for it, but the parent is the one who should see that it happens.

Teens need the structure of knowing someone is looking out for them, and providing meals for a teenager lets them know that in a very powerful way. They probably won't thank you and may even complain when you insist they show up for meals, but they *will* benefit. They will benefit, that is, unless your meals are

27

unpleasant times when everybody jumps on everybody else or when none of you speaks to each other. Then *nobody* will benefit, and the problems are a whole lot deeper than just meal planning.

Teens will take care of their own snacks, either by raiding the refrigerator or by hanging out at the pizza parlor with friends. But you can still say to them, "you're eating too much for snacks because you're not eating your dinner." Teens will have their own schedules, and you may move mealtimes around or, at times, cook early and eat in shifts. Keep in mind, though, that there is a difference between being considerate and letting the teenager run the family.

The basic division of responsibility holds true throughout the growing-up years. Parents need to provide the food, but kids have to eat it. If either of you gets started doing the others' job, there will be trouble.

Your children *will* grow up with eating, but I would recommend that you not get too eager about it. You will have a long wait.

References

1.   Olson, D. H.: Circumplex model VII: Validation studies and FACES III. Family Process 25:337-351, 1986.

2.   Bell, S.M. and Ainsworth, M.D.S.: Infant crying and maternal responsiveness. Child Development 36:57-71, 1972.

3.   Birch, L.L. and Marlin, D.W.: I don't like it; I never tried it: Effects of exposure on two-year-old children's food preferences. Appetite 3:353-360, 1982.

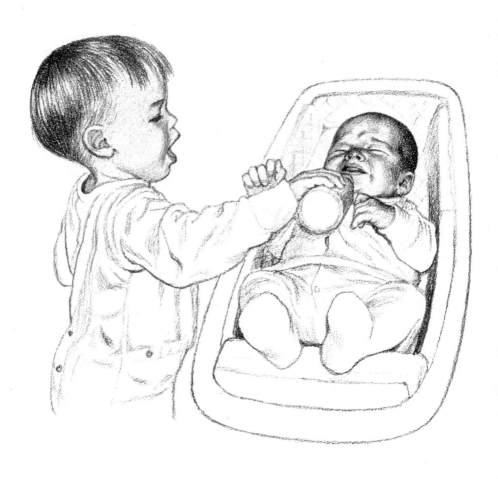

3

Pressure Doesn't Work

The way to get a kid to eat is not to try. You have to let it be her idea. YOU SHOULDN'T FORCE YOUR CHILD TO EAT (OR RESTRICT THE AMOUNT SHE EATS). It is the most unhelpful thing you can possibly do. To either of you. Pressuring your child to eat can make her eating worse, and make her grow poorly, and make her feel bad about herself and her body and her eating. Forcing can make YOU miserable. It can make meals and feeding degenerate from a fun and satisfying process into a battle in which nobody wins.

Parents (and children) get into trouble with feeding when they cross the lines of division of responsibility: When they do what they shouldn't, and fail to do what they should. You are crossing the lines when you try to control the amount your child eats. Any direct control on the amount a child eats amounts to pressure—from then on, it's just a matter of degree. You are also crossing the lines when you fail to take responsibility for planning and preparing meals and snacks and for making them important.

I am fully aware that you are probably pressuring, because almost all parents do, just like their parents did before them. Parents pressure from good intentions—because they want the best for their child and because they want her to grow up well and strong and well-formed and lovely. They think they *need* to put on pressure to get their child to eat enough (but not too much) and to eat the right stuff.

Wrong, all wrong. This most logical and pervasive of presumptions just does not hold up when you look at it closely. Research has shown (as I will elaborate later) that when adults put pressure on eating, children don't eat as well and grow as well[1]. Period.

I am not advocating letting kids do exactly what they want with eating and food selection. That is called anarchy. And neglect.

There is a difference between putting on the pressure and setting limits. If you fail to set limits you won't like what happens, and your child will not do well. You have to find the middle ground between being too rigid and controlling and letting things get out of control. We'll wait to talk more in other chapters about finding that middle ground. The message here in this chapter, Pressure Doesn't Work, will get you generally oriented, combat all the misinformation out there, and get you ready to take a look, in some of the other chapters, at some of the tactics that DO work.

Let's start out by looking at some of the many ways you can get into forcing with feeding.

Forcing Can Take Many Forms

Starting with the assumption that parents have to CONTROL eating, I have seen people get into horrendous struggles with their children. Often the problem starts with a child who eats funny or is sick, and parents and advisors get scared and put on the pressure. The child resists and parents get even more scared and put on even more pressure. Eventually it gets to the point where the situation is so bad that everyone is afraid to change it, because, as bad as it is, how much worse would it be if everyone stopped doing what they were doing?

32

Pressure Can Be Forcing Food In

Brian provides us with a good example. Brian's mother was perfectly furious with him. It seemed that, no matter how she tried, he simply would not eat. As she told it, she had to stand over him for an hour to get him to eat a piece of french toast. She had to tell him to put it in his mouth, to chew it and to swallow. And, as she told it, if she didn't go through all those steps with him, he simply would not eat and she was afraid he would die.

His growth pattern supported her worry. (Brian's growth chart is Figure 13-3 in The Child Who Grows Poorly, Chapter 13.) In the six months since his third birthday Brian's weight had remained the same, and he had fallen off his growth curve*. Now, instead of being average weight he was thin. Rather alarmingly thin. There was nothing wrong with him, the doctor said. Mother wanted some more tactics to use to get him to eat.

There were just two times in Brian's life when he had grown well. One was when he was a new baby and being breast fed. But when he had started eating solids the fight had begun— he just wouldn't eat from the spoon unless mother forced. The other was when mother had been sick with her second, very rough, pregnancy. During that time she just hadn't had the energy to devote to Brian. But now the baby was ten months old, and things were getting back under control again. And the fight was on.

It is funny how, if you have a different slant toward a situation, it can seem entirely different to you. Brian's mother was convinced that her pressure was the only thing that was keeping Brian eating and alive. It hadn't occurred to her that Brian did better with eating when she wasn't so forceful. I can understand why. The fight can develop so quickly, that you don't realize it's happening and don't catch what leads up to it.

I had this point brought home to me by a fun TV program I did a couple of years ago. Dan Smith, the host for a local talk show, invited me to be on *Madison Magazine* to talk about feeding children and about *Child of Mine*. Dan wanted to jazz the topic up for his audience, so he named the segment "Preventing

---

*I'll explain growth charts in the next chapter.

Family Food Fights," and we came up with some feeding vignettes that illustrated common feeding situations in families. Then he recruited his two-year-old daughter, Lindsay, to be our star.

Before I tell you what happened, let me give you some background. Dan says that he has absolutely never forced Lindsay to eat. He doesn't believe in it, we have talked about it over the years and he has gotten support from me for his view, and he has gone to some trouble to avoid it.

However, for the program, the first segment was planned to have Dan force feed Lindsay. He was funny and charming, but he *was* forcing, and Lindsay knew it. She was seated at the table. He walked up to her and she held up her arms to get down. He said, "No, no, no, you have to eat that. Here, have a spoonful. Here comes the airplane, into the hangar. Mayday! Mayday!"

Meanwhile, Lindsay wasn't waiting to hear about airplanes and hangars. The instant he started with the pressure, she had her hands over her mouth and began squealing. She continued throughout the sequence.

Lindsay had had absolutely no coaching in reacting this way. But her response was immediate and emphatic. She fought back. That's just how easily and quickly distorted feeding can get started. From that moment the situation can go either way— it depends on the parents' reaction. Dan backed off, she went back to her own way of doing business, and at last report she is eating and growing normally. If he had seen her reaction as a sign of trouble to come and had increased his pressure to get her to eat, she would likely have continued her resistance and the struggle would have been on in earnest.

Brian's mother hadn't backed off, and that is exactly what had happened, probably from the time they had tried to get started with spoon feeding. He had gagged and that probably was what had frightened him. He could have used more time and patience to get used to the idea. He had only been four months old at the time, and undoubtedly would have been better at living up to his mother's expectations if she had waited until he was five or six months old to introduce solid foods.

Mother was such an intense and hard-driving woman, it was likely she wasn't able to be very patient. She had some pretty high standards of what her mothering should accomplish, and Brian's poor eating didn't live up to those standards.

34

I tried, as diplomatically as possible, to tell Brian's mother that she should back off some and put less pressure on his eating. But she couldn't accept that from me. She left, and went off to find a dietitian who would tell her how to get Brian to eat. So I don't know how it turned out. It could have degenerated into an even worse situation, like a Louisiana boy whose parents were feeding in the bathtub. They pressured him so hard to eat, and he fought back so hard, that between them they made a terrible mess. So they fed him in the bathtub and just rinsed him off afterward.

Pressure Can Be Withholding Food

Pressure on eating can also take the form of withholding food. Todd was a robust three-year-old whose parents came to see me because he was so greatly interested in eating. He demanded big helpings at mealtimes, even though his parents tried to get him to settle for less, and he insisted on seconds and threw a fit when they refused him. He would finally get his way, but still get down from the table and want a snack right away.

He was "always" panhandling for food and his parents kept trying to stave him off, though eventually they almost always gave in and gave him more to eat. Whenever they had company and put out the cheese and crackers, Todd wouldn't even go off and play with the other kids. He stood right by the coffee table and ate as long as the supplies held out.

As you can see by Figure 3-1, Todd's weight fluctuated modestly, and MAY have been increasing more than it should have. But to his parents, his weight pattern was beside the point. They saw his EATING as being abnormal, and that is where their major concern lay.

Todd's parents were tired of this struggle with him and they could tell it made him feel bad when they tried to get him to go without eating. But they were afraid to stop because if he ate that much when they were withholding food they were afraid he would REALLY eat if they stopped.

His mother also felt sorry for him. She knew what it felt like to be deprived of food and upset about eating, because she was bulimic. She was always trying to diet, and periodically giving in to her hunger and eating a lot and then feeling terrible about it, and generally forcing herself to throw up. She was

35

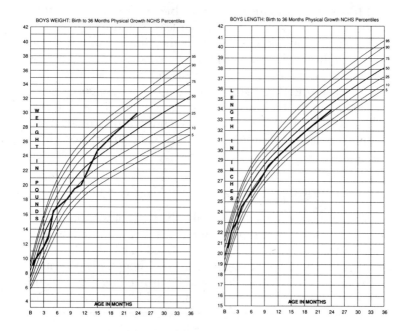

Figure 3-1   Todd's Growth Chart.

frightened that her eating would get *really* out of control, and was becoming more and more rigid and depriving with herself, trying to bring order to the chaos that was her eating.

I explained to the parents that Todd was putting so much pressure on eating because he was afraid he wouldn't get enough to eat. Children whose parents withhold food from them, or adults who withhold food from themselves, become preoccupied with it and are prone to overeat when they get a chance or when their (or somebody else's) willpower runs out.

The way to get a handle on the problem was not to increase the controls or to plan menus that were lower in calories, but to reassure Todd that he would get enough to eat. He needed to know that he would not have to go hungry.

But we were not simply going to throw open the refrigerator door. We were going to reestablish the division of responsibility for feeding. Parents were to take more responsibility for

36

offering regular meals and snacks and for controlling Todd's access to food between times, but they were not to try to hold back on how much he ate at meals and snacks.

While the parents were not to tell Todd *how much* he should eat, there were some other controls they were to impose. They were the ones who were picking out what they all were going to eat. They were to put the meal on the table, and let Todd choose from what was available. I suggested they put bread on the table so if the main dish or vegetables or salad didn't fill him up, he could fall back on bread.

They were to keep some structure in his eating. He was to have meals and snacks, but not to be allowed to panhandle. At mealtime, they were to tell him he could have as much as he wanted but that he had to stay at the table to do his eating and that once he got down, that was all until snack time.

I reassured his parents that it was all right for Todd to have snacks—he really did need them. Like every other child that age, his stomach was small and his energy needs were high, and he really couldn't get from one meal to the next without refueling. But I encouraged them to make planned snacks, where he sat down to the table and had something that they had helped pick out.

At snacks, as at meals, he was to be allowed to eat as much as he wanted. To keep from having his snack spoil his next meal they were to offer it mid-morning or mid-afternoon, far enough away from mealtime so he'd have a chance to get hungry again.

As I said, I encouraged them not to let him panhandle. When he got right down from the table and asked for something to eat, they were to tell him he had just had his meal, that he could have a snack before too long, and now he could run along and play. When he got hungry just before the next meal, they were to tell him that he was going to get all he wanted to eat then, and that he could wait.

At first he ate a lot whenever food was available and had a lot of crying fits when they didn't give in to his panhandling. I expect he was still afraid they wouldn't deliver and still stocking up in case they really didn't mean it. It was hard for his parents, because they didn't trust his internal food regulation process. His bulimic mother had long since lost touch with the process within herself, and his father had a hard time dealing with feelings of all kinds.

Part of the treatment was working with his mother on her eating, and keeping the father involved in the parenting of his son.

In any event, they were able to persist in giving Todd permission to eat, at the same time that they maintained some structure. And he relaxed about his eating. Eventually he got over eating as much as he could get his hands on, and began responding to his own hunger and appetite rather than to what was available. He became less likely to demand second helpings, and even stopped, at times, before he cleaned his plate. At other times he was more hungry, and his parents went along with him when he asked for more. (Although that was hard for them, and I have since wondered if they were able to persist in that without my reminders.)

You may remember the story they told initially to illustrate his uncontrolled eating: how he would clean up all the hors d'oeuvres when company came. At last report, they had had company, Todd had helped himself to a couple of cracker sandwiches and gone off to play. Once he was relieved of the necessity to fight for food, he had been able to go back to being a kid again. And his growth continued in an appropriate fashion. (In retrospect, I wondered if the fluctuations in his weight were a result of their being over-managing with his food intake—kind of like the swerving you get when you over-steer a car.) If I had had a chance, I would have worked with Brian in much the same way: controlling his mealtime and snacktime behaviors, and then leaving him to take over with his actual eating. If we had simply presented the food and left him alone to figure out that he was hungry, I think his own interest in food would have kicked in and he would have been all right. I'm not sure, because I didn't get a chance to try it.

But I'm not advocating the old "Leave them alone, when they get hungry enough, they will eat." In some cases children are so turned off to eating that they have to be worked with in a special treatment process to help them get back to it. I'll talk about that in Feeding the Child with Special Needs (Chapter 16).

Pressure On Food Acceptance

People get into forcing when they try to get a child to eat more or less than she really wants. They also do it when they try to get a child to finish a vegetable that she doesn't like (even if she simply doesn't like it just *that day*), or to eat in a manner that is not comfortable. It is also forcing to short-order cook, because that makes it very important to you that your child EAT and removes not-eating as an option. It is forcing when you try to get a baby to nurse faster or more slowly than at her natural tempo, or to eat on a schedule that is yours and not hers. It is forcing to keep a child from exploring solid food with her fingers or to stop her from trying to feed herself. It is forcing to bribe a child with a cookie or praise for eating certain foods, or to give a child "a look" when she turns down something.

It's Hard Not To Force

Forcing comes in many different forms, and ranges in intensity from the subtle to the vehement. Children are not innocent bystanders in the process. They do things that bring out the forcing tendencies in us adults, who are, after all, concerned about their welfare and *do* want the best for them.

Small Children Are Neophobic

In the first place, small children are neophobic: they fear anything new. Leann Birch[2], a child psychologist at the University of Illinois, found in her research that most two-year-olds routinely refused to taste new foods and did not like them when they tasted them. It took several exposures to the new food for them to get ready to taste it, and once having tasted it, it took a lot of tastes for them to get to the point where they liked it. (I hope you are getting the message that it is not wise to hold your breath while all this happens.)

Children's first reaction to a new food is negative and suspicious. In a word, "Yuk!" (And they also learn very quickly that that "Yuk" can run a thumbnail up the spine of any but the most placid of adults.) And most of us are at least tempted to respond, "Oh, it's Yuk, huh, well, we'll see about that!"

Forget it. You'll only embarrass yourself. She's in charge. When it comes to putting food in her mouth, chewing it and swallowing it, she is the one who is calling the shots. YOU got the food in front of her, and once you did that, you were out of a job.

(However, I must admit that I respect my own aggressive impulses enough to enforce a rule in my home against anyone saying "Yuk!" about anything I have prepared. They can refuse to eat it, but they must be polite about it.)

So we have actual research to prove what we have suspected all along: Generally toddlers turn down new food flat. (In this regard, anyway, common knowledge is right on the button.) But there is hope. Neophobia peaks out in two-year-olds and is much less of a problem with three- and four-year-olds, and five- and six-year-olds.

Knowing that helps us to recreate some scenarios with people like Brian, our reluctant french toast eater, or almost any finicky eater you know. Suppose in either situation a parent came along and started to put on pressure when they were just getting warmed up to try something new. What do you think would happen?

Right, they would balk. Or suppose that the parent provided an alternative food whenever the child showed the slightest hesitation about eating? Right, they would learn that the food wasn't worth considering in the first place. And they wouldn't get the chance to get used to the food and to grow out of the two-year-old neophobia. And, most limiting of all, they would learn to pay more attention to the parent's moves than to their own internal reaction to the food.

As generations of parents before us have wailed, "Why is my child behaving like this?" It doesn't seem like much of a survival tactic for a child to behave in a way to enrage her parents. There is a kinder interpretation. It could be that neophobia is an instinctive self-protective mechanism—how is a barely-talking two-year-old to know that something is good and safe? Until she gets older and develops some judgment in the matter, you wouldn't WANT your two-year-old to go around eating everything that is left sitting out.

Children Vary In How Much They Eat

Children also bring out forcing tendencies in parents because of the big variations in the amount and type of food they eat. Combine that with adults' tendency to manage quantities, in both themselves and their children, and you have trouble. I guarantee it!

Struggles over quantity are so common that I am spending the whole next chapter on it. I will summarize here. You can't predict how much a child will eat. From birth on, children vary a lot in their day-to-day food intake. They may eat half again one day as the next, and may go for several days eating relatively little, and then make up for it. They also eat differently from year to year. They generally eat relatively large amounts during infancy, then when they hit about age two they fall off on their food intake. That happens at about the same time that they get into neophobia, which *really* sets the stage for battles over eating.

It's easy to fall prey to this variation, especially if there is anything about your child's growth that is concerning you. I can easily understand how a parent of a small and thin child would get frightened and try to get a little more in on the small-eating days. I can also understand how the parent of a fat child might be tempted to restrict on the big-eating days. Add to those feelings the very common attitude (even among health professionals) that parents SHOULD manage amounts, and you have a lot of pressure–and it's on YOU.

Children Vary In What They Like

Children vary in what foods they find appealing. They love green beans one day, and you make more the next time, and then they aren't interested. Your mother will ask, "do the children like peas?" and you will be stumped for an answer because sometimes they do and sometimes they don't. Now the pressure is on *you* to be able to predict and produce pea-eaters. It's not your mother's fault—she just wants to know what to cook.

Children Vary In Their Love Of Eating

Everyone feels different about eating. Some children get a big kick out of eating, and others seem like they couldn't care less. A young mother in Louisiana (who looked like she was about 16 herself) had two of each, and two were twins. Louisiana has some great story tellers, so let's let her tell it.

"My daughter is 12 now, and she has always been chubby. She has always liked eating a lot, and at first I went along with her. I enjoyed it when she appreciated her food so much and got so excited when I fed her. But then I got started worrying that

41

she would get fat. So I tried to get her to eat a little less, and then when she did start getting fat I tried even harder. But she likes eating a lot, and she is always begging me for food and eating it when I tell her she can't.

"She has an eight-year old brother who is just the opposite. He doesn't like to stop what he's doing to come to dinner, and when he is full, he's full and I can't get him to take another bite.

"Now I also have twins and there is one of each. One of the little boys just LOVES to eat and he always pays attention to every spoonful and would eat forever if I kept on feeding him. When anybody else is eating, he wants some of it, whether he's just eaten or not. The other lets me know when he's hungry and eats as long as he's hungry, but once he's full, he completely loses interest. He won't even swallow if he gets full in the middle of a bite. When others are eating and he's full he just wants DOWN, and he'll yell until you let him."

So, which of the children have the "right" attitude about eating? Both, all of them, and everything in between. People feel a lot of different ways about it, and all feelings are acceptable. Our thinness-conscious times tell us we're not to be too hooked on eating. But some of us just are, and we'll get lots further if we work with those feelings rather than battling against them.

Since children are a lot smarter than adults in the area of feelings and interactions, I won't be able to list ALL the ways they arouse us to use forcing tactics. I think you'll get more clues from the age-related chapters in the middle, numbers 7 through 12.

Forcing Doesn't Work

If you feed (or try to feed) a child less or more than he really wants, it can produce the opposite of what you want. Children who are overfed become revolted by food and prone to undereat when they get a chance. They also become skillful at manipulating their parents to do what they want them to do by refusing to eat.

On the other hand, children who are underfed become preoccupied with food and prone to overeat when they get the chance. The more parents try to restrict children's eating the more pressure children put on eating. They feel like they have to put up a struggle to get food.

In the struggle with their parents about eating, children learn that there is something the matter with their bodies, and with them. Since their desires are so often in conflict with what their parents seem willing to give to them, eventually they become embarrassed at their needs. Later, when they grow up, children enter into the struggle with themselves. They feel a great deal of conflict between what they want and what they think they should want. And they continue to be ashamed of their desires.

You, as a parent, may get into problems with feeding because you have a lot of pressure on YOU. Part of that pressure comes from "common knowledge." People have a lot of opinions about what it takes to make a child eat well. If feeding is not going well or if a child is growing poorly, they are quite willing to offer their advice, "for whatever it is worth," they often say. Usually it isn't worth much. In fact, it is worse than worthless; it is downright destructive. Fortunately, we have more to go on than opinion. There has been quite a bit of good research on effective feeding, and we can use it to guide us.

Pressure Can Make A Child Grow Poorly

A nutritionist in Texas, Ernesto Pollitt[3], wondered specifically if mothers' behaviors could produce underfed children. He was working with Puerto Rican children who were not growing very well. In fact they were growing so poorly that they were classified as "failure to thrive," a diagnostic term that refers to serious growth failure. Pollitt compared their mothers' feeding techniques with techniques of mothers whose babies were growing well, and observed that the mothers of the poorly-growing babies were very active during feeding. They did a lot of nipple-moving and wiping and arranging of their babies and generally disrupted the pace of the feedings.

Children Can Call Out Forcing

A researcher in Scotland, Peter Wright[4], wondered if there were characteristics of certain babies that encouraged their mothers to be overactive in feeding them. Wright compared the mothers of low birth weight babies with those of normal weight babies and further subdivided the groups into bottle-fed and

43

breast-fed babies. He found that the bottle feeding mothers were more active with low birth weight babies. And the more active they were, the less the babies ate. Mothers would ignore their baby's responses and screw the nipple into the baby's mouth whether or not she was turning toward the nipple or rooting for it.

The less active bottle feeding mothers in both low and normal weight groups had babies who grew better. On the other hand, all breast-fed babies grew about the same, whether they were low or normal weight. Even the babies' smallness didn't (or couldn't) encourage overactive breast-feeding. One of the advantages of breast-feeding is that it is lots harder to be over managing. You have to share the responsibility for feeding whether you want to or not.

In short, Wright found that parents' concern about their children's nutrition and growth often showed up as pressure tactics in feeding. Tiffany Field[5], a specialist in infant-parent interactions, observed the same thing, both with parents of premature babies and with those who were post mature (born considerably after their due date). She observed that after babies were designated as being "at nutritional risk," pressure tactics in feeding began to emerge. Parents (and health workers) did more jiggling of the bottle and pulling the nipple in and out and jostling the babies.

We can understand why they did that—when someone seems to need help it is natural to try to help. But, ironically, the "helping" tactics backfired—the children ate less, rather than more, when feeders got pushy.

Even Subtle Forcing Backfires

If you do anything with feeding that even remotely feels to them like forcing, most children will do the exact opposite of what you want. Leann Birch[6], our Illinois psychologist-of-the-neophobia, tried it, in the nicest possible way. In her preschool laboratory, she rewarded children for trying a new food. *Rewarded* them: gave them something nice. Another group she did not reward, but simply let them approach the food in their own way; no comments, no facial expressions. The children who were rewarded were *less* likely to go back to the new food than children who were left alone. Children are not dumb: They know when they are being forced, even when it is done in the nicest possible way.

Other research findings are consistent. Martha Kinter and her colleagues[7] at the University of Wisconsin found that children had poorer diets when their family tried too hard to control their behavior *in general*, not just their eating behavior. Years ago, Mary Hinton[8], a home economist, found that teenage girls' diets got WORSE the more their families criticized and interfered with their eating.

I don't have any research on toddlers, but it doesn't take a research project to know that if you try to get a toddler to do anything she doesn't want to do you have a fight on your hands. And you'll lose. Since I don't like to lose, I have learned to pick my battles: I can stop a toddler from doing what I don't want her to do, but I can't get her to do what I want her to do. I won't short-order cook for her, but neither will I try to force her to eat her peas. Withholding food can make matters worse.

Forcing doesn't work with fat children, either. The tactic of withholding food from a too-fat child can not only make her feel bad about herself, it can also make her eat more. In my practice, I have observed children getting fatter, starting from the time their parents instituted a weight reduction regimen. The children have been frightened that they won't get enough to eat, and apparently ended up eating more than before.

My clinical observations, however, hardly qualify as research. As a consequence, I was extremely interested in a study of overweight children by two psychologists at Duke University[9] that showed that the more parents had controlled and restricted the children's food intake, the fatter they were. (The Duke psychologists also pointed out that lots of studies in areas other than eating have shown that children don't do as well when their parents are too controlling. Children grow up to be less self controlled, more dependent, less persistent, and do less well in real-life situations.)

With respect to eating, when parents over manage, it takes away their children's ability to manage themselves. So when you are not around or when you relax your supervision, children don't have themselves to fall back on, and they may eat too much.

Where To From Here?

I have said pressure is out in child feeding. What does that give you as an alternative? LOTS! We'll be spending the rest of this book talking about thinking, approaches and attitudes you can use in helping your child learn to eat well and, more importantly, to grow up with healthy *attitudes* about eating.

Throughout, we'll talk about division of responsibility in feeding: The parent is responsible for WHAT, the child is responsible for HOW MUCH and even WHETHER.

As I said earlier, parents get into trouble with feeding because they fail to do what they should, and do what they shouldn't. They fail to put themselves in charge of the menu, and short-order cook, or fail to get a meal on the table at all. Then they get after their child for the amount she is eating or the type of food she is digging out of the refrigerator.

Why Do Parents Force?

Parents cross the lines of division of responsibility in feeding for a variety of reasons. The reason I run across most often is simple misunderstanding about food regulation or food selection. Parents don't know that children have the built-in capability to choose a nutritious diet (assuming a selection of generally-nutritious food is offered) and to eat the right amount to allow them to grow well. Both are much-misunderstood topics, so we'll spend whole chapters on them in How Much Should Your Child Eat? (Chapter 4), and Nutritional Tactics for Preventing Food Fights (Chapter 6).

In many cases there is something about the child that brings out pressure tactics in the parent. We'll talk about that in lots of places, most notably Feeding the Child with Special Needs (Chapter 16). Sometimes a child has had an interruption in feeding, and problems develop when you try to get back to normal feeding. I'll talk about that in the chapters I just referred to. Sometimes health workers give bad or misguided or tactless information, and it puts pressure on feeding. I will try to protect you against that, throughout. I might add that health workers are only human, and have been subjected to the same myths and misconceptions about eating and feeding as everyone else.

Finally, to be brutally honest, sometimes feeding is distorted because parents aren't doing a good job of parenting—in general, or with food in particular. To learn from this or any other book, you have to be functioning pretty well. If you are having a really difficult time, you need more help than I can give you in a book. You need counseling to be able to look at your situation and come up with solutions that work for you. I hope you'll get it—it can make an enormous difference.

Do You Really Want To Know All This?

As a medical student said to me the other day (in reaction to my sterling lecture on feeding), "Why do we have to know all this? Feeding is just instinctive. It isn't that important, and it doesn't have to be so complicated." I reacted calmly and persuasively (I thought), and told him what I summarize below.

• The world is full of dumb ideas about feeding, and they can mess up parents who are trying to do a good job.

• When feeding is done poorly, children eat and grow poorly.

• Feeding is a metaphor for the parent-child relationship overall. Parents will probably treat a child in other areas the way they learn to treat her in feeding.

• Children learn from feeding what to expect from the world. It teaches them about themselves and about other people.

Enough said and on to our how-to!

References

1. Satter, E.M.: The feeding relationship. Journal of the American Dietetic Association 86:352-356, 1986.

2. Birch, L.L. and Marlin, D.W.: I don't like it; I never tried it: Effects of exposure on two-year-old children's food preferences. Appetite 3:353-360, 1982.

3. Pollitt, E. and Wirtz, S.: Mother-infant feeding interaction and weight gain in the first month of life. Journal of the American Dietetic Association 78:596-60l, 1981.

47

4.   Wright, P., Fawcett, J., and Crow, R.: The development of differences in the feeding behavior of bottle and breast fed human infants from birth to two months. Behavioural Processes 5:1-20, 1980.

5.   Field, T.: Maternal stimulation during infant feeding. Developmental Psychology 13:539-540, 1977.

6.   Birch, L.L., Marlin, D.W. and Rotter, J.: Eating as the "means" activity in a contingency: Effects on young children's food preference. Child Development 55(2):431-439. 1984.

7.   Kinter, M., Boss, P.G., and Johnson, N.: The relationship between dysfunctional family environments and family member food intake. Journal of Marriage and the Family 43(3):633-641, 1981.

8.   Hinton, M.A., Chadderdon, H., Eppright, E. and Wolins, L.: Influences on girls' eating behavior. Journal of Home Economics 54:842-846. 1962.

9.   Costanzo, P.R. and Woody, E.Z.: Domain-specific parenting styles and their impact on the child's development of particular deviance: The example of obesity proneness. Journal of Social and Clinical Psychology, 3:425-445, 1985.

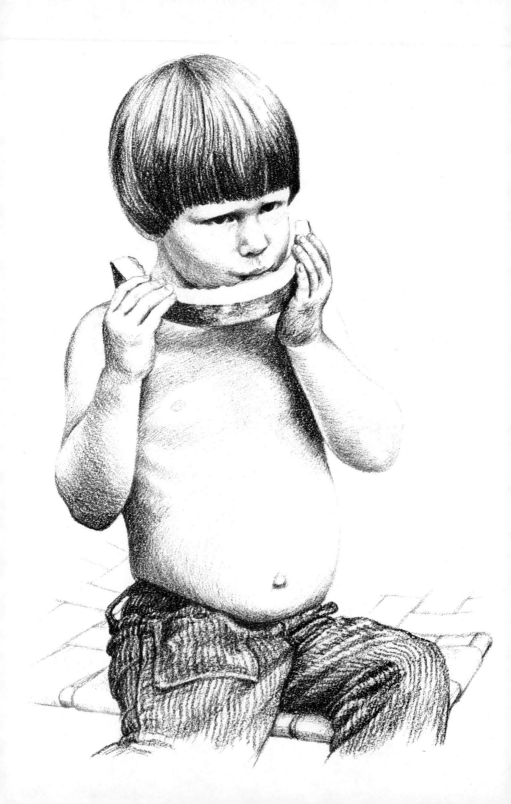

4

How Much Should Your Child Eat?

Don't try to control the amount your child eats. There is nothing that will get you into struggles about eating faster, unless it is fighting about *what* your child eats. We'll get to that soon.

Your job, as parent, is to help your child eat in a way that allows him to grow up with the body that is right for him—and feel good about it. Your child has within him the genetic blueprint for his height, weight, growth pattern and physical capability. You won't know what the blueprint says until it is all over. You can modify the course of his growth somewhat with feeding and training, but only a little and with a lot of effort (and trauma) on all sides. It's pretty risky to try to change a child's growth pattern, because that pattern is changing all the time even *without* your help, and you have no way of knowing what's normal for him in the first place.

You can help your child grow up appropriately by following his lead and playing a supportive role. I will talk more about your role in other chapters. Here, I will tell you some things about food regulation and growth and try to steer you in a direction that, I hope, will get the pressure off you to try to make things turn out the way you think they ought to.

51

You Can't Predict How Much Children Will Eat

Children know lots better than their parents do how much they need to eat. If you try to help in that area it *won't* help, and may only cause a lot of trouble. Wiser heads than yours and mine have found that out.

Children Vary Day-to-Day

Back in the thirties, when people were first beginning to bottle feed, they tried very hard to learn how. This was the "scientific age of feeding." A formula based on evaporated milk had just been perfected. Supplemented with vitamin C in some form, it finally solved the age-old problem of babies' getting diarrhea from artificial feedings, and opened the door for bottle feeding. And people switched from breast to bottle feeding in increasing numbers. Bottle feeding was "modern," but nobody really knew how to do it.

Unfortunately, to begin with, nobody asked the babies. The then-new professions of pediatrics and nutrition attempted to fill the gap with scientific reasoning. They figured out how many calories babies "should" be having per pound of body weight, weighed them and measured them and calculated their total allotment. Then they divided that into six equal feedings (every four hours, you know) and instructed parents to give the babies just that, no more, no less, at exactly those intervals around the clock.

If parents failed to follow the regimen, there were dire warnings about the physical and emotional distortions that would result. Like the feeding recommendations, these were largely the product of someone's imagination, and had very little to so with knowledge of how babies really operated.

But at the Gesell Institute, Arnold Gesell and Frances Ilg challenged these assumptions[1]. They said, essentially, wait a minute, that's not the way babies really are! If feeders are that controlling and ignore information coming from babies, it is going to cause a lot of problems, and both parents and babies are going to suffer.

52

By way of backing up their contention, they did a series of bottle feeding experiments with babies, where they fed them when they were hungry and as much as they were hungry for. They let them go to sleep when they wanted to and sleep as long as they wanted to. And when they woke up they fed them whenever they asked for it, even if they wanted to eat twice in a row after a long nap.

They kept track of how much the babies ate and weighed them every day. Figures 4-1 and 4-2, show what happened with one little boy, Baby "J."

The only thing that was consistent about J's intake was its inconsistency. One day he ate a lot, the next day not so much. His intake from day to day varied by about 20 to 30%. During the third week of the study, when he was eight weeks old, he had a cold and his intake varied even more. One day, for example, it was only 20 ounces, the next day it was 32. But his growth was perfectly smooth, even during that third week when his food intake varied so widely. Little "J" knew what he was doing.

Children Vary Child-to-Child

Babies are not weird about eating. In fact, it seems to me they demonstrate normal eating for us in the purest form, before it is all distorted by funny ideas.

Babies are not the only ones who vary in their food intake: Older children and adults do the same thing. We just aren't aware of it, because we don't hover and measure food intake in ounces and count carefully numbers of feedings per day. Let's go back to babies to start discussing how people vary in their overall calorie intake.

Figure 4-3, "Variation in Food Intake—Light Babies Were Heaviest Eaters," illustrates graphically a rather routine feeding study that gave some rather remarkable results[2].

Researchers talked to the mothers of 650 children up to a year old to find out how much their children ate, and calculated the children's average 24-hour intake. The researchers then separated off the 35 who ate the most and the 34 who ate the least. The contrast was startling. The lightest-eating children, who consumed only 550 calories per day, were the heaviest—they weighed on the average 20 pounds. The heaviest-eating children ate 1100 calories per day weighed an average of 14½ pounds.

53

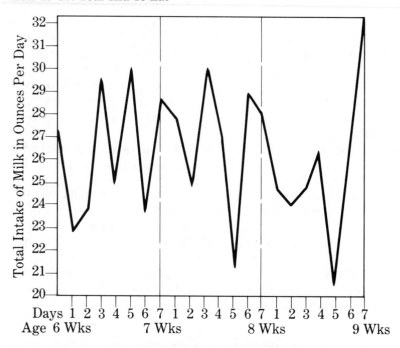

Figure 4-1 **Formula Intake Chart of Baby J** *(Courtesy J. B. Lippincott)*

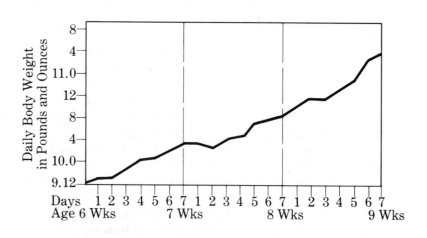

Figure 4-2 **Growth of Baby J** *(Courtesy J. B. Lippincott)*

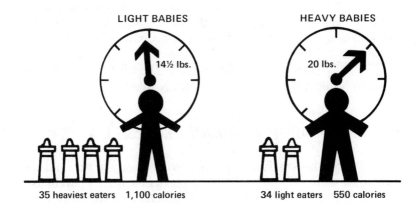

LIGHT BABIES — 14½ lbs. — 35 heaviest eaters   1,100 calories

HEAVY BABIES — 20 lbs. — 34 light eaters   550 calories

Figure 4-3   Variation in Food Intake—Light babies were heaviest eaters.

There is some question about this study because the researchers got their data by talking with mothers, who could have distorted the information. If a mother was self conscious about having a thinner-than-average or fatter-than-average baby, she could have fudged the information a bit to make it look like her baby was eating more or less than he really was. (I'm not accusing the mothers of lying—in most cases this fudging is done unconsciously.)

But there was another, more-carefully controlled study done by two Harvard nutritionists that showed essentially the same thing[3]. They actually recorded and measured what the babies ate. They also found out how much they exercised, by strapping tiny pedometers to their arms and legs. Like the study above, the Harvard people noted that the fattest babies were the least active and ate the least. And the leanest babies were the most active and ate the most.

All of this is to demonstrate that you *can't* do what they tried to do in the thirties: look at a baby, or even weigh him, and decide how much he needs to eat. There is too much variation, day-to-day and baby-to-baby. And that variation persists beyond

55

the baby stage. Statistics about children of all ages (and adults) show that one person may be eating twice as much as another who is the same height and weight and seemingly exercising the same. Figures 4-4 and 4-5, "Range of Recommended Calorie Intake at Different Ages for Boys and Men/Girls and Women," respectively, show in graph form information from the National Research Council's Recommended Daily Allowances[4].

Controlling Amounts Doesn't Work

People think they can get their child's body to turn out the way they want it to by feeding in a particular way. A psychologist in Minnesota told me about a young mother who was so determined that her children were not going to get fat that she frankly underfed them. The children were thin and short. They were eating too little to grow properly in any way.

The mother used only low-fat recipes and foods and would not allow them to have butter or margarine or salad dressings (even though they needed *some* fat to keep them healthy—see Nutritional Tactics for Preventing Food Fights, Chapter 6). She was very stingy with breads and other starchy foods (although, as I'll explain in the nutrition chapter, starchy foods are not really all that fattening). And she *certainly* would not let them eat candy. Or any thing sweet.

Not only was all the food low in calories, she also restricted the amounts they ate. She would let them eat only so much at mealtimes, even if they said they were hungry and begged for more. And she would absolutely not let them eat between meals. She left instructions with all the baby sitters she hired that they were not to feed the children. It was hard on the sitters, because the children were hungry and couldn't get their minds on playing. But the sitters didn't dare feed them, because the mother could tell by the satisfied way they behaved if they had been fed. Most sitters wouldn't work for her any more, because they felt so sorry for the kids.

This is an extreme case. So extreme, in fact that I called it child abuse and advised the psychologist to report it to the proper authorities. Failing to give a child enough food is fundamental neglect.

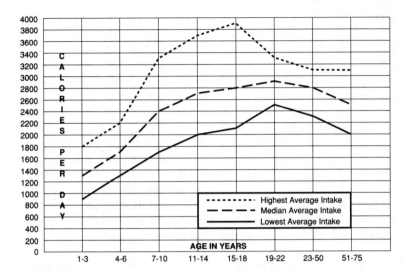

Figure 4-4:   Range of Recommended Calorie Intakes at Different Ages for Boys and Men

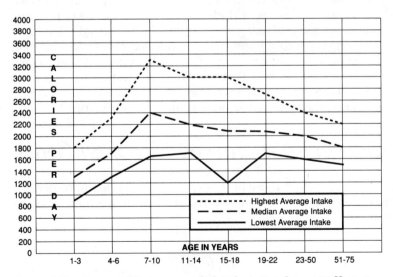

Figure 4-5:   Range of Recommended Calorie Intakes at Different Ages for Girls and Women

Happily, parents' attempts to control amounts are generally more benign, although not totally so. As with the Minnesota family, often over-control starts out with concern about a child's body build. There are all sorts of variations on the theme of parents wanting their children to turn out a certain way: Fathers who want a petite and slender daughter who is pretty and appealing; mothers who want a robust and muscular son who is strong and forceful; parents who want their children to be great soccer players or gymnasts or dancers. And, consciously or unconsciously, parents put pressure on children's eating to get to get the reality to fit the dream.

It is better for you to be curious about how your child will turn out than committed to a certain outcome. We all have our fantasies about our children. If we have the ability to let them grow up to be their own people, the fantasies get replaced by the reality, which, while it may not be as ideal, is a lot more entertaining. But if we let the fantasies (and our own egos) take over, it can result in a lot of pressure and frustration and disappointment on all sides.

The child who grows up in a family with over-controlling parents has a hard time knowing if he is making choices based on what he wants and is interested in, or whether he is just going along with (or rebelling against) what his parent wants for him. Many psychological studies[5] have demonstrated that when parents are too managing, they interfere with a child's developing ways of managing *himself*. Our underfed Minnesota children, like "overfed" Brian and "underfed" Todd in the last chapter, are going to have a difficult time detecting and respecting their own senses of hunger and fullness. They have always been forced to depend on their parents to manage their eating for them.

Growth Is Determined Mostly By Genes

Your child is more likely to grow and develop in response to your genes than to your wishes. There is such a thing as body type. You have it, I have it.

Body Type

There are three basic body types: The ectomorph, the mesomorph, and the endomorph. Translated into plain English, the types are: Slender and linear, muscular and blocky, and broad and, well fat. Soft, maybe. Slender and linear is popular right now—for women and, some for men. Mia Farrow is an ectomorph, as is Anthony Perkins. Pete Rose is a mesomorph, and so is Mary Lou Retton. Michael Caine is an endomorph, and so is Bette Middler.

A child who is an ectomorph will probably weigh relatively little compared to his height on the growth curves: He would have a higher percentile ranking for height than for weight. (More about growth curves later in the chapter.) The mesomorph is likely to be heavier than he is tall on the growth curves and, when an adult, may even weigh in the obese range on the height-for-weight tables, even with very little fat on his *or her* body—some *women* are very muscular, too.

The nutrition textbooks give the example of the football players who were rejected for the military draft on the basis of their "obesity," when actually they weren't obese at all but very muscular. They compare the physically-fit football player with a ribbon salesman, who weighed in the "normal" range but actually had a higher percentage of body fat.

The endomorph might or might not be heavier than average. Fat is fluffier than lean, may look bulkier but doesn't weigh as much. Endomorphs have pear-shaped bodies—relatively narrow shoulders and broad hips. They have more fat layered over their muscles than the other types, so they feel and look softer.

Hardly anyone is a "pure" body type, but we all have our tendencies. Children inherit body types from their parents. And parents are not always happy about that, particularly when they would rather their child would inherit something other than their body type, like intelligence or charm, maybe.

I know an attractive couple with two attractive children. The father is a mesomorph—broad and strong in face and body and hands and arms and feet and legs. He's about average height. The mother is short and slender with a narrow face, and slender body and limbs and hands and feet. And the children take after them. The boy is built like his mother and the girl is built like her father. The boy is over six feet tall and slender and linear. The girl is about her mother's height, and blocky.

Both children describe their ideal bodies as what they would have had if nature had switched the genes around and

59

made her more slender and him more solid. But they laugh about it—it's a family joke that they all enjoy. It certainly is hard to pity them—the kids are strong and healthy and talented and resourceful and popular.

Bodies And Performance

Let's face it, body type is not just an *aesthetic* concern. It is a concern about *performance*. We learn that tall people do better in business, and we certainly don't know any mesomorphs who are ballet dancers or ectomorphs who are weight lifters. To a certain extent, your body can determine your destiny.

The same holds true for kids, and they start finding that out in middle school and high school. Kids' bodies determine their opportunities in sports. There was a article in the paper the other day about a 76-year-old-man who is very active in community recreational sports. He said he had been playing in community rec ever since he was a sophomore in high school because he couldn't make the school teams. He was too short for basketball, too light for football, and his legs were not long enough for track. But he loved sports, and he had to find his outlet wherever he could. So he turned to recreational sports, and has been at it ever since. He is probably playing and contributing long after his super star associates have hung up their jock straps.

My daughter Kjerstin got into the same thing with her body, and she is typical of a lot of other kids. She wasn't light enough for track, was too short for basketball, and didn't make the soccer team. She finally went out for high school crew and did very well at it, because she is strong and coordinated.

But now she is in college and competing against kids who are strong, coordinated and TALL, and she has lost out in crew also. For a while, she kept measuring herself and hoping that she would GROW. (She thought she had gotten taller, but it turned out she had found a defective height measure, and she was still having to look way up to talk to some of her teammates.) So she decided she would be the team manager. She travels around with the team and makes things work for them and is a part of all the fun and trauma. She trains with them, but only competes in the games, not in the real competitions. And she's having a good time.

60

These situations get resolved, but in the process we are talking real adolescent tragedy. It is hard to be philosophical when your child spends the whole weekend crying because he is too small and light to make the hockey team. And you *shouldn't* be philosophical. You should be sympathetic and understanding and accepting of the way he feels. You'll feel bad, too, but as an adult you'll know that other opportunities do present themselves.

Keep things in perspective for yourself, but keep it *to* yourself. There is nothing worse than having a *parent* come along and advise you to take a more dispassionate point of view when your world has *ended*! Eventually, he'll recover, and then could use your support in finding some other outlet for his talents.

Those who got the luck of the draw got a body type that is currently fashionable and one that lets them do what they want to do. The rest have had to learn to live with it. When it really comes right down to it, most of us don't have the most fashionable physique, but we manage to do very well in spite of it. We've all known successful short business executives.

Changing Your Child's Body

Some people try to change their body types by dieting or working out with weights or having plastic surgery. There is probably nothing wrong with that, for adults who have their opinion of themselves pretty well formed. Nothing wrong, that is as long as the people don't end up making such horrendous sacrifices of time and emotional and physical energy that it impairs their ability to live their lives.

But, with children, it is a different story. If you keep after them to diet or to eat more or to exercise more (or less) than they really want to, they are going to get just one message from it: There is something wrong with their bodies the way they are. And for kids, it is a very short step from your saying something is wrong with *them*.

Kids don't need that. It is pretty alarming for a child to grow up and find out what his body holds in store for him. Teenagers, especially, are so body conscious and have such fixed notions about the "ideal body." The girls wait for breasts and hope that they won't get too tall or too fat and hope that their

61

legs and hips and waists will be nice and slender. Boys watch some of their friends growing taller and faster and becoming muscular and see themselves still being short and slender and wait for the day when they will start to grow—and fear that it will never come. Who said the teen years were the best years of life?

If parents are caught up in body consciousness for their child, it makes it even harder. If parents impose diets or health foods, or pressure a child to eat certain foods to become "big and strong," there is nobody around to help the kids hold steady. What parents need to do is remind their kids to keep their nerve and keep eating sensibly, to wait for time to pass and to adjust to whatever nature has to offer.

Helping Your Child Like His Body

Your attitude about your child's appearance makes all the difference. If you truly feel your child is attractive and competent, he will feel that way about himself. If your attitude is positive, you will be able to help him deal with problems his body presents. On the other hand, if you can't have a positive attitude toward your child you had better get some help with it. Don't be like the mother who hauled her chubby three-year-old in to me and said, "I will NOT have a fat child!"

One good example of how you can help is with appearance. You can encourage your child to find clothes that are truly flattering. Short T-Shirts don't look good on little kids who have a roll of fat around the middle. Skinny stretch pants and tight T-Shirts don't look good on people who are very thin. "Floods" (a term applied to too-short jeans) accentuate tallness and thinness (and are also not cool—right now).

The way a skirt or a pair of pants is cut can make all the difference in how attractive they look on someone. And *everybody* but the most perfectly-built person has to put some time and energy into finding clothes that fit and look good. Your attitude about doing that will make all the difference. I have so often had my obese adult patients tell me about how their mothers would run out of patience with shopping for them, and tell them, "If you would just lose some weight, it wouldn't be so hard to buy clothes for you."

Understanding Kids' Growth

To understand normal growth, it helps to understand growth charts. I talked about growth charts in detail in *Child of Mine*[6], and I have included growth records of the children I have talked about. There are several in The Child Who Grows Poorly (Chapter 13).

To summarize the principles of growth charts, children usually grow in height and weight in predictable ways that you can plot out on standard growth graphs. There are graphs for height and weights of boys and girls of different ages. I have included copies in "Tools and Strategies" in the Appendix.

The graphs, most importantly, allow you to observe your child's growth over time to see if it is following one of the percentile lines on the charts. When a child fails to follow the channel he usually follows, especially if he diverges significantly (like Todd did in figure 3-1 in Pressure Doesn't Work, Chapter 3) we can catch it and try to figure out what is causing the growth to vary.

You can also use the charts to compare your child's shape and growth with that of other kids. This is strictly for entertainment, however. Kids vary enormously in the way they grow and, as far as the charts are concerned, it is all normal.

Most doctors' offices use growth charts for plotting children's progress in height and weight. You can ask to see them, but do get help from your health worker in interpreting them.

Surprises In Growth

While it is all very predictable, kids' growth still does some alarming things that might make you lose your nerve about letting them grow up on their own. Normal growth during the first year includes putting on a considerable amount of fat. The average newborn infant has about 11% body fat, the year-old infant about 24%. That percentage decreases to 21% by age two and 18% by age three[6].

Children generally slim down as they get older. Curtis, my youngest child, is the chubby 2-year-old at the beginning of this chapter (page 50), and the lean teenager on page 236.

Children sometimes get chubby during the winter (at least in the upper midwest, where the winters are long and the out-

63

door sports limited by endurance and frostbite). Both boys and girls gain in percentage of body fat just before the growth spurt of puberty. It is like they have to store up extra energy to provide for the demands of sudden growth.

On the other end of the spectrum, often children grow very slowly and appear very small and slender. In most cases, this is normal for them. Trying to determine that is what makes everyone so nervous: *Is* this normal growth for the child, or is there something wrong? We'll struggle with this in The Child Who Grows Poorly (Chapter 13).

To repeat, most cases of slow growth are normal for the child. A child who grows slowly early on is not necessarily going to keep on growing slowly. Children do catch-up growing. When they get through a period of illness or a slow start for whatever reason, they will often grow faster for a while.

Normal Growth

As a general rule, the newborn doubles his birth weight by four months and triples it by one year. During the first year the average gain is about 15 pounds; during the next two years it slows to five or six pounds a year. Then for the next two years weight gain levels off at around five pounds annually for boys, four pounds for girls. Then it starts to climb again to the growth spurt of adolescence.

The growth patterns of boys and girls diverge as they get into the accelerated growth of adolescence. On the average, boys grow most from ages 12 through 16. During that time they have a good chance of getting 12 inches taller and 50 to 60 pounds heavier. They achieve *most* of their height by the time they are 18 to 20 (but they might be as much as an inch taller by their late 20s), and they continue to put on weight from added muscle for about two years after that[6].

Girls grow the fastest from ages 10 through 14, during which time the average girl gets 10 inches taller and 40-50 pounds heavier. After that time, they grow slowly in height and put on weight, primarily in the form of fat[7].

Sexual maturation signals the near-end of the rapid growth of adolescence. When girls get breasts and body hair and their periods and boys develop body hair and adult-type genitals, they can assume that they are almost as tall as they are going to get.

Girls And Dieting

Girls often dread putting on weight, and try to prevent the weight and fat gain that is a normal part of maturation. It's not surprising that they feel that way. The partly-mature teenage girl has the body build that tends to be idealized by the fashion and advertising industries. Fat accumulation supposedly spoils that body. Girls need real encouragement to allow themselves to grow up. It they get caught up in vehement dieting to try to prevent that normal fat accumulation, they will waste a lot of perfectly good energy and creativity and postpone having to deal with what it means to be a woman.

Girls are all too ready to diet. My children's girl friends in the sixth or seventh grade began to talk about being "too fat," and to discuss their diets. For the most part it was what everyone else (and their older sister) was doing. Typically, the diet was initiated at breakfast only to be scrapped when something good showed up on the line at school lunch. They shelved the diet whenever it was convenient and ate just the same at parties as they always had. They shrieked and giggled and groaned about their eating and weight and, generally, acted like adolescent girls.

But some of them (and not only the chubby ones) were dead serious about it. They truly starved themselves. A medical center study has shown that some girls diet with such dedication they don't grow very well and even delay puberty[8]. Some sports make that worse. Girls who are very active in gymnastics and figure skating and ballet have a special pressure on them. The successful gymnasts and skaters, particularly, have prepubescent body builds.

Sadly, body build has a real impact on the performance of the sport. Once a girl starts to develop and gain weight, it changes the balance of her body and the amount of strength it requires to maneuver. Consciously or unconsciously, many girls involved in there sports restrict their eating to delay puberty. Some develop anorexia nervosa in their determination to control their body builds.

Parents' Role In Girls' Dieting

Generally, when the situation gets really serious the girls aren't getting much help from their parents. The parents are

65

often very concerned about their own weight and not very supportive about encouraging their children to take their chances with growing up. Some parents have a very hard time letting go of their dreams about their child's performance or appearance, so they don't help their child in changing directions, either. Sometimes parents are just plain not available to help, and the kids get frightened and diet to try to provide structure and safety for themselves.

Your attitude as a parent can make all the difference. One of my friends told her girls when they wanted to diet, "you're not fat. You are getting hips and you are getting breasts. That's normal and it's sexy and you're growing up to be a woman. You are not fat." Your daughter will probably deny you know anything about the subject, but secretly she will listen and be helped by your conviction and reassurance.

Even if your child is fat, don't promote or even support dieting until he or she gets through puberty. You really don't know what is normal growth for your child, you don't know how it is all going to turn out. If you intervene, you could screw up the natural growth process and just make matters worse.

I am not saying you should ignore the whole process. In Helping All You Can to Keep Your Child from Being Fat (Chapter 14), I talk about some indirect methods that can be helpful in allowing your child to achieve normal growth. You need to do what you can do to support normal growth. But you mustn't try to do too much, or you will get a physical or emotional reaction that could end up making your child fatter rather than thinner.

Once your child is well through the rapid growth of puberty, he may get to the point where he wants to diet to lose weight. That's a different matter. Diets at that point can be helpful. Maybe. If they are conducted very carefully. It's a pretty touchy subject, and I am going to wait before getting into that, too. Chapter 14 is a good place for that discussion.

What have we really said in this chapter? Your child will eat and grow according to his or her own constitutional blueprint. If you don't like the way things are going, you'll be better off learning to live with it rather than trying to change it. In the long run, you could make matters worse. Lots worse.

References

1.   Gesell, A., and Ilg, F.L.: Feeding Behavior of Infants. Philadelphia: J.B. Lippincott, 1937.

2.   Purvis, G.A.: Infant Nutrition Survey. Gerber Products Company, 1979.

3.   Rose, H.E. and Mayer, J.: Activity, calorie intake, fat storage and the energy balance of infants. Pediatrics 41:18, 1968.

4.   Committee on Dietary Allowances, Food and Nutrition Board, National Research Council, National Academy of Sciences, Recommended Dietary Allowances. U.S. Government Printing Office, 1980.

5.   Costanzo, P.R. and Woody, E.Z.: Domain-specific parenting styes and their impact on the child' development of particular deviance: The example of obesity proneness. Journal of Social and Clinical Psychology 3:425-445, 1985.

6.   Satter, E.M.: Child of Mine: Feeding with Love and Good Sense. Palo Alto, CA: Bull Publishing, 1983. Expanded edition, 1986.

7.   Christian, J.L. and Greger, J.L.: Nutrition for Living. Benjamin Cummings, Menlo Park, CA 1985.

8.   Pugliese, M.T., Lifshitz, F., Grad, G., Fort, P., and Marks-Katz, M.: Fear of obesity; a cause of short stature and delayed puberty. The New England Journal of Medicine 309:513-518, 1983.

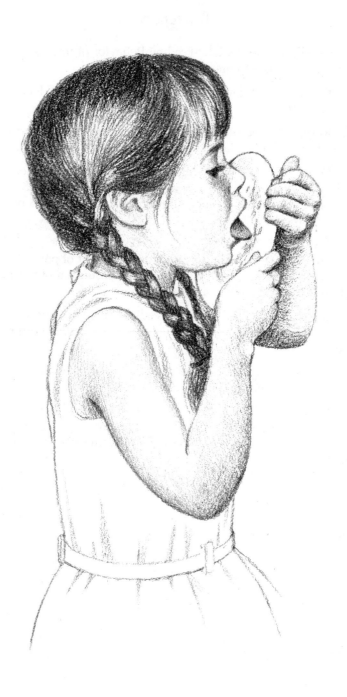

5

What Is Normal Eating?

Before we are going to be able to talk about normal eating for your child, we have to talk about normal eating for *you*. Dieting is so prevalent, and puritanical attitudes about eating are so common, that people have gotten some very restrictive ideas about what is normal and natural in eating. Normal eating is, essentially, positive and flexible eating that depends on internal cues to regulate it.

Let me share with you a handout that I give to people whose eating problems I treat:

Normal Eating

Normal eating is being able to eat when you are hungry and continue eating until you are satisfied. It is being able to choose food you like and eat it and truly get enough of it—not just stop eating because you think you should. Normal eating is being able to use some moderate constraint in your food selection to get the right food, but *not* being so restrictive that you miss out on pleasurable foods. Normal eating is giving yourself permission to eat sometimes because you are happy, sad or bored, or just because it feels good. Normal eating is three meals a day, most of the time, but it can also be choosing to munch along. It is leaving some cookies on the plate because you know you can have some again tomorrow, or it is eating more now because they taste so wonderful when they are fresh. Normal eating is overeating at times: feeling stuffed and uncomfortable. It is also undereating at times and wishing you had more. Normal eating is trusting your body to make up for your mistakes in eating. Normal eating takes up some of your time and attention, but keeps its place as only one important area of your life.

In short, normal eating is flexible. It varies in response to your emotions, your schedule, your hunger, and your proximity to food.

With children, especially with babies, we are ahead of the game. They already know how to eat normally; they were born with the ability to take in food and to regulate it, and they haven't had a lot of outside influences disrupting that ability. I have learned a lot about normal eating from babies, because I always think, if babies do it, it must be normal! In fact, I often teach my eating-disordered adolescents and adults about normal eating by talking about how babies do it.

Older children are pretty good at eating normally, too, but since they have had time to learn strange ideas and habits from their elders, they aren't as good at it as babies.

The key word, when you talk about normal *anything*, is flexibility. Whenever I observe feeding interactions, I am always struck by the great variability in the positive interactions and the rigidity of the negative ones. When things are going well, parents and children have many different, and often surprising, ways of working it out. When things are going poorly, there is a rigid sameness about the way people operate.

I'll tell you more about infant artistry in eating in The Newborn and The Older Baby (Chapters 7 and 8). Right now I am making the point that the way your family works out eating is a very individual matter: there are no hard-and-fast rules. In this chapter, in fact, in this whole book, I am trying to free you up so you CAN work it out.

Let's take a look at some of those variations in normal—in children and in eating.

Temperament

The way a child eats has everything to do with how she operates as a person. There are intrinsic variations in babies, and those variations affect their eating. When children get older, the way we react to them begins to moderate their behavior. When they are babies, we just have to go along and be as accommodating as possible.

Some babies are easy, some are hard. You don't get to choose. Not too long ago, we invited a young couple to our house for dinner. We wanted to see their new baby and to give them a break from cooking. They came with their four-year-old, Alex, and their new baby, Sarah, and a very large bag. We dug out the toys and the high chair, and waited to see what would happen.

The little girl was just beautiful. Like her handsome brother, she had lovely dark hair, dark skin and dark eyes. Her parents were quite smitten with her, and it wasn't long before we were smitten, too.

But did she keep them going! They took turns being on their feet the whole evening, holding her and jiggling her and rocking her back and forth. They held her, face down, across their forearm, with her face looking down from their elbow.

I stress the exact position, because it appeared to be *very* important to Sarah. As long as they kept moving and held her in that position, she was relatively quiet and only gave out an occasional squawk. But when they shifted her around or sat down, she put up an enormous fuss. She cried and threw herself around and generally let them know how unhappy she was and how unsatisfactory they were.

Once, something about the way she operated must have changed, and they fed her. I think she squawked a little more loudly, or wouldn't let herself be comforted by their rocking. She seemed hungry, and ate, took a three-minute catnap, and then they all went back to what seemed to me like an exhausting routine.

Apparently this went on most of the time. The mother took her to her laboratory where she was a graduate student, and she said some of the time she got some work done. But she also spent a lot of time holding and rocking from side to side. One of her colleagues commented he was going to get her a rear-view mirror so she could see when the little girl's eyes fell shut.

71

They were quite cheerful about it, and simply kept talking and working in shifts. The mother commented that she couldn't remember Alexander's being that fussy. She was so calm about it, I could see that there was nothing remarkable about it to her—no wonder she didn't remember! By the time the evening was over, I was exhausted from just watching them, whereas they were still bearing up very well.

I thought of Sarah when my son Luke and I were waiting for our pizza at the local pizza place the other night. There was a baby there, too, a really cute little boy about the same age as Sarah. But what a difference!

It was so noisy in there, and he was at a table with eight adults—grandparent age, most of them. They were passing him around and taking turns holding him. They jostled him as they passed, the women cuddled him and rocked, the men held him out in front of them in their hands and his arms and legs dangled down and they talked to him. There was smoke curling around his head, and they were laughing and talking to each other. And he was just as calm and relaxed as ever you please. He didn't make a peep the whole hour and a half he was there. If that had been Sarah, she would have been a mass of nerves and screaming at the first stop around the table.

I don't know how he ate, because he didn't. I would guess that he is a regular little baby who gives clear messages about what he wants, and who eats well and then goes off for a satisfyingly long nap, when his parents can scurry around and get all their work done.

Through no fault of their own or anybody else's, some children are just hard to please. And hard to predict. And hard to do anything with. Some children are positive and attracted to other people. They wake up happy and greet the world with a smile and just seem to be wondering what delightful things are in store on still another wonderful, satisfying day. They are regular in their habits—you will both fall into a fairly predictable feeding and sleeping schedule that allows you to do your grocery shopping and know you are not going to have to leave your shopping cart in the middle of the store while you go off somewhere and attend to a screaming baby.

Others are profoundly irregular in their habits. They sleep for five hours at a stretch and then take 15-minute catnaps. They want to be fed after four hours and then after an hour. Some wake up angry and don't want anything to do with anybody. I know a little boy who served his parents notice about his black mood for the day by crawling down the stairs and over to his high chair *backwards*. They knew not to look at him or to talk to him—just to give him his breakfast.

I have had both kinds, and with one I felt like the most wonderful, successful parent in the world, and with the other I felt like I was always struggling to work things out. My first, my daughter Kjerstin was so positive and regular and easily pleased. With my two boys, it was a *whole* lot harder. It seemed like something always had to be going on. They were awake all the time and wanted to be entertained constantly. They weren't especially angry or fussy—all I had to do was hold them practically all the time and feed them very frequently, always at irregular intervals.

While I enjoyed them a lot and thought they were just the nicest babies ever, I was just not temperamentally able to sit around and hold them. Much of the day I kept them in a backpack and did my work with them perched on my back. I had a pack like the little cloth front packs people use nowadays, except I perfected a method for getting it on behind so I could do my work without bashing them into things.

It worked fine. It calmed them to be back there; they seemed to enjoy looking around and liked being close to me. I liked it too—I enjoyed the feeling of having them back there, and, as they got older they peeked over my shoulder and we talked and they kept an eye on what I was doing. All I had to do was keep moving. The minute I sat down, it was all over. Fortunately with two and then three little children to care for, sitting down was not often a problem.

We wouldn't want to deceive ourselves on this touchy topic, so you will be glad to know there is research by a disinterested outside observer who confirms our suspicions that, indeed, babies are different. We can even quote statistics[1].

About 40 percent of children are positive and regular. They adapt well to change, they are responsive and interested and are generally agreeable. They take to most new foods and new situations easily, and can accept frustration with relatively little stress. They are regular: they sleep and eat regularly.

Fortunately, a considerably lower number, 10%, are at the opposite end of the temperamental spectrum. These unlucky

73

young people are irregular in sleeping and eating, they react negatively to new situations instead of approaching them, they hate change and get very tense when they are exposed to new things. They are slow to accept new foods and new people and new situations. They cry loud and long and have violent tantrums if they are frustrated. They also laugh, loudly.

Somewhere in between the two extremes, which the researchers label "easy" and "difficult" (might as well call a spade a spade), is the "slow-to-warm-up" child. About 15 percent of children belong here. They are less negative or positive than either of the two groups I just described, their reactions are mildly negative, and if given time to get used to something they generally come around and enjoy things all right. But they do not wax enthusiastic.

That adds up to 65 percent. Other children show a mix of traits and reactions to new situations. They are negative sometimes and positive at others, mildly reactive sometimes and extremely responsive at others.

You have to take what you get. Sometimes what you get is so hard to understand and work with that you get into trouble and need help with it.

A young woman from the west coast called me, desperate about her six-month-old baby's eating and growth. The little girl was falling off her growth curve and had been for the last two months. At that time, the mother had been breast-feeding her, and the pediatrician had become alarmed at the baby's poor growth and had told the mother to "Feed her, I don't care *how* you do it." (Sad to say, I have heard that destructive bit of advice more than once.) Thinking the problem was her breast-feeding, the mother weaned the little girl from the breast and started her on a bottle.

Things weren't any better with the bottle. At the time the mother called me, she was, as I said really desperate. The little girl's growth had continued to fall off, and feeding had become a nightmare. The mother was trying, every two hours, to get her daughter to take her formula. The baby would take about an ounce of it, then throw herself backward, and squirm and fuss. The mother said she felt wiry and "not cuddly," and it was so frustrating to deal with her when she was like that, that she found it hard to warm up to her.

It had gotten to the point where the mother was afraid the

little girl would not survive. Her growth was below the charts, but most alarming was her reluctance to eat.

We had a conference on the phone about her eating, and I advised her to, first of all, hook up with a pediatrician she trusted to help her through this. Then, working with the doctor, I suggested she make some feeding changes. Essentially she was to back off and let her daughter take the lead. She was to feed her daughter when she was hungry and stop feeding *immediately* when she indicated she was full.

The baby was taking some infant cereal, as well, and Mother was to do the same with that. She was to wait for her daughter to pay attention to each mouthful and open her mouth before she gave it to her. If the little girl didn't indicate any interest, she was to stop feeding. When her daughter ate, she was not to be excited about it or to praise her lavishly. In that case, even acting pleased could feel like forcing.

She could offer finger food, but the mother was to be very neutral about whether the little girl ate it.

About a month later, the mother wrote back and said things were going better. As she said, "I have seen her be hungry, and eat willingly and gain some weight. She looks happier and seems healthy. She still isn't too cuddly, and she is hard to figure out."

The mother went on to say that the last couple of days before the letter was written the little girl had been fussy and refusing food and drink. At that point, they had gotten into their old struggle again. Sort of. The baby had squirmed and fussed when the mother sat down to feed her. But the mother was quitting earlier. "There's no use fighting. It seems like the whole day goes by in this useless cycle of preparing food, warming food, throwing away food."

I asked the mother how things were going with her husband, and never really got an answer. That could have been part of the problem. It is a whole lot harder to do well with a child if a spouse isn't being supportive.

It may also be the little girl is a "difficult" child, and it's hard to feel successful with her. Once we got rid of the force feeding, those difficult-child characteristics seemed to appear. I suggested to the mother that she and her husband see a baby psychologist to get some help figuring out how to feel more satisfied and successful with their daughter.

Your child's characteristics will not necessarily persist. As an older child or an adult she could be quite different from what she is as a baby—provided you are willing to forgive and forget, that is, and keep trying. If you hold it against her for being a negative baby or keep reminding her what a pill she is, she likely will continue to be a pill. Don't give up on her.

Difficult, nervous babies are approachable, but it takes the patience and persistence of a saint. Which is surprisingly normal parent behavior. You keep the environment quiet, you approach them slowly, you hold them tenderly and keep hanging on tenderly, even when they throw themselves around and react. You talk to them soothingly, and help them get through their reacting. You wait to make eye contact with them, and can even work toward getting eye contact before you feed. You can help a child with his temperamental characteristics. You don't just have to put up with them[2].

You can use these same gentle and persistent tactics for the colicky baby. We still don't know what causes colic, but it's not hard to understand that a baby with colic feels *awful*: He may be nauseated, and probably has a stomach ache. How would you like to be treated if you felt that way? Probably very gently, with a reassuring person there to keep you company.

Hunger

Not everybody feels the same about hunger or about being full. Not everyone expresses their feelings the same way. Your particular baby may have very clear feeding cues, or more subtle ones. It will take you a few weeks to get so you can read your particular baby's signals, but if you work at it and pay close attention, you will be able to produce what she wants.

Some babies seemingly get hungry suddenly and are immediately desperate to be fed. Those same babies often are extremely unwilling to eat unless it is their idea, first. Some babies get hungry slowly and are more tolerant of waiting to be fed—it seems like their hunger is not so pressing. Those same babies will allow themselves to be persuaded to eat, even if they aren't particularly thinking about it.

The same thing goes for getting full. Some babies get enough abruptly, and stop nursing with no uncertainty. Others

76

kind of drift into satiety, nursing more and more slowly. They can always be persuaded to take a couple more sucks, and often the feeder quits because of mutual lack of interest rather than because of any clear signal from the baby.

What is common to all, however, is their primitive and pressing need to be *fed* and relieved of their hunger. Imagine what it would be like for you to be totally dependent on another person for food (perhaps you only have to go back to the last time you hungrily waited for a flight attendant to serve you on an airplane), and not to know whether that person will deliver or not. There is a fearsomeness in that, a reaction that can only be relieved with time and repeated good experience.

As children get older and their experiences with eating are positive, they get better about waiting. Their brains develop so they can remember earlier feedings, they have trust that some-one will provide, and they are able to calm and reassure themselves while they wait.

Parents worry if their children's hunger and satiety behav-iors seem odd. A little boy in Wyoming had been the object of great concern on the part of his parents. He was born prema-turely, had been on tube feedings for the three months he was in the hospital, and once he got off tube feedings he was very hard to get on bottle feeding. He was reluctant to take the nipple, and did a lot of choking and gagging. It was only with the utmost patience and persistence, and the help of a dietitian and an occupational therapist, that this little boy was finally able to get enough control of his mouth muscles so he could nipple feed.

They got into the same resistance introducing him to solid foods. And table foods. They waited until he was older to start, which they should have, because with premature babies you start counting their maturity from when they *should* have been born, not when they *were* born.

He was tiny and didn't eat very much. He grew, but he was always below the fifth percentile on the growth chart. He ate, but his mother still didn't feel comfortable with his eating. She was concerned that his eating always had to be her idea. She had to interrupt his playing and remind him that it was meal or snack time. Once she did that, he was interested in eating and ate very willingly. But she wished HE would think of it. He just never seemed to think about eating, and, to her, that was still too much like that early behavior that had been so traumatic for her. It still just wasn't "normal."

I reassured her that his behavior *was* probably normal for him. He was showing signs of hunger that she could pick up: he would become listless and cross and just run out of steam when he got hungry. In time, he would be able to detect those signs in himself and identify them as needing food. For now, he was too little to do that.

Some people are just plain interested in food. Some people are not. My eating-preoccupied patients remember themselves as being the first to come to dinner when their mother called: "The other kids would keep on playing, but I was always right there." Sometimes that behavior is innate to them; other times they appeared to have developed it when their parents deprived them of food on the misguided notion it would help them to stay thin.

I am not saying your child will get fat or develop an eating disorder if she is super interested in eating. She *might*, if she is super interested in eating and you deprive her of food or teach her there is something bad and awful about feeling that way. But if you are accepting of the way she operates, she will be, too.

Let's keep this in perspective: Some kids are just easier to get to the table. For other kids you have to develop tactics to get them away from their playing so they will come to eat. (The best bet is to separate *coming* from *eating*. They'll say, "I'm not hungry." You say, "You don't have to eat, but you must come and keep us company at mealtime.")

Many children get so engrossed in their playing that they forget to notice what is going on with their bodies. Then suddenly they run out of gas and get crabby. They also get stubborn, so if you try to get them to eat, they won't. Just ask them to come to the table and sit for a few minutes—they may settle down and get hungry.

Some people feel excited when they get hungry. Eating is really very exciting business, and if it is generally pleasurable, then eating gives you something pleasant to look forward to. A little boy I observed being spoon fed by his mother cried real tears, but happily, between bites while he ate. It was puzzling to us observers, but the way his mother behaved gave us a clue to what was going on. She just kept feeding him very nicely, talking calmly and enjoying the process. Eating must have been painfully pleasurable to him.

78

I see this same conflict between positive and negative feelings toward eating in my patients. They feel anxious when they get hungry, because their eating experiences have been so negative and conflicted, but at the same time they feel very attracted to food and eating. Unlike this little boy, they are unable to tolerate the conflict, so they have resolved it by feeling nothing at all—they numb themselves to the feelings, and eat chaotically and only THINK they enjoy their eating. In reality, they are hardly even experiencing it.

If they work on it, people can bring those feelings up to a conscious level, learn to tolerate them, and eventually, become less anxious and ambivalent about their eating. To achieve that, they have to be very reassuring with themselves about eating, and not do anything that raises those old fears of having to go without.

Love Of Eating

I talked about this before, in Pressure Doesn't Work (Chapter 3). It's worth talking about it again, even if it seems repetitive. People sometimes feel embarrassed about the way they feel about eating. In our eating-conscious society, liking to eat almost seems like a prurient interest. It's not. Eating is one of life's great pleasures. Some people take more pleasure in it than others.

I often think of the parents I met at a workshop in California. Their three-year-old daughter, Marion, was chubby, and just loved to eat. In fact, she loved it so much that she **moaned** when she ate, looking forward expressively to the next bite and responding to it with intense pleasure. All the adults thought it was hilarious, and made a special effort to show up when Marion was eating. Her mother was mortified.

Marion had a special kind of sensitivity, but she was learning to be ashamed of it. Those feelings can go underground, and cause people a lot of pain. One of my woman patients was an obese compulsive eater who had dieted and failed at dieting throughout her growing up years and adulthood. After lots of retraining and reassurance and encouragement to let herself enjoy her eating, she admitted to a very powerful, sensual response to eating good food. I say admitted, because she was

79

mortified by the way she felt. Her early history had been very like Marion's.

When I tell the story about Marion, it usually frees someone up to confide their own child's "oddity" about eating. A wonderful, expressive mother in Louisiana announced that her six-year-old daughter "...is just the same way. She just loves anything to do with eating. She always wants to go to the grocery store, and when she is there she is just like a little fairy. She skips up and down the aisles, saying 'I want this—can we have that?' Whenever I cook, she is right there helping, and when she eats she keeps up a running commentary, yumming and saying how good everything is.

"She moans when she eats, too. Every night before she goes to bed she wonders what we are going to have to eat the next day. (That can be kind of annoying, because I don't always *know* what we are eating the next day.) She is slender now, but I wonder how long she is going to stay that way when she is so enthusiastic about eating."

I reassured her that even though her daughter loved eating a lot, she also apparently had an excellent ability to regulate her food intake: She knew how much she needed to eat, and had a stopping place within her that let her know when she had had enough. I would expect that ability to continue. It is, after all, more normal to regulate than *not* to regulate.

Unless, that is, someone gets frightened by her "excessive" interest in food and tries to put some curbs on her opportunities to work with food or to eat good food. Then she is likely to feel a lot of conflict and anxiety about this wonderful sensitivity she has. She will want to gratify her pleasure in eating, but will feel guilty when she does, and this basic conflict will interfere with her detecting her food regulation cues.

The ability to eat well and enjoy good food is another of those qualities that make people distinctive. Some people become great gourmets, and do reviews of restaurants and go on vacations where their main recreation is eating wonderful food. Or they cook for their own enjoyment and spend lots of time and effort at it. They delight in entertaining their friends and introducing them to new taste sensations. Like other special sensitivities, the love of good food can afford someone a considerable amount of joy—and even money.

Food Preferences

Parents worry that children are trying to "pull something" when they express their food dislikes, and that, unless they are forced, they simply won't learn to like a variety of food. Quite the opposite is true. Kids expect to grow up with their eating the same as with every other activity. Adults just have to provide them with opportunities.

Not too long ago as I ate lunch with a friend I told the waiter that I did not want the peppers on my enchilada. As I told my companion, peppers are one of the few foods that I truly do not like. My friend laughed and said, "Don't tell your kids that, or they'll think *they* can get away with not liking foods, too."

Well, I have confessed to my children that I do not like peppers, and they eat them none the less. There are things they don't like, but for the most part they are very accepting of foods. In fact, sometimes they do better than I do, like when I brought home three selections from the Cajun restaurant. It was pretty hot for me, and I was reaching for the water. But they loved it. They considered it a positive challenge to eat the hot food. At the Greek place, it was another story: I ate, they were turned off.

As teenagers, my children all behave very similarly in the way they approach new foods. When they were younger, they were quite different from one another. Curt was enthusiastic about almost every food, and ate it. Luke was more suspicious of new foods, but gradually, as he got older, he has eaten more and more. And Kjerstin ate a very limited assortment of foods until she got in high school, and then she expanded her food choices considerably. A study on feeding larger groups of children shows the same three types of eaters: The enthusiastic, the steady accumulator, and the late bloomer[3]. Reassuring, isn't it?

The whole topic of approaching new foods brings up the intriguing question a reporter asked me on a radio broadcast: Is the finicky eater born or made? He told the story of his recent dinner guest. The reporter and his wife had made a lovely casserole and salad. The guest, commented the reporter, was "...just like a roto rooter. He said, 'what's this, what's that?' and went through his plate, using his knife and fork to sort through his food and put it into edible and inedible piles." Finally the reporter's wife had had enough, and shouted, "Why don't you just shut up and eat your dinner!"

81

That was the end of the story, and it was up to me to answer. On live radio. I said I thought it was probably both. Sometimes parents make their children react against food by putting too much pressure on them to eat it. Sometimes people over-baby their children, and if the children express the slightest hesitation about trying something, the parent is right out in the kitchen getting out the peanut butter and jelly.

But some people have naturally sensitive palates or over-developed gag reflexes and there are foods that make them react. Actually, being finicky can be quite a handicap. People who are finicky just really never know if they are going to be able to eat, and sometimes food is so unpleasant to them that it makes them downright nauseated. Which can be very unhandy in a social situation.

But whether my reporter's guest had been born or made finicky, his parents certainly hadn't given him much help in learning how to deal with it. They should have reassured him he didn't have to eat what he didn't want, but they also should have taught him how to be tactful and *discreetly* to eat what he liked and leave the rest. They shouldn't have let him get away with the kind of behavior that my reporter and his wife found so objectionable.

A woman called me from Indiana, worrying about her four-year-old son John's finicky eating. John's mother said he had a very short list of foods he would accept, and if they didn't appear at meal times he became very upset. His mother limited her menus to foods that he liked, and if he didn't want to eat something, she immediately offered him a substitute.

It worked all right as long as they were at home, but John's inability to eat a variety of food was starting to bother his parents. They rarely went to a restaurant or out to eat at someone else's house, because John got into such a state, worrying if he would be able to eat what was served. His parents had catered to him for a long time, but now they were getting tired of it and angry with him. They were even fighting with each other about it.

The mother said she, too, was a finicky eater and on a weight reduction diet to boot, so her food selection was *really* limited. The husband was a gourmet cook and concerned that his son would turn out to be as finicky as the mother. (I asked the mother why her acute sensitivity to food made her *finicky* whereas her husband's made him a *gourmet*, but she was stumped for an answer.) Frequently the family had two meals, the mother and son eating one and the father eating another.

John's eating was becoming even more of an issue because the mother was thinking of going back to work. If she did, John would be at a day care center over the noon hour. Already he was worrying if he would get what he wanted to eat. He asked his mother if they could go out to lunch every day after she got off work, and she was seriously considering it.

I told the mother that the primary problem was not how to get John to accept more food, but to keep his eating from being such an issue. To do that, she would have to help John become more comfortable with his feelings and reactions toward food. He needed to learn to come to the table and be polite and pick and choose from what was available. Sometimes he might not eat anything at all, but that is really not so terrible. There would be another snack or another meal, and he had a good chance of getting something he liked. They always had bread on the table, and if he couldn't eat anything else he could eat that.

I discouraged her from further short order cooking for him. (You know what that is—they say "I won't eat that," and you say, "OK, what will you eat?" And then you get up and make it for them.) I pointed out that short order cooking was teaching him that it was of desperate importance that he eat and if he didn't it was a real calamity. THAT was the real problem, not his lack of food acceptance in the first place.

The day care situation offers John an opportunity to be exposed to different foods and to children eating them. If he's lucky, he'll be in a center where the grownups don't put pressure on eating. In many cases children do better with eating when they get out with other children, and away from their parents and the tensions at the family table.

Reading between the lines, it seemed there were tensions at home. The parents were disagreeing on how the son's eating should be handled and he was getting some attention for NOT eating. He was clearly taking mother's side (he was eating her food), and father didn't like it. It wasn't just John's eating at stake here—it was the whole battle between mother and dad. They couldn't even work things out with each other enough to choose a family menu. Until they settled their battle, they weren't going to make much progress with John's eating—or with allowing him to grow up.

I told John's mother they should see a family counselor to take a look at how she and her husband were operating—with John, and with each other. Their relationship with each other was really the issue. They weren't getting along, and they weren't behaving effectively with John. As the mother said, they didn't expect enough of him with his eating. They couldn't, because they were so busy undermining each other's efforts with him.

Tempo

One of the places you may find yourself having conflict with your child is with tempo. We move faster than children do. Small children eat slowly. Small children even prolong meals, at times, way beyond limits that adults find reasonable. You'll need to go by your particular child to judge what is enough time, but not so much you lose your patience.

Little children, in general, take a LONG time to eat. They are particularly slow when they first start feeding themselves from the table and learning to use utensils. They get the greatest amount of entertainment from getting a pea or a piece of grated cheese in their mouth. They love to explore the colors and textures of food. They chase food from one place to another on the high chair tray. They bite a piece off from a cracker and then can't chew it, so most or all of it falls out of their mouth—and then they take another bite and do the same thing with it.

They STRUGGLE to load up their spoon and lift it up to their mouth, and turn it upside down just when it gets there. And then they do it again, working in a dedicated way to LEARN. It's enough to drive you wild.

It doesn't bother them to be slow and inept. They just keep working away at it, experiencing the greatest amount of pleasure and challenge from the whole thing.

They need *time* to do all this, and you mustn't interfere. You can take the spoon away and do it so much faster and more efficiently, but that is *your* tempo, not *theirs*. Remember, it's *their* food, not yours. But don't underestimate the importance of your simply being there. Babies do more when their parents remain

84

nearby and take a casual and sometimes admiring interest, but don't take over.

You will be better able to enjoy the magic of this laborious process if you don't hover. Eat your own meal. Start meals early enough so you don't have to rush off in ten minutes. Learn to eat more slowly, yourself, so you can be companionable. Do stay available, for sociability's and safety's sake, but don't be in a hurry to get eating over with.

Here is something you can learn from your children: *Effective eating takes time.* Find out how good it feels to sit down to a meal hungry and to have good food and to take your time with it. You will end up truly satisfied and able to forget about eating between times. Your children can do that—watch them.

If you learn from your children to take your time with meals, they won't learn from you to rush through meals. They will grow up thinking that slowly and attentively is the way to eat.

Capability

Some children give you more help with feeding than others. Sometimes you have to temporarily take over part of their job to get things going. If you do that, though, it is important that it only be temporary.

It can cause problems, especially with nursing, if children aren't demanding enough about asking for food. Rose's baby was active and awake and not easy to satisfy. He wanted to nurse "all the time," and when he ate he latched on to the breast and sucked strongly and acted like he was starved. He wanted to eat about every two hours, and between times he was mostly awake and wanting her companionship.

Margie's baby was just the opposite. She was sleepy and compliant and SO easy to be around. She quickly got herself on an every-four-hour schedule, and sometimes went for five hours before she ate again. She didn't really cry to be fed, but fussed a little, and her mother checked the time to know that she was probably hungry, and fed her. Margie's baby nursed ever so politely, and didn't seem like she spent much time at the breast at all.

85

The upshot of the first month with these babies was that Rose felt like a frazzled failure and Margie felt like a calm, cool and collected model mother.

The scales in the doctor's office told another story. Rose's son had gained two and a half pounds in the first month. Margie's daughter had barely made it back to birth weight. The little boy was giving his mother the sucking stimulation and frequent breast emptying she needed to develop and maintain her breast milk supply. The little girl was not.

For some unknown reason, she was one of the occasional newborns who are so sleepy and placid and so immune to their hunger feelings that they don't demand to be fed much. It may not have been all the baby—there might have been something about the way Margie was dealing with her that was making her behave that way, like not taking enough time with her or not looking at her or not talking to her, or perhaps doing the opposite and coming on too strong so the baby withdrew.

There are lots of things that can happen that have an impact on breast-feeding, and since I didn't observe the feeding relationship, I don't know where the problem lay. (I'll talk about the topic more in The Child Who Grows Poorly, Chapter 13.) Margie's baby was undereating right from the first, under-stimulating her mother's breast milk production, and the breast milk supply fell off. So a downward spiral set in, where her undereating made her sleepy and undemanding. She ate less and less, and ended up doing poorly.

In the first case, there was nothing to be improved upon. Rose and her baby were having a busy and somewhat frustrating time of it, but they were actually doing very well. (Although reassuring Rose that everything was going well represented a *very* significant improvement for her.) On the other hand, Margie had to give her baby supplemental bottles, and wake her up to feed her while she worked on increasing her breast milk supply. Unfortunately, the little girl developed a preference for the bottle, and Margie had to discontinue nursing.

We generally recommend that breast-feeding pairs get in to their doctor's for a feeding check about 48 hours after they leave the hospital and then again when the baby is about a week old. That way you can catch problems like Margie's early enough to turn the situation around. Rose could have used some reassurance, too, instead of feeling like she was doing so poorly all that time.

Not only does it take two to breast-feed, there are some real individual differences in children's ability to take nourishment. Even though Rose was feeling so frazzled, her baby was giving her a lot of help with feeding—he was letting her know in no uncertain terms when he was hungry, and he was keeping after her when he wanted MORE. Margie's baby, on the other hand, gave up more easily, and her demands for food were so subtle, that her mother had to supplement the information she was getting from her. She had to weigh her regularly to make sure she was getting enough.

Difficulty Learning To Eat

If children have a difficult time learning to eat, don't automatically assume they are being resistant. There could be something going on that is making it hard.

Children can have problems with the nerves and muscles in their mouths, and sometimes those problems first become apparent with their eating. I know a boy who didn't do much mouthing when he was little, and he had a very difficult time learning to eat solids. He gagged so much on solids that it scared him, and he didn't want to try again. His mother finally taught him to mouth other things, like his fingers and toys. She even gently used her own fingers to rub the inside of his mouth and "walk" along his tongue. He gagged when she did that, but eventually the gagging decreased and he was able to approach food more confidently.

That same little boy had a lot of difficulty adjusting to increased lumpiness and thickness in his food. His mother followed my advice (standard for any baby, whether he's gagging or not) and kept him on iron-fortified baby cereal mixed with milk as his first solid food for a month. After that time she decided to diversify a bit, to get him accustomed to some new flavors and textures.

Because he had had problems to begin with, she decided to go the most conservative route, and give something really smooth and thin like commercial strained baby food. She was wise to do so—he had trouble with it.

87

His first taste of baby carrots came as quite a shock to him. He reared back in his high chair and looked at her with surprise. He would not accept the next spoonful she offered, but instead looked at it closely and felt of it with his fingers. His mother let him take his time, and eventually his carrot-laden fingers found their way to his mouth. This time it wasn't such a shock, and he explored a bit more with his own fingers before he let her give him another spoonful.

And that was the end of the feeding. He had done pretty well, for one so cautious, and she recognized that. Another time he was willing to take more, and eventually added carrots to his repertoire.

Another baby was considerably more adventurous about accepting cereal. From the first, she yelled between bites, and her clever mother figured out that she wanted more—faster. The baby *loved* the cereal, and had no problem with gagging. Because she took the solids so readily, her mother decided to increase their texture and thickness when she progressed from baby cereal. She fork-mashed cooked carrots for her daughter. And the little girl took the grainy new food with enthusiasm.

Miscellaneous Glitches

You can't really make hard and fast rules about what to do with kids' eating, because there are always exceptions. Instead, you need to pay attention to your child and keep track of what works and what doesn't.

People ask me, "Should I make my child taste everything?" I always answer, "You have to know your audience." Lucas, for instance, was very cautious about tasting new foods. If he saw something he did not recognize, he automatically decided he didn't want any. But he could also be persuaded. I would say, (and we did this many times), "Why don't you just taste it to see if you like it?" He would do that very willingly, and generally he would like it and eat a bunch.

Curtis, on the other hand, was more adventurous. He tried most things and liked most things. But if he made up his mind not to taste something, it was MADE UP, and there was no changing it. *One time* I suggested to him that he try something, and he turned me down flat and looked me straight in the eye

88

with a glint that let me know that if I went any farther it would be disaster. So I quit while I was ahead.

Kjerstin ate bread and vegetables in *very* small amounts, then filled up on several glasses of milk. We finally told her she could have only one glass of milk at a meal, because she wasn't eating much of her other food. That helped. Different kids, different tactics. (It's always been puzzling to me, but children often appear to prefer drinking to eating. Very occasionally, you have to limit beverages to encourage children to eat their food.)

At times, you have to be a darned good detective. Babies are especially challenging to decipher. A colleague of mine told about his adventures with his two boys, one of whom has safely survived his infancy, the other who is still in the midst of it. In both cases, the boys were breast fed from birth, and in both cases, about the time his wife was getting ready to go back to work they started trying to teach the boys to drink from a bottle. Jerrod, the older one, had a problem with a collapsing nipple. He would suck all the air out of the bottle, the nipple would collapse, and his father would take the nipple out of his mouth to let the air go back into the bottle, intending to let him go back to eating.

Jerrod did not know that. Since human nipples do not collapse when you nurse from them, he hadn't a clue as to what was going on. To him, losing track of the nipple meant the feeding was OVER, and he certainly did not go along with that idea. So he yelled. And screamed. And kept it up until the nipple recovered and he could go back to eating.

So the pattern repeated, until Jerrod began to notice that he wasn't being deprived of food when he was still hungry. He began to get the rhythm and trust his father to keep feeding until he got done. Eventually, he got to the point where he voluntarily let go of the nipple when it collapsed. They worked it out. The father was a patient and perceptive observer and Jerrod, in his own way, was equally so.

Eric presented a problem of a different sort. They got Eric well-established on bottle feeding, and he began to put up a fuss about breast-feeding. His mother would get started nursing him and he would start fussing. He would fuss and fume for quite a long time before he finally settled down to nursing. With bottle feeding, he was fine—he ate like a little lamb.

His mother was upset, because she thought his behavior

89

meant that he didn't want to nurse any more, and she was nowhere near ready to give it up. They couldn't understand what was going on, so they called in an outside observer: a nurse practitioner in their pediatrician's office. And the nurse did a marvelous job of sleuthing. She asked about schedules and formulas and what was going on around Eric when he was eating.

Finally she asked about position: How was Eric's father holding him when he got his bottle? Aha! He was holding Eric stretched out in front of him on his lap, with Eric's head on his knee. They were face to face, Eric could watch his father while he ate, and he preferred it that way. He wasn't being a pill, he was merely telling his mother to follow suit.

It should be apparent to all but the most disinterested observer that his mother couldn't follow suit. So father had to change. He had to cuddle Eric in the crook of his arm to have his bottle. And Eric didn't like it one bit. He fussed and fumed and threw himself around and spit out the nipple. It took over half an hour, that first feeding, before he finally settled down and ate something. After that, he gave up his preference, and breast and bottle feeding both went just fine. But the father never dared feed him the stretched-out way because they would have had the whole struggle to go through again.

Clever little bodies, aren't they? We couldn't possibly deal with all the variations in this book. To help you with all your child's weird behaviors, why not do a couple of things: First, assume that they're normal. They probably are, anyway, and usually, if you don't overreact to a behavior and make it a problem, it will either come to seem normal to you or go away of its own accord.

Second, if something is *really* being a problem, try to figure out what is going on. Look at what leads up to the behavior, and what happens afterward. What is it getting for her to operate this way? Are you doing something that encourages or rewards your child when she does what she does? (For instance, with Marion, our chubby little girl who *loved* to eat, I wondered if she got so much attention from other people for her enthusiasm about eating that she started to eat to show off, rather than to satisfy her hunger and appetite.).

90

But remember, the norm is to vary. There are as many approaches to food and ways of dealing with eating as there are children. Every kid is different—and entertaining.

References

1.   Thomas, A. and Chess, S. Genesis and evolution of behavioral disorders: From infancy to early adult life. The American Journal of Psychiatry, 141:1-9, 1984.

2.   Greenspan, S. and Greenspan, N.T.: First Feelings: Milestones in the Development of Your Baby and Child from Birth to Age Four. New York: Viking, 1985.

3.   Davis, C.M.: Feeding after the first year. IN Brennaman's Practice of Pediatrics. Hagerstown, MD: W.F. Prior Co., 1957.

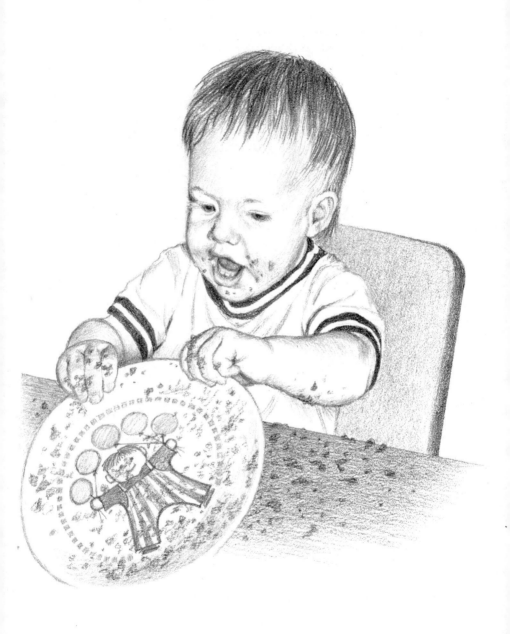

6

Nutritional Tactics For Preventing Food Fights

Many an eating battle between parent and child has been waged in the name of good nutrition. Parents want their children to eat their vegetables, or get concerned that they are eating too many junk foods, and try to get them to change. The battle lines are drawn, and the outcome is all too familiar: bad feelings about eating, and about nutritious food, and mealtimes that are tense and stressed.

It needn't be that way. A theme I stress throughout this book is the utility of a division of responsibility in feeding—Parent:what/child:how much. Restated, it's the old horse-to-water adage: you can get your child to the table, but you can't make him eat his vegetables. You can *try*, but the results will disappoint you.

In the other chapters, I talk in detail about doing your parenting job with feeding, and outline ways of keeping from intruding in your child's area of deciding how much (or even whether) he eats. The object of this chapter is to help you to do your job of choosing and preparing food.

If I had to tell you to do ONE THING to enhance your child's eating behavior and nutritional status, that one thing would be having family meals. Having the structure and relia-bility of family meals is essential to your child's nutritional and emotional health. Without meals, you haven't a chance of enhancing your child's food acceptance and teaching him to behave appropriately with food. I am very concerned about the trend away from family meals.

A study done in the seventies indicated that at that time 43% of parents espoused dietary individualism, meaning they believed their children should be free to make their own food choices. The good news is that leaves over half of parents doing their traditional job of picking out and providing food. The bad news is that almost half of parents do not consider that a priority.

In this chapter, I'll talk about having meals and snacks, and about choosing food for those meals and snacks that will allow your child to grow and develop to his greatest potential. Toward the end of the chapter, I'll talk about disease prevention. The first is the priority, although it need not rule out the second.

Choose Age-Appropriate Food

In the chronological chapters in the middle of the book I will discuss the specifics of feeding children of different ages. I touch on food selection for these children, but I'll talk about it more here. There is still more to know, particularly for infants.

The child under a year of age has specialized food needs, and the more you know about those needs and the foods that can satisfy them, the better able you will be to provide nutrition-ally for your child. Medical people will advise you, and many of the nurses are very good at it. But since their priority is caring for your child in areas other than nutrition, there may be some gaps in the information you get. You'll get accurate and com-plete information if you get to see a registered dietitian (RD), but most people don't get that opportunity.

You can fill those gaps, or at least question them when they occur, if you know more about the topic. I talked about infant nutrition and food selection in detail in *Child of Mine*. The three chapters there, The Milk Feeding, Breast-feeding How-To

and Introduction of Solid Foods to the Infant Diet have a lot
of information I consider very valuable to you that I won't
try to go into here. This book is about *feeding*—it's not about
food selection.

I will summarize. The newborn needs breastmilk with
certain nutrient supplements, or a specially prepared infant formula (with careful attention to sanitation), for most of the first
year. Your baby should be on one of these milk feedings, or a
combination of the two, exclusively for most of the first six
months. He should continue to get one of these milk feedings
as his primary food source until he is well established on table
food. For most babies, that will be when they are between eight
months and a year old.

As a general rule, you should start solid foods for a baby
who was born at term at around six months of age. More importantly, though, before you start solids he should be able to sit up
with minimal support, follow the spoon with his eyes, and open
his mouth when he sees something coming. When he can do
all these things, you will also find he'll be able to learn to
swallow solids.

His first solid food should be iron-fortified infant rice cereal
mixed with formula or breastmilk. He should continue to eat
that iron-fortified cereal throughout his first year, and even into
his second year.

Once he is well established on baby cereal (taking at least
½ cup per day, divided into two or more meals) you can start
introducing fruits and vegetables—pureed, fork-mashed or
milled. If you use home-prepared, be careful about sanitation,
and don't add any salt or sugar.

Finger foods follow soon after—usually in the bread and
cereal category—and when he gets so he can manipulate his
fingers and bite off and chew reasonably well, your child will be
able to sit at the table and eat soft and cooked foods with his fingers. (Again, it is important to take out the baby's portion before
salt or sugar is added.) That's the time to add meat to his diet—
either finely diced or ground—because his formula or breastmilk intake will start to drop with all the other food he's taking
in, and he'll need the protein source.

Once he's taking about three ounces of solid foods, three
times a day, it is all right to start giving *pasteurized whole* milk
instead of formula or breastmilk. That is also a good time to

start weaning, at mealtimes, from the breast or bottle and instead give milk in a cup (although I wouldn't both introduce cow's milk and stop nipple feeding at the same time).

For eating purposes, your baby will be a toddler starting with making the transition to table foods somewhere between eight months and a year. He'll be able to eat most soft and cooked foods from the family table. He'll be even more successful with eating if you make the simple food modifications I talk about in Is Your Toddler Jerking You Around at the Table? (Chapter 9). Check Figure 9-2, "Making Foods Easy to Eat for Toddlers," page 185.

There is a safety concern with making the transition to table foods. The danger of choking is greatest with toddlers, but it continues to be a concern throughout the preschool years. You can greatly reduce the risk of your child's choking by taking the simple precautions I have outlined in the Toddler chapter, Figure 9-3, "Preventing Choking," page 186.

Preschoolers and young schoolagers continue to have some limitations in their chewing and swallowing. You'll still see a six-year-old get overwhelmed by a piece of dry meat and take it back out of his mouth. It's best to overlook those lapses in etiquette—and pay attention instead to cooking meat so it is tender and moist. Children do better with swallowing when food is moist—the dry stuff seems to get stuck in their mouths.

Older children can fit right in with family fare, the same as everyone else. They'll prefer the more familiar, but even the occasional gourmet production (or "crummy meal") shouldn't throw them if you teach them how to tactfully turn down food they don't find particularly appealing. (I will touch on that topic repeatedly.) Just be sure there is bread and a starch like rice or potatoes on the table—they won't starve.

Having made the transition to table food, we will spend the rest of the chapter talking about feeding children who are eating from the family table.

Have Regular Meals and Snacks

You must be reliable about feeding. If you plan and present your meals in a responsible and matter-of-fact fashion, you will reassure your child that he will be cared for. You will also avoid a lot of struggles about eating. The food you cook and serve will simply be a fact of your child's world, and he'll get accustomed to it like he does everything else in his world.

You can go a long way toward helping your child have a nutritionally optimum diet by taking seriously your function of planning and preparing meals. If what you have on the table and what you prepare for snacks is generally desirable, your child can have the occasional meal or snack that isn't so wonderful (or that may even be disgusting), and he will still be all right nutritionally.

You are the gatekeeper: the one who controls what foods come, in quantity, into the house. Don't underestimate the enormous influence managing the source of supply can have over your child's eating. Even if he doesn't initially accept everything you offer him, eventually he will, because that is what's familiar and that is what he sees people who are important to him eating.

Israeli children, for instance LOVE vegetables. They even eat them for breakfast. An Israeli mother asked her daughter while they traveled in England what she was hungry for—what she was going to eat when she went home. "A salad," she said, "a wonderful salad with all the fresh vegetables and greens you always put into them." She had developed her food preferences from those of the people around her—they valued their vegetables, and she did, too.

When dietitians do nutritional analyses of children's diets, they ask parents to record not only what the children *eat*, but also what is being *served*. They know that the total family food supply is a much more accurate representation of a child's nutritional status than what he happens to eat during an isolated three or four days.

You take your gatekeeper function seriously not only when you buy good food, but also when you generally keep foods out of the house that you don't approve of. You needn't apologize for not buying pop or potato chips if you don't want those to be a staple in your child's diet and if you don't want him hounding you for them all the time.

You also take your gatekeeper function seriously when you allow less-nutritious foods to come into the house once in a while, just for variety. It's a matter of the law of averages, and generally emphasizing high quality in what you prepare and

97

present for meals and snacks can cover for the periodic food or meal that isn't as good.

Learning to eat meals is an important part of children's maturation. There is a whole set of accomplishments associated with coming to the table and behaving pleasantly there, with being able to manage utensils reasonably well, and with accepting most foods and politely rejecting others. Without meals, your child won't learn those skills, and he won't be able to manage his eating in a matter-of-fact way. If you find yourself hesitating to take your child along when he has been included in a dinner invitation, then you have some work to do.

Meal Planning

In your meal planning, give your child the same consideration as you do everyone else in the family—prepare his favorite foods some of the time, but don't do it to the exclusion of what everyone else likes.

Offer a variety of food at the meal. Put it all on the table, so there are several dishes from which your child can pick and choose. That way he can express his likes and dislikes and you can respect them without having to resort to short order cooking. Don't make the mistake of presenting foods one at a time, because that will seem like his refusing and your offering alternatives. If you have offered a variety, and he still chooses not to eat anything, that is his choice. You needn't feel responsible or apologetic.

You also need not give in to his panhandling when he comes around right after the meal wanting something else to eat. He can wait for the next planned snack—we'll discuss that soon. If you give handouts, he won't learn to eat his meals.

Clearly, like everything else, you can take firmness about food selection to sadistic excess. Planning a meal of liver and onions, cooked cabbage and boiled potatoes would be my idea of sadistic menu planning, because those are foods that children generally dislike. More charitable menu planning might be liver and onions, corn and soft mashed potatoes with butter or margarine. And bread. And milk.

Try to have something on the table your child generally likes. If you have an unpopular meat, try to have a popular starch or vegetable. And for sure have bread. Children will generally eat that if nothing else pleases them.

A meal should provide:

- Protein: Meat, fish, poultry, egg, cooked dried beans.
- Bread and/or cereal: Bread, buns, noodles, spaghetti
- Fruit or vegetable or both
- Milk

A meal could be hamburgers, raw vegetables and milk; roast beef, mashed potatoes, vegetables, bread and milk; stir-fried chicken with vegetables, rice and milk; spaghetti with meat sauce, french bread, tossed salad, and milk; burritos with cheese, chopped lettuce, and tomatoes and milk. It can even be hot dogs, potato chips, raw carrots and milk, and EVEN pizza from the frozen foods case at the grocery store—and milk.

Let's face it, most of us wouldn't want to invite Gourmet magazine out to review most of our family meals. But we like them, just the same. The important ingredient is you taking the trouble to get a meal on the table, regularly and reasonably on time, and letting your family know that you want them there at meal time. If you do that, your child will benefit from your reliability and he will feel provided for. It doesn't have to be fancy, it just has to be THERE.

Do some advance planning for your family meals. In the long run, it will save you a lot of time and money, and help you when the crunch is on and everybody's hungry and you're tired and don't feel like cooking. Get things lined up for dinner the night before, while someone *else* does the dishes, so you don't have to tackle it when it's late and you're tired.

Don't make the mistake of routinely planning things that are too elaborate. Unless you take positive pleasure in making wonderful things from scratch, you probably can get along very nicely on simple foods, and even take advantage of some of the good quality mixes and pre-prepared foods that are on the market today.

Don't feel like you have to do it all yourself. In The Industrious Schoolager (Chapter 11), I point out that children take real pleasure in accomplishing tasks. Even starting as young as six or seven, children can make a contribution to preparing family meals, and take a lot of pride in it. If you make it fun, it is something you and he can enjoy together.

As he gets older, one of the after-school chores your child can do is getting dinner started. If you think through your menus and develop simple procedures and teach them to him, I expect you'll find he can be a real help to you, and he'll be proud of making a contribution.

Take Snacks Seriously

Most children can't last from one meal to the next without a snack. Take snacks just as seriously as you do meals—they are an important part of the day's food supply.

A snack is not a food handout. A snack has a planned time and place, and, like a meal, represents food that you more-or-less control. Most people go along with children's food preferences more at snacks than they do at meals. You can do that, but you can still limit snack options to the generally nutritious foods that you are comfortable about having in the house. There are suggestions for snacks in the "Tools and Strategies" section in the appendix.

Snacks should be spaced far enough before meals to allow your child to be hungry at the meal. If you find your child eats so much at a snack that he isn't hungry for his next meal, then present it earlier, before he gets so hungry. That way he'll control the amount automatically, instead of your having to do it. If your meal interval is particularly long, like the one between lunch and dinner often is, then have two snacks. Or make the one snack very substantial, so it is likely to stay with your child longer and keep him comfortable and satisfied.

Day care providers could do parents a big favor by having substantial afternoon snacks, and by having them rather late. Most children leave day care positively ravenous and unable to wait for dinner. They have a snack when they get home, and are so hungry they can't stand to just have something small. They eat so much they spoil their appetite for dinner.

As an alternative to (or maybe in addition to) a substantial afternoon snack, a solution to this problem might be to give your child a piece of fruit or a can of juice in the car on the way home. That will take the edge off his hunger by the time he gets home so he can get his mind off eating and keep himself entertained until dinner time.

Keep in mind, though, being hungry is not such a terrible

thing if the timing is right. An older child can learn to tolerate moderate hunger, particularly if he knows there is a tasty and satisfying meal in the offing. You want your child to come to the table hungry, so he is interested in eating and so his appetite encourages him to be more adventurous in trying new foods. You don't want him to come to the table starved, so he is either too cranky to eat or so famished that he simply wolfs down his food and gets a stomach ache.

As with meals, your child should have a snack, and be done with it. He shouldn't be allowed to run with food or get food handouts whenever he wants them. That kind of eating tends to be less nutritious and leads to misuse of food for entertainment or distraction. If you give a child a cookie (or even carrots) to amuse or divert or calm him, he will soon learn that strong feelings are not to be tolerated or dealt with, and that eating can be used as a panacea.

Make Eating Worthwhile

To do his best job with eating a nutritious diet and regulating the amounts he eats, your child should come to the table hungry and eat slowly until he is satisfied. At mealtime (and snack time, for that matter) he should be allowed access to an adequate amount of food to fill him up. That food should be easy enough to eat so he can manage it, it should feel good in his stomach and should have enough calories so it will satisfy his energy needs and keep him comfortable until it is time to eat again.

Children Need Modifications

You'll save yourself a lot of guarding-the-kitchen type hassles if you make your meals and snacks filling and satisfying. While it's not necessary to cater to all of your child's whims about eating, some ways that you cook for yourself have to be modified when you cook for children. Until they are eight or nine years old, children simply aren't as efficient at handling utensils, and chewing and swallowing. Particularly for the toddler and preschooler, the minor modifications in texture and

101

consistency of foods that I talked about earlier can be very helpful in allowing your child to accept food well and to be successful with his eating.

Meals that provide for your child's nutritional needs and
are tasty and satisfying need to have a reasonable distribution of
protein, fat and carbohydrate in them. If you are on a diet yourself, you may be making some modification in your eating
pattern that shorts one or the other of these major nutrients.

Some kinds of cooking, like weight-reduction or some vege-
tarian cuisines, are so low in fat and in calorie concentration
that children simply can't eat a large enough volume to meet
their energy needs. Adults can eat larger volumes and get by on
relatively low calorie foods. Children can't. If your general diet is
pretty austere, you had better give some attention to making
some modifications so your child gets enough calories.

Fat in moderate amounts is an essential part of the diet,
particularly for children. No less than 30% of the calories in a
child's diet should come from fat unless a child is on some sort
of specially-modified diet. That means a child taking 1800 calories per day should use at least 12 teaspoons of fat per day. Of
course, that includes fat in food, like whole milk and fatty meats,
as well as fat in the form of spreads on bread and oil in salad
dressings. If your child is eating a lot of fried foods, potato chips,
heavy desserts and rich candies, however, it is likely his diet is
too high in fat and that fat could be replacing other essential
nutrients.

The key, of course, is moderation—neither being too liberal
nor too restrictive with fat. I'll be talking later in this chapter
about figuring out how much fat you are eating. If you think you
may be going to one extreme or the other—providing a particularly high fat or particularly low fat diet—I'd suggest you make
some changes to get back more toward the middle.

Meals have to have carbohydrate—starch is the best
kind—in order to get a feeling of fullness and substance from a
meal. Children like their starchy foods, and generally don't have
to be persuaded to eat breads, noodles or potatoes. A very high
carbohydrate diet, however, is likely to be unsatisfying because it
is low in fat. It is important to offer fat and also appealing
sources of protein at meals. It may be wise in some circumstances to take care to put some butter or margarine on the rice or a
spread on the bread.

102

During the early years, milk is the primary source of protein in a child's diet. If you use 2% or whole milk, it is an important source of fat, as well. For the child under two years old, in fact, it is best to use whole milk, because young children have difficulty getting enough fat in their diets. Protein adds to the satisfaction and staying power of the diet, particularly since most protein foods also have significant fat in them.

Toward the end of the first year, when a child makes the transition to table food, he starts to get meat, fish, poultry or other protein foods in his diet. These foods begin to supplement milk as a source of protein and need to be offered on a regular basis.

Putting It All Together

It's really not that hard to provide an adequate diet. You simply have to supply a variety of foods daily in adequate amounts, including selections of fruits, vegetables, whole grain and enriched breads and cereals, milk and other milk products and meat, poultry, fish and other protein foods. Your children have probably been exposed to the basic four food plan in school, and whether you know it or not, you probably use it as the basis for planning your meals. I have outlined nutritious patterns of eating for different age groups in the "Recommended Daily Pattern of Food Selection" in the "Tools and Strategies" section in the appendix.

The Recommended Daily Pattern outlines amounts of food needed from each food group for a nutritious diet. For ease of translation for different age groups, I have taken two different approaches to stating requirements. For meats and milk, I have recommended total quantities. To make substitutions within these groups, see the tables, Milk Group Portion Sizes, and Meat Group Portion Sizes. As you can see from the Recommended Daily Pattern, young children have the same requirement for milk as adults, but about half the requirement for meat. Adolescents and teenagers need more milk to satisfy their increased protein and calcium requirements.

In the fruit and vegetable and bread and cereal groups, I have outlined requirements in terms of numbers of servings per day. Serving sizes, however, are smaller for children than they

103

are for grownups. As a rough rule of thumb, the toddler and preschooler will be well nourished eating about a tablespoon of fruit or vegetable per year of age. They might need a bread or cereal portion a fourth to a half what an adult would eat.

Your child can eat more than that if he wants to, and he probably will, at least at times. What the chart is telling you is that once he has eaten the stated minimums he has had what he needs for a nutritionally adequate diet. That is the point at which you can relax and stop worrying about it. Those minimums won't add up to enough calories, so he likely will eat more from one of the other food groups, or will get some of his extra calories from butter or margarine, or sugar in desserts. Often children fill up on bread, and that's OK. As long as he doesn't consistently slight one or another food group, his nutritional status will be all right.

Don't let him overdo it on the liquid foods, though, or he won't eat his solids. Like some adults, children would rather drink than eat, and if allowed unlimited access to juice or milk, they'll not eat their meals and snacks. Give water for thirst and use juice and milk as foods as a part of meals and snacks.

There is a point embedded in what I just said, and it's important: Serve small portions and let your child ask for more. If you put a lot on his plate, it can overwhelm him and make him give up before he has ever started.

On The Matter Of Vegetables

I don't know of any definitive research on the matter, but I would wager that parents and children have more struggles over vegetable consumption than over any other item in the diet—and maybe more than any other item, period.

It's hard to know why vegetables are the perennial problem. It could just be tradition—parents have grown up having vegetables pushed on them by anxious parents who assume they won't like them, and they pass the same attitudes on to their children. With the possible exception of having an innate preference for sweets, children approach all new foods pretty much the same. Don't forget that children in some cultures love their vegetables!

Another possible explanation for the concern about vegetables is that without them it is difficult to get enough vitamin A in the diet. Vegetables *are* important, and the perennial question is, how do you get children to eat them? In several of the chronological chapters, I have talked about the importance and utility of simply matter-of-factly presenting vegetables (and all other foods) to children, eating the food yourself, and letting children approach them on their own. In that way, eventually they learn to like them. If you try to force vegetables on your child, about the best you can hope for is that eventually he will grow up and eat his vegetables because he *should*, just like you do.

While you are waiting for your child to learn to like vegetables, you can offer other foods that have vitamin A in them, like milk and dark orange fruits. Check the appendix under "Tools and Strategies" for a list, "Vitamin A in Fruits and Vegetables." Peaches, apricots and watermelon, for instance, have vitamin A in them. If you offer substitutes, though, do it matter-of-factly. Don't make it look like you are short order cooking.

If you can keep from putting pressure on his vegetable consumption, left to his own devices, one fine day he may even begin to LIKE vegetables. (Ah, the little triumphs that bring tears to parents' eyes!)

About Milk

Milk provides important amounts of protein in most children's diets, and is everybody's primary source of calcium and vitamin D. Studies of children's diets indicate that calcium is one of the two nutrients that is likely to be low (the other is iron)[1]. The issue with calcium is bone health.

Recent research on osteoporosis tells us childhood is the time to get bones well-mineralized. Once you become an adult, it is all down hill as far as bone mineral is concerned. Very little is deposited after that time and, worse, mineral is slowly lost as we age.

Milk consumption is a particular concern for teenage girls, who begin to skip their milk in order to save calories. They couldn't do it at a worse time. The teen years are a time of particular calcium need as they grow taller and mineralize their bones in the process.

105

Kids do better at drinking milk if you drink milk yourself. If you can't stand to do that, at least restrict yourself to water. If you are drinking pop or juice your child will naturally want that.

Kids go through stages where they don't drink much milk. Parents often complain about decreases in milk consumption after their child is weaned and before he gains facility with the cup. Don't worry about it, and don't make a big fuss about it. Continue to offer milk at meals, don't give substitutes, and your child will likely go back to drinking it. He will, that is, unless you make such a big fuss about it that he will lose face if he starts drinking milk again.

On The Matter Of Meat

The meat group includes meat, fish, poultry and cooked dried beans. This group is important in the diet for protein and for trace elements like iron and zinc. Iron and zinc in animal protein are particularly well absorbed. As I said a moment ago, iron is one of the two major nutrients that are most likely to be low in children's diets. It is hard to have optimum iron nutrition without including meat, fish or poultry regularly.

Young children often don't eat meat too well, so it's a good thing that they don't NEED that much to get their protein requirement. If he is drinking two cups of milk a day, a toddler can get by on an ounce of meat a day, a preschooler on two ounces, and a schoolage child on three. It isn't until the rapid growth period of puberty that children's protein requirement goes up—at that time they need three or four glasses of milk a day and four ounces of meat.

Offer children meat or meat substitutes at least twice a day, and let them eat as much or as little of it as they want. Even if they eat only small amounts, a little meat, fish or poultry eaten with a meal will help the absorption of iron from all the food in the meal. (So will including a vitamin C source.) If you are serving a variety, and if the meat is generally moist, tender and easy to chew, your children will do all right with their meat intake.

If you have chosen to exclude meat from your own diet, consider offering it to your child anyway. If you don't want to do

106

that, see a registered dietitian to make sure you are compensating adequately for the nutrients he'll be missing.

On Breads And Cereals

It is important to choose enriched or whole grain breads and cereals. These foods have the B vitamins and iron we count on getting in the bread group. Whole grain also has the extra added benefit of vitamin E, trace elements like magnesium, and fiber, all important components of the diet.

While it is helpful to include whole grain in the diet, it is unnecessary in the usual mixed diet to have all grain products be whole grain. Too much fiber can interfere with absorption of other nutrients and cause fullness and gas. Try for an average of about half whole grain—that will give the advantages without the shortcomings.

Margin Of Error

As kids get bigger, their appetites get bigger and their nutrient needs go up. But they always have some leeway between the calories they need to use up to get their needs satisfied for protein, fatty acids, vitamins and minerals, and the total calories they can eat to satisfy their energy needs. I call that gap the margin of error.

In "Tools and Strategies," the chart, "Calorie Requirements Compared With Basic Needs," shows you in picture form how the margin of error principle works in nutrition. Not every food has to be nutritious for total food intake to add up to a nutritionally adequate diet. The margin of error allows you to relax and take a philosophical approach to your child's eating.

If you don't, you could end up in fights like the parents who called me, upset about their teenage son's eating. As they saw it, his eating was really awful. He liked pop and potato chips and candy. And they were adamant that he shouldn't be consuming any of it. Very adamant. The struggle had escalated to the point where the whole family was in an uproar.

They came in for nutrition counseling, but they were having such a hassle about the topic that just talking sense to them about nutrition wasn't going to solve anything. But I did that anyway, and went on to wonder why they had to be so preoccupied with their son's eating.

107

I told them what I just told you: their son had such a high calorie requirement that he could eat everything he needed to eat in order to have a nutritious diet and still have calories left over for foods that were really pretty worthless nutritionally. I went on to say that it was pretty hard to find foods that didn't have *some* nutrients. While pop was one of them, it really wasn't going to be that harmful for him to have pop as long as he also ate regular meals and got the other nutritious food he needed.

I don't know whether he was eating very well in general— he said he was and his parents said he wasn't and I couldn't get any actual food reports out of any of them. But I do know that his parents were having such a fit about his eating that it was increasing the chances of his eating poorly just to spite them.

I told them that, and I also told them he was old enough to take responsibility for his own nutrition. I said I didn't know why they had to get in such a fight about his eating, but it was definitely outside the range of normal struggles with a teenager. I suggested they consider getting some family counseling, because if they didn't, the next struggle that erupted would be worse. As yet, their teenager was being pretty easy on them. If they didn't react positively to his efforts at this level to manage his own behavior he would simply escalate his strivings for independence, and do something that was REALLY a cause for concern.

They couldn't hear me, but I expect that someone else farther down the road will tell them essentially the same thing, and I hope then they'll hear it.

Teach Them To Eat What's In The World

I know a mother who boasts that her six-year-old has never been to McDonalds. When I told my son Curtis that, he was disgusted. "What is he going to do when the other kids talk about going to McDonald's?" he asked. "He won't have anything to talk about. He won't even know anything about it!"

Curtis, like most children, has the disconcerting habit of hitting the nail on the head. Food is culture, it's part of knowing what's going on in the world and feeling like a part of it. Fast

108

food franchises are a fact of life, and parents are not going to get them to go away by refusing to let their children eat at them.

The mom's concern was nutrition, but as a long-term method for protecting her child's nutritional status, her tactic won't work. That six-year-old will grow up eventually, and go out on his bicycle with his friends, and they just might take some money along and he just might stop by at McDonalds. I wonder what that mother will do then—will she stand by the door and examine his hands for catsup stains and smell his breath for french fries?

But one thing is for sure: until that fateful day when he takes matters into his own hands, he isn't going to learn anything about managing foods that are not nutritionally optimum.

If you deprive your child of something other kids enjoy, he will want it. If you forbid certain foods, his interest will be heightened in those foods, and he will want them. It is better to include less-desirable foods occasionally and matter-of-factly, and to talk about your philosophy about them: they aren't as good as some of the other choices you make, but an occasional use won't interfere with getting a good diet.

A periodic trip to the fast-food franchise for the entire family, even if you miss out on your vegetables, can be a pleasant and reasonable choice for you all. You can always make up on your vegetables another time, and an occasional high-fat meal will not clog your arteries, zap, just like that.

When your child gets into middle childhood and adolescence, he may develop quite a preference for foods you consider to be nutritionally undesirable. All you can do is talk about it, and keep preparing nutritious foods for family meals. Read the two chapters, The Industrious Schoolager (Chapter 11) and the Individualistic Teenager (Chapter 12), for more suggestions on dealing with older kids and their eating.

Eating For Prevention

I'm going to start out by talking about prevention for you, because your ideas about diet will shape your child's eating environment. I'll make a more direct connection with your children and their eating toward the end of this section.

109

The Dietary Guidelines

The Dietary Guidelines for Americans[2], put out by the U.S. Departments of Agriculture and Health and Human Services, states that to maintain health, we should all:

- Eat a variety of food

- Maintain desirable weight

- Avoid too much fat, saturated fat and cholesterol

- Eat foods with adequate starch and fiber

- Avoid too much sugar

- Avoid too much sodium

- If you use alcohol, do so in moderation

Earlier in this chapter, I talked about eating a variety of food. The Guideline principles for eating a good diet are the same.

The role of obesity in disease is debatable. Certainly, "Maintain desirable weight" is self explanatory but, as I'll point out later, may need some modification based on a more realistic health picture and a more practical view of how people operate.

The usual level of fat in the American diet is around 40%. The Guidelines recommend reducing it to 30 to 35% (for children, the higher level is desirable). Fat modification is based on the belief that high blood cholesterol promotes heart disease, and that high blood cholesterol, in turn, is caused partially by a high saturated fat, high cholesterol diet. There is also evidence implicating excess fat in some types of cancer.

The reasoning behind increasing starch in the diet is to encourage an alternate, fat-free source of calories. If you choose whole grain, it can also be a source of fiber. Adequate fiber in the diet improves colon function and may reduce the risk of colon cancer.

The major problem with excess sugar intake is that it satisfies hunger and displaces sources of important nutrients in the diet. Sugar that comes in contact with the teeth over an extended time can contribute to tooth decay (particularly with sugary foods that stick to your teeth, like caramels or raisins, or sugary foods or beverages that you consume slowly over time, like pop or fruit juice).

Limiting sodium intake may reduce blood pressure for some who are susceptible, which may, in turn, reduce incidence of heart attacks and strokes. Just on general principles of moderation, Americans eat more sodium than they need, so the guidelines recommend cutting down.

Alcohol calories replace calories from nutritious foods. Excess alcohol consumption can impair the nutritional quality of the diet—and produce another whole set of problems. I hope drinking is not an issue for your child—either directly, or because of *your* habits.

The Guidelines In Perspective

Research continues, and the answers are far from complete. The Dietary Guidelines represent a moderate attempt to deal with the uncertainties of nutrition and its relationship to disease, and make recommendations for today. They are debatable in some circles. If followed, they won't do you any harm, and may even do some good.

Keep in mind that there is probably much about your usual food intake that is worth preserving. Most people eat an adequate diet, as attested by the increases in life expectancy, achievement of good average body size and general good health of the American population.

Foods we have to choose from are varied, plentiful, and wholesome. The incidence of heart disease has declined markedly in the last 20 years, and no one is quite sure why. Like all issues of prevention, it is difficult to decide what, if anything, is helping. How does one research a question like that? We can't ask, "Check this box if your eating methods kept you from having heart disease."

However, even though the general health picture is good, questions continue to be raised about the American diet and its relationship to certain chronic diseases: heart disease, high blood pressure, strokes, diabetes, osteoporosis, cancer, tooth decay. Research on these topics is, by and large, in the early stages, and so far the results only support modest dietary modifications. Evidence is not strong enough, however, to make hard and fast recommendations about major changes for the general population[3].

Dietary guidelines don't resolve all the dilemmas in food selection and preparation. Research continues to be done and reported in the media, and, based on that research, people continue to tinker with their diets. There is room for caution, however; some tinkering may be premature. Even with seemingly authoritative and conclusive studies, some experts raise issues that call the results into question. There are so many divergent points of view, for instance, in the area of nutrition and its relationship to heart disease and cancer, that about all that the experts can agree on is that they disagree. The evidence, at this point, is contradictory and inconclusive, and you will even have a hard time finding two people to agree on *that*.

If you would like to get into this topic in more detail, *The Nutrition Debate*[4] makes fascinating reading. The authors have selected the best statements from each side on the eating questions of the day, and reprinted them. They intend it for their readers as a "resource for personal decision-making."

At this point, there is general agreement that people who have risk factors for heart disease should make some modifications in the type and amount of fat they use and in the amount of sodium in their diet. The debate is whether these changes should be made for the general population.

There is general agreement that obesity can be implicated in heart disease, diabetes, and possibly, cancer. The argument is about what really constitutes obesity. Some authorities say there is consistent health impairment only for the severly overweight[5] whereas others say that even five pounds of excess body weight can be a problem[6]. No doubt the biases of experts come into play, too. They can be as prone to lipophobia* as the population as a whole.

The only disease that can be linked to excess sugar intake is tooth decay. Only flimsy, speculative, or anecdotal research evidence supports the idea that excess sugar has an effect on mood or emotional stability[3]. At times, parents who reduce the levels of sugar in their children's diets think it helps considerably, but the active ingredient might actually be parental firmness in refusing food handouts or their consistency in offering more nutritious, and more filling alternatives to sugary foods.

---

*Lipophobia: The irrational fear of fat.

We read that people with low levels of vitamin A and vitamin E in their blood (presumably from poor dietary intake) have increased risk of certain types of lung disease, and that adequate fiber in the diet may be protective against colon cancer. People are beginning to think that increased calcium in the diet can help hold blood pressure at a normal level and that, in turn, helps prevent heart disease[3].

The good outcome of these kinds of studies, and publicity, is that they encourage some people to take their nutrition seriously and going to the trouble of seeking out and preparing good foods.

The Problem Of Excess

The bad outcome of nutritional speculation—and enthusiasm—is that people are going to excess. They are dosing themselves with large quantities of nutritional supplements that they think will be protective (the research really isn't good enough yet to dictate that—there is *more* research to demonstrate harm from supplements). There is a certain excitement in that, and people run out and buy calcium that doubles as an antacid or take big doses of vitamin C and vitamin E (which may or may not be harmful) or vitamin A (which certainly *could* be harmful, if you take enough of it). One of the nutritional principles that we *know* is that overdosing yourself with one nutrient can cause deficiencies in another. In the long run, over-enthusiastic attempts at prevention can do more harm than good.

Along with excess comes more excess. People go gung-ho on getting their weight down or the fat level of their diet down, and they use such extreme measures that they take all the joy out of cooking and eating. They can stand the austerity for only so long, and then they fall off their regimen and overeat, and their extremes flood their bodies with all the fats and sugars they are trying to avoid. Is this progress?

The extremes are particularly characteristic in the area of weight management. In my view, the last thing people need is more pressure on them to lose weight. In the name of achieving thinness, many people do things to themselves that are more harmful than the condition itself.

Harsh and nutritionally inadequate weight reduction diets take their toll on health and fitness. So does regaining weight

113

after a failed attempt, which is much more typical than atypical. The weight losing and regaining process is harder on the body than maintaining a high but stable weight. While the question is unresolved of how bad it really is for you to be obese, there is no doubt that the yo-yo syndrome is *not* good for you.

Set Reasonable Goals

The key to avoiding ricochetting from one excess to another is setting long-term, reasonable and personal goals. If you feel your diet is too high in fat and salt and sugar, and too low in vegetables and fruits and whole grains and milk, and you want to change it, then you should. But the way you make the changes can make all the difference.

You need to start where you are, and make changes gradually. If you are now having fried food five nights a week, you can begin by cutting down to four. If you are now having heavily salted foods, you can start by tasting your food before you salt it. If you now have rich desserts every night, you can gradually cut the portions smaller and smaller, change occasionally to something less rich, or substitute fruit one night a week.

It is even better to start by adding on desirable foods, and letting them crowd out the less desirable ones. You can make it a point to buy an occasional loaf of whole-wheat bread (or start with a loaf of part whole-wheat), and make vegetables a part of your dinner. And when you achieve your goals, you can pat yourself on the back and compare yourself with, not Jane Brody, but with yourself where you were before. You'll get further if you give yourself encouragement rather than criticism.

Give yourself time to get over the shock of those changes before you push on. If you make modest changes and do it over time, your new eating style will feel familiar and comfortable to you. If you try to change too abruptly, it will always be a struggle, and you will periodically fall off and go back to your old way of eating, which will seem all the more desirable because of the deprivation you will feel you have just been through.

Weight Loss

Many of my patients have found that the solution to the weight-loss, weight regain struggle is to set aside weight loss as the primary (or only) goal, and set other goals that *are* more reliably achievable. Even if you can't get your weight to go down, you can develop and maintain an enjoyable and nutritionally sound diet, a fulfilling and healthful exercise program, and let weight do what it will in response to clean living.

Sometimes it goes down, and that is wonderful—I wish it for all my patients. But sometimes its doesn't, and then the task is to learn to live with it. My patients find it easier to accept their weight if they can respect the way they manage their eating and exercise—if they are able to eat and exercise in an orderly and positive way.

The Impact On Children

Which brings us back to children's eating. You are providing for your child's continued good health by making wise choices in the kinds of foods you offer. Let that stimulate you, not to nutritional perfection, but to nutritional constancy. Your child will be exposed to the same excesses and frustrations and inconsistencies in eating that you expose yourself to. If your eating is erratic and emotionally charged, for whatever reason, your child's will be too. If you diet all week and relax by going to a huge brunch on Sunday where you load up on all the things you have deprived yourself of all week, your children will, too. And they will experience the same ambivalence about eating that you do.

Also keep in mind it is possible to make too much of a good thing out of being disciplined about your diet. A study in New York found several children who were growing poorly because their parents restricted their food intake or had them on low-fat diets.[8] As I said earlier in the chapter, children have high energy needs, and they just can't eat enough to grow well on some of the restrictive regimens that adults follow.

Eating is, after all, one of life's great pleasures. If your health measures are taking the joy out of eating, you are going too far. You may be able to get yourself to eat unattractive food because "it is good for you," but your children won't, and your family mealtimes and ultimately the quality of their diet will suffer.

You can read about this topic, and that is helpful. You can get the Dietary Guidelines booklet and its backup series of mini-

115

bulletins[7] from your local county Extension agent or public health nutritionist. The individual booklets in the series talk about the specifics of changing the diet. You'll be able, for instance, to estimate how little fat is little enough, and be able to get a realistic estimate of the percentage of fat in your diet.

In addition to the above information, it seems to me that getting a dietary evaluation and some nutrition counseling from a registered dietitian is often money well spent. The results might surprise you. In my years as a clinical dietitian in a medical practice, I often found my patients to be too restrictive rather than too liberal. Wherever you find yourself along the continuum from overly-restrictive to appropriate to overly-liberal, I think you would benefit from knowing more about making appropriate food selections and putting together a healthful diet.

The food your child eats during his early years can have a major impact on his lifelong health. The first priority is adequate calories and nutrients to allow him to grow and develop optimally. The second priority is prevention of disease. Efforts to manage weight or control blood cholesterol must never be so vigorous that they keep children from growing properly.

Unless he makes a real concerted effort to change, the nutritional habits your child learns at home are the ones he is likely to carry with him for the rest of his life. He will develop his habits more from the way you handle feeding and from the foods you present to him, and consume yourself, than from anything you say about nutrition and eating. His early conditioning will work for him if you are consistent and positive about eating. It will work against him if you are erratic and negative.

References

1.   Christian, J.L. and Greger, J.L.: Nutrition for Living. Menlo Park, CA: Benjamin Cummings. 1985.

2.   U.S. Department of Agriculture, U.S. Department of Health and Human Services: Dietary Guidelines for Americans. Home and Garden Bulletin No. 232, Hyattsville, MD. 1985.

3.   Pariza, M.W., Task Force Chairman, Council for Agricultural Science and Technology: Diet and Health, Report No. 111, Ames, IA, 1987.

4. Gussow, J.D. and Thomas, P.R.: The Nutrition Debate: Sorting Out Some Answers. Palo Alto, CA: Bull Publishing, 1986.

5. Stunkard, A.J. Editor, Obesity. Philadelphia: Saunders. 1980.

6. Health Implications of Obesity National Institutes of Health Consensus Development Conference Statement 5(9). February 11-13, 1985.

7. U.S. Department of Agriculture, U.S. Department of Health and Human Services: Dietary Guidelines for Americans. Home and Garden Bulletins No. 232-1 to 232-7, 1986.

8. Pugliese, M.T., Weyman-Daum, M., Moses, N. and Lifshitz, F.: Parental health beliefs as a cause of nonorganic failure to thrive. Pediatrics 80:175. 1987.

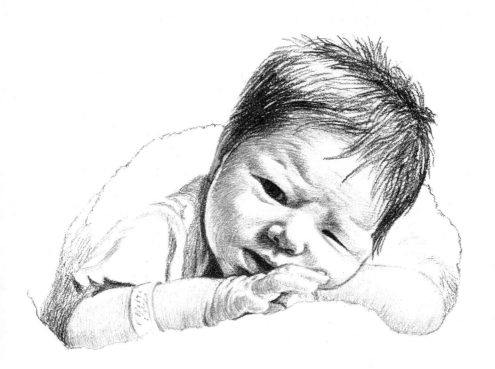

7

The Newborn

Working out a positive feeding relationship with your baby can make a significant difference to both of you. Whether your baby grows well or poorly—and both of you come out of infancy feeling good about yourselves and the relationship or feeling bad—is determined to a large extent by what happens in feeding. Children and parents do best when parents recognize and respond appropriately to babies' needs. But babies can be difficult to decipher, or parents can be insensitive in detecting and responding to their cues, and parents and babies end up not hitting it off. When that happens, babies don't do as well, either emotionally or physically, and parents don't feel as successful. When you feel attached to your baby and gratify her needs, you gratify your own.

I'll be telling you in this chapter how to work things out with your baby in feeding. You may find you have some room for improvement. If you are like most parents, you are operating on the basis of some faulty attitudes or information. Please, *please*, PLEASE don't get down on yourself if you are doing something that I tell you is not a good idea. You have to learn. Babies are resilient little things, and if you change the way you

119

operate, in most cases you will find your baby will change right along with you. You may have never been a parent before, but she's never been a baby before, either. . .you can learn together.

The Process Of Attachment

Feeding provides you with the best opportunity you have during the early months to get to know your baby. Feeding provides your baby with powerful messages that you see her as being a valuable person, and that you respect her and are willing to go to some trouble to work things out with her. The easy respect, and give-and-take, and working things out between parent and child has been termed synchrony. Establishing synchrony between you and your baby has everything to do with parenting in an emotionally healthy way.

In the process of applying yourself to figuring out your baby, you will establish the attitude and relationship you need to allow you to be a good parent. You need to feel attracted to your baby, to become preoccupied with her, to be sensitive to and aware of her special characteristics, to feel like she is the world's first perfect baby, and to get to the point where you feel lonely for her when she isn't there and miss her when you see another baby.

That attachment, and those feelings, don't develop automatically. There is no maternal or paternal "instinct." You develop the feelings as you take care of your baby, as you spend time around her, and as you take pride in being important to her[1].

Fathers, as well as mothers, can become engrossed with their baby. In fact, they NEED to, if they are to avoid feeling jealous of their baby and competitive with the relationship that mother and baby have with one another. In one study, fathers who helped care for their babies in the hospital became fascinated with their newborns. Being present at the birth helped engage fathers with their babies[2].

That early time after birth is helpful in establishing the parent-child bond, but not essential for most people. It's wonderful if you have the opportunity to be with your child early on, but you needn't feel you have missed something irreplaceable in

120

your relationship if you haven't. With healthy mothers* and healthy babies, immediate contact doesn't seem to make any lasting difference in the relationship[3]. However, early contact is important if there are limitations in infant or parent—if baby and/or mother are sick or if the mother is young or under stress[4].

It is important for you to see your baby as a small person and for you to find out that *you* can provide what this small person needs. A tall order, but it can all take place during feeding time.

Understanding The Newborn

Despite the besotted way we all behave around them, the beauty of most newborn babies must really be in the eyes of the beholders. They just kind of lie there and don't do anything. They can't even hold up their heads. We deceive ourselves that they smile at us—but at the very first it is just gas (or whatever). No matter—it entices us anyway.

But people, especially parents, find a wonderful kind of beauty, and are remarkably good at doing so. What they have is entirely sufficient for the task of getting their early relationship established with their baby. Newborns *do* respond to the people in their environment. They brighten when they see a face, they calm when they are cared for by someone they are accustomed to, and they become more or less engaging and involved with the world, depending on how engaging and involved their caretakers are with them.

They know when they are hungry and let us know with methods ranging from squirming to screaming, and know when they are full and communicate that with tactics ranging from sealing their lips to throwing up. They do things that make them engaging to adults: They can examine images that are close to them, echo sounds, and imitate facial expressions. They know how to eat and how to grow and do it with great dispatch. Many a mother has commented with awe that she is glad that all that amazing growing waited to take place until AFTER her baby left the womb!

---

*With apologies to fathers—most studies observe *mothers*.

121

The newborn has very limited feeding skills, but they are entirely sufficient to get the job done. She is equipped with a rooting and suckle reflex so she can turn toward the nipple when it touches her cheek and can open her mouth. When a nipple is presented she knows, for the most part, how to latch on to it and suck (or suckle, which depends more on stroking the nipple with her tongue than on suction) and swallow. She can take nourishment, but needs a lot of help to do it.

It is the most natural thing in the world to cuddle a newborn and to feed her in a way that fits with cuddling. Ergo, the nipple—either the human one or one that comes on a baby bottle.

The newborn's ability to digest food is as limited as her ability to ingest food. We used to start them early on pasteurized milk, but now we know that's not good for them. During the first six months, she needs breast milk (with some extra vitamin D and fluoride) or a specially-prepared formula that has been exquisitely concocted to make it nutritionally appropriate and easy for her to digest.

With only one food to worry about, it might seem that infant nutrition would be simple. It's quite the opposite. Because that one food item has to be so absolutely appropriate for the baby's needs, infant nutrition is a highly technical area. Not so technical, however, that you can't understand it, even if you know little about nutrition. In fact, it's helpful to know something about the topic so you can follow along and check to see if there is logic in suggestions you are being given about feeding. I'm not going to go into the topic here, but I wrote about the milk feeding in detail in *Child of Mine*: you can read it there.

Your newborn will gain skills rapidly during the first six months. She will learn to smile, and if all is going well, she will become a even more engaging and sociable person. But until she learns to sit up, she still has to be held in a semi-reclining position to be fed, and her mouth muscles still only know a primitive suckle-swallow pattern. The way to feed a child for most of the first six months, then, is by nipple.

Simple as it seems, nipple feeding can go well or poorly. The way you and your newborn work out nipple feeding can make an enormous impact on her physical and emotional health.

Feeding The Newborn

Feeding demands a division of responsibility: You are responsible for *what* your child is offered to eat, and for offering it in a positive and supportive fashion. She is responsible for how much she eats, and for when, where and in what manner. Figure 7-1, "Division of Responsibility in Nipple Feeding," outlines some of the basic points in that division.

Feeding will go best when you pay attention to your baby to figure out what is going on with her, work to calm her, and for the most part, conduct a smooth, uninterrupted feeding time. You'll need to depend on messages coming from her about amount, timing, pacing and eating capability.

You'll need to work with her to understand what you do that makes her alert and organized and comfortable enough to eat well, and follow through with those behaviors. You have to pay attention to how she reacts to your voice, your gaze, the way you touch her, move her around, the position you hold her in and how tightly you hold her.

It sounds very complex, but most of us "read" our babies all the time, and do it intuitively. We notice, maybe even on a subconscious level, that our baby quiets when we talk or sing to her softly and steadily, but not when we talk very loudly or in a particular tone of voice.

You may also notice that talking "wakes her up," or helps her to get organized so she can get ready to pay attention to the feeding, rather than drifting off to sleep or getting upset about something else going on within her or around her. (Of course, the most effective method of allowing your baby to be relaxed and alert for the feeding is letting her determine the feeding schedule.) Once feeding starts, most babies will stop sucking when you get active—when you talk to them or jiggle the bottle or even look at them. You need to experiment and observe to see how your baby responds.

At the risk of belaboring a point, let me underscore: *Your baby is an active participant in the feeding process.* To get feeding to go well, you *must* let her be in control of it. She is the one with all the information about how much she needs to eat to grow well, when she needs to eat and in what fashion she can manage to eat and still remain comfortable. Your baby will give you little signals that let you know what she wants. Your job is to decipher what those signals mean, and go along with them.

123

Parents are responsible for what is presented to eat and the manner in which it is presented

- Pick out the right milk feeding
- Hold her securely but not too tightly
- Touch her cheek to get her to root for the nipple
- Hold the nipple still at a comfortable angle
- Feed at her times
- Keep it smooth—don't burp or wipe unnecessarily
- Check her out after a pause to see if she's still hungry
- Talk and smile, but don't be too entertaining

Children are responsible for how much and whether they eat

- Use trial and error to find out what her signals mean
- Let her decide how much to eat
- Let her decide how fast to eat
- Let her tell you when she's hungry

Figure 7-1   Division of Responsibility in Nipple Feeding

Even though it is very important, don't expect to do it right the first time. We have all had to learn. Some babies are easier to learn with than others. As I pointed out in What is Normal Eating (Chapter 5), babies vary in their temperament and their ability to take in food. But you *can* be successful with even the most challenging baby. And if you are successful, you will likely call even a difficult baby "good." But no matter what you call her, it takes a while to know what your baby likes.

Feeding doesn't take an expert (even though a knowledgeable consultant can be very helpful when you get stuck). You have within you the ability to pay attention to your baby and to collect all the information you need to establish a nice feeding relationship.

124

Learning How Babies "Talk"

Dr. Gail Price, a clinical psychologist, demonstrated in her research on feeding[5] that mothers could learn how babies "talk." Dr. Price videotaped forty mothers and divided them into two sets: one set she worked with, one she didn't. She did three tapes on each feeding pair: the first in the hospital, the second in the home at age 10-12 days, and the third at age four to six weeks.

As part of her work with the first set of mothers, after she did the second taping she showed them both the first and second tapes. While the tapes were being shown, she encouraged the mothers to discuss their observations about the way they were feeding. For the purposes of the study, she was careful not to come across as an expert. She wanted to see if the videotaping, and having her to talk to, was helpful to the mothers in figuring out what was best for their babies. She suggested that she was studying how babies "talk" to their mothers, what signals they give to the mothers of what they like and dislike. She then asked the mothers to tell her what they observed about how babies "talked" to them.

During the interviews, Dr. Price found that most mothers caught on very quickly to the idea that their babies were communicating with them. They were also usually open about critiquing themselves—in deciding when they were being effective or not effective in responding to those messages. Most times they were pleased by what they saw. They could tell that they had done something that helped their baby calm down or attend to her eating better. At other times they were uncomfortable while they watched the interaction. They felt like they were doing something that their baby didn't like. For instance, one mother commented: "I'm burping him so hard I look like I am killing him. Oh, you poor baby. Why didn't you tell me?"

While the mothers felt bad about doing things that their babies didn't like, they could handle it as long as they could develop something else to do that DID work. Even when they were making mistakes, they were able to relax with their babies when they realized they could find a better way.

Along those lines, one mother observed that her sleepy baby opened his eyes and sucked when she talked with him, and when she touched his fingers, but not when she jiggled his body.

125

The mother had been doing that consistently, even though she hadn't been consciously aware of it. (That was the same mother who burped so vigorously that "I look like I'm killing him." She was behaving effectively in one area, but not in another.)

The final tapes, done at age four to six weeks, were analyzed to compare the relationships between mothers and babies in the two groups—the one which had seen tapes of the earlier feedings, and the group which had not. Mothers who had seen the videotapes and gone through the exercise of looking for communication signals from their babies showed an increase in synchrony with their babies. That is, they had realized their babies could communicate with them, and they had adjusted their own behavior to accommodate to their babies and let them be more effective with eating.

The mothers who only saw the tapes at the end of the project and hadn't had any encouragement to think about how their babies "talked" to them (the "controls"), showed less sensitivity to their babies, and a decrease in synchrony during the study. They also reacted very differently to the tapes. Those mothers were generally interested in how the babies looked and how they, themselves, looked, but they didn't pick up on the interactions. Generally, the control mothers saw their babies as being set in their ways, and didn't think that their own behavior affected their babies one way or the other.

In the case of the mothers who had been helped by the videotapes to improve the way they related to their babies (the "experimental" group), the improvements in the relationships had lasted beyond the newborn period. Once the mothers came to see that what they did gave their baby pleasure—or displeasure—they continued to adjust their behavior to that of their babies. They also liked mothering better because they felt more effective and important to their babies.

I wish someone like Dr. Price had been around with her videotape equipment, or at least with her ability to help people be successful with their babies, when my children were tiny. My most vivid memory of meeting my first, Kjerstin, for the first time was of alarm—I was so afraid that if she cried I wouldn't know what to do for her. She was so lovely and appealing, and I was so touched by my love for her. I wanted to just hold her and watch her. But I was also afraid to do that. Whenever she squirmed or wiggled or gurgled, I tensed up, because I was afraid she was going to cry and I wouldn't know what to do about it.

I learned, but I was lucky. She was an easy baby to care for, and only cried when she was hungry. Even though we got along all right, I am sure I could have been more sensitive. And I am also sure that it would have been a lot more fun if I could have been more confident in my abilities to work things out with her.

Observing A Spitting-up Problem

Since then, I have been around for some other people, and have played that magical role of helping *them* to feel successful with *their* baby. Let me tell you about an experience I had with one young mother.

The parents had been in couple therapy with me during their pregnancy, and had taken leave while Marie was born. The mother returned when Marie was 10 days old. When they came in, Marie was already crying and showing by the restless way she was throwing her arms and legs around that she wanted to eat and that she wanted it *right now*. We hurried and got her bottle warmed up for her, and she started nursing in a very effi- cient manner. The feeding went smoothly. Her mother held her well-supported and cozily and held the bottle nice and still, and Marie sucked steadily. While Marie ate, her mother explained that they were having a lot of trouble with feeding. Marie had been throwing up a lot, they had been back to the doctor several times, and they had already changed her to a soy formula to see if that would help. However, it didn't seem to, and Marie had continued to throw up.

About five minutes into the feeding, the mother pulled the nipple out of Marie's mouth, even though she was still nursing steadily and showing no apparent discomfort. She abruptly put Marie across her shoulder to burp. "The doctor told me I was to burp her often," she explained. "He says she is probably filling up with air, and that is making her throw up." She burped Marie energetically for a few minutes, then sat her up on her lap and rocked her quickly back and forth across her hand. "Josh [the older brother] always burped when I did this with him." (Still no burp.)

127

She then laid Marie back down on her lap and attempted to feed her again. This time Marie didn't take the nipple voluntarily, but did accept it when her mother pushed it between her lips. "The doctor says to get her to take enough so she doesn't eat so often," she explained. "She's only taken two ounces, and she won't last long if I let her stop now." Marie took an apparently reluctant few sucks, then stopped nursing completely. Whereupon her mother again put her across her shoulder and again patted her back energetically. "She must have air," she said. "I didn't get it up before." At this point, Marie did throw up. A lot.

Watching from the outside, it was easy for me to speculate that Marie's throwing up was coming from all that rough handling. The mother couldn't see that, however, because she was so involved in the process, so tense, and so preoccupied with following all the instructions she had been given. My task became, in a tactful way, one of interrupting those instructions, and helping the mother to tune in on information coming from her daughter. I got my opening when Marie threw up.

I volunteered to hold Marie while her mother cleaned herself up. Once I took the pressure off her for Marie's care, the mother relaxed and got interested in what Marie was doing. And what Marie was doing was fairly alarming. I could feel by the way she tensed her body and arms and legs that there was one position she liked to be in, and one only. She liked to be held fairly securely against my body with her arms and legs supported. And she liked to be held at an angle. A certain angle.

Even when she was held in this fashion, she still got restless at times. Periodically, she would seem to get jittery, and her arms and legs would go, and her face would pucker up like she was going to start to cry. I restrained my impulse to move her, and she calmed herself down, and went back to resting quietly again.

And she gurgled. Every so often, this little bubbling noise would start in her throat, and you could just visualize her lunch rising up in her esophagus. That too, was alarming. I had seen how Marie could throw up when she got going. Again, I restrained myself from protecting either my chair or my best suit and just sat there holding her, and she again calmed herself down.

While all this was going on, the mother and I shared

impressions about Marie. I commented to her that she was getting a lot of instructions from other people about what to do, and that that was making it hard for her to pay attention to information coming from Marie. It seemed to me, I said, that Marie was a little fooler. She looked calm and restful, and she certainly was a nice size and well-developed. But she was actually a somewhat jittery baby, and reacted to sudden movements and became startled when she felt unsupported.

That one observation opened the door for the mother to do her own observing. She was able to see how Marie got agitated, then calmed herself. I let her know when I could hear those alarming little sounds starting in Marie's throat, and let her know when they went away again. I told her I found Marie pretty alarming, too, and that I had to restrain myself from taking evasive action when the gurgling started.

Even though faced with this extreme feeding behavior, Marie's mother only had to make modest changes in order to respond in a way that was more helpful to Marie. But she shifted her whole emphasis. Instead of going by the advice and the mechanics, she went by Marie. I did the same thing. The only piece of advice I gave her was to cut back on burping. I suggested she wait until Marie stopped nursing or in some way indicated she was uncomfortable before she burp her. If Marie didn't show any signs of needing it, I suggested she skip it. (Marie didn't seem to need burping while I watched. The mother was very good at adjusting the ring on the baby bottle so the air bubbles could go into the bottle while Marie nursed, and she didn't have to suck so hard that she took in air.)

Things went better with Marie's eating after the mother got the idea of watching her for answers. The mother went home and told her husband what we had observed about Marie, and they both started going by Marie's reactions to determine how they handled her, and started ignoring the outside advice. Marie's incidence of throwing up decreased a lot, even though she still threw up occasionally. They didn't get as upset about it, though, because they had some sense of control over it.

The experience with Marie demonstrates what to do and what NOT to do in working out how to feed your baby. When things go wrong with feeding, it is very typical to discuss the problem with someone and for that someone to give advice. It is much LESS typical to have someone sit down with you and

129

observe a feeding and try to figure out what works with your particular baby. From my own observations and experience and from all the reading I've done and stories I have heard from people about how things go wrong with feeding, I would say observing and problem solving based on those observations are the only ways that one can be really helpful in solving feeding problems.

Problem-solving With Feeding

Too often when feeding is not going well, advisors look for mechanical explanations, like the wrong feeding or the wrong schedule or poor burping. Too seldom they look at the interaction between baby and mother to find out what is actually *happening* at the feeding.

When a baby is growing poorly or has digestive difficulties or is eating poorly at a feeding and wanting to eat right away again—all these situations call for taking a close look at feeding. It is, in fact, ESPECIALLY important to look at feeding when things are going wrong. You can be scared by your baby into doing counter-productive things. People tend to get overactive with feeding when babies are tiny or seem to be having trouble with eating. They jiggle the bottle and jiggle the baby, and try to feed the baby when she isn't interested in eating or try to feed her past the point where she indicates she has had enough. They check the level of formula in the bottle, push the nipple into the baby's mouth when she is indicating no interest in eating, and burp frequently for no apparent reason.

Ironically, these very common and natural attempts to "help out" actually backfire. Babies eat more when feeders work to calm them, trust their feeding cues and develop methods that promote a smooth and uninterrupted feeding. They eat less well when feeders are too active[6].

Peter Wright, a physician working in Edinburgh, Scotland, observed in a research study that parents were more active with smaller, bottle-fed babies than they were with smaller, breast-fed babies. The smaller breast-fed babies grew better than bottle fed babies, probably because feeders were not as able to be overactive[7]. (It *is* possible to force with breast-feeding, but considerably harder.) Parents *weren't* over active with normal-sized, bottle fed babies, probably because they didn't feel like the babies needed as much help.

130

Tiffany Field, a specialist in parent-child interaction, points out that parents become more active when children are designated as being *at nutritional risk*[8]. Undoubtedly, parents try to help out with feeding the fragile baby. Ironically, what helps most with feeding is patience and self restraint—your taking time to observe and try out options, follow your baby's lead, and be careful not to take charge or overwhelm her.

It may help you in figuring out your baby to have someone you trust sit down with you and help you understand what your baby is like and what works with her. It may help to use Dr. Price's approach, and video tape yourself and observe the tapes. Video tape long enough so you get over being self-conscious, and try to get tapes of both effective and ineffective feedings. You'll get clues both from when feeding is going well and when it is going poorly.

Work with your spouse in figuring out your baby. I have observed that fathers may, at times, find a way with babies and are more effective with them than mothers are. Often mothers feel offended and defensive about that. But rather than perceiving their greater success rate as a threat, why not take a close look at what they're doing and get some more information about what works and what doesn't with a baby?

It's always possible to change your behavior and learn a new way of operating. And, of course, the same advice holds true for fathers who want to learn from mothers to be more effective with their babies.

Get Professional Help

If you can't make any headway with correcting your feeding problems, get professional help. It can make an enormous difference to sit down with an accepting and supportive person who is trained to be a good observer, who can give you guidance in improving your relationship with your baby. Ask for help observing and interpreting your baby. Ask for feedback on what you are doing that is helpful—and what is not. And take advantage of the opportunity to talk about the feelings and attitudes that make you operate the way you do.

You may have pressures on you that make you insensitive to your baby. The first and most important consideration is the relationship with your spouse. Things have to be going well

131

between the two of you in order for things to go well with your baby. Family therapists often say that the child is the barometer of the relationship between the parents. This rather esoteric statement simply means that as parents fail to resolve the tensions that build up between them, the child will get upset and act out in some way.

Another family therapy axiom is that children serve their parents in whatever way they can. Children who show problem behaviors, like eating upsets, allow their parents to get their minds off the conflict with each other—and on to the child's problems.

Being stuck in the relationship with your spouse can keep you stuck with other things, as well. If you can't deal with a critical mother or mother-in-law, and you can't seem to get control of a schedule that is too busy, it might be because you're not getting any support or cooperation from your partner.

Allow me a final axiom from family therapists: Parents are the architects of the family. Your children can't function any better than you do. You can't do your best job of parenting if things are not good with your partner. First you must get your relationship in order, then you can improve your parenting.

Guidelines For Feeding

This section will give you more ideas about what to look for as you work on improving your feeding interactions. I will generalize, at first, and then I will put together a set of observations about feeding—illustrations of positive and not-so-positive feeding interactions.

If you want to be more systematic about your observations of feeding, take a look at Dr. Price's feeding scale, AMIS (Assessment of Mother-Infant Sensitivity)[9]. This usable and understandable scale describes in detail the way feeder and infant behave with each other.

General Observations

Observe how your baby reacts to the way you hold her and move her around. See what she does when you speak or remain quiet, or when you use one or the other tone of voice. Position yourselves so she can look into your eyes, and let her be the one to look and look away.

You will probably observe that your voice will calm and quiet your baby when she is agitated, or it may wake her up when she is dozing off. Pay attention to your manner of speaking—a friendly, animated tone of voice will probably bring out a different response than a quiet, soothing tone. Even if you are trying to keep her awake, don't use a sharp or loud or abrasive voice—just a regular voice will do it.

If you speak in an unpleasant tone of voice to get her attention or to wake her up to feed, she'll associate that with feeding and have some negative feelings when it is time to eat. That can confuse her feelings about eating. You want her to feel good and positive. The same advice holds true for tactics that people sometimes use for waking up sleepy babies so they can eat, like unwrapping them and flicking their feet or washing their face with cold water. You don't want your baby to have the feeling that something unpleasant is going to happen when you are around.

Observe how she reacts. What works with one baby won't work with another. What is over-stimulating to one baby will be under-stimulating to another. If babies are over-stimulated they can withdraw—they can become less sociable and maybe not eat as well as they should. If babies are under-stimulated, they can do the same thing. Do some observing to see what it takes to draw your baby out and let her play with you and enjoy talking and smiling and making faces with you without getting her so agitated she seems uncomfortable.

Hold her so she can look in your eyes, and observe how that helps her to stay involved with the feeding. If your baby won't look at you or respond to you or make eye contact, it is cause for concern. *Do* get professional help if your baby won't be drawn out. Connecting with you is a vitally important part of her emotional development.

Observations About Feeding

To help make this discussion about feeding more concrete, I have put together a set of observations of mothers and babies in the feeding situation. Again, I apologize for the fact that they are all *mothers*—they have been the ones who showed up for the

133

studies and the appointments. Always remember, however, that the father is VERY much a part of the picture, however invisible to the observers. When mother and baby are doing well with each other, in most cases there is a supportive father. Dr. Price asked her mothers, on a scale of one to ten, how supportive their husbands were. She found that when the husbands were more supportive, the mothers were able to be more sensitive with their babies.

At times that supportive person is an important someone other than the father. Mothers need to be getting their emotional needs met in order to have the energy to be caring with their babies. (But it's not a one-way street. Fathers need to be getting *their* emotional needs met, too, so they can be supportive and available to their families.)

The observations I will share with you (with the invisible-but-present-fathers) come from my own experience as a mother, neighbor and practitioner, some from the studies of Dr. Mary Ainsworth, a well-known child psychologist, some from Dr. Price's videotapes.

Some mothers were very sensitive to their babies' signals and skillful about their feeding. They didn't wait for their babies to cry before they picked them up, but picked them up when they started to squirm or snort or show by little signs that they wanted some attention. They presented the food so the baby could take it easily, and they and their babies enjoyed each other in the feeding situation.

They held their babies facing them, so the babies could look into their mothers' eyes. They nestled them firmly, close to their bodies, and at the same time, they gave them a little freedom to move around. The babies could wiggle and move their arms and legs without feeling frightened that they were going to fall. The mothers paid attention to the babies' positions so their necks were straight while they ate. The bottle feeders held the bottle up at an angle so the nipple was filled with formula all during the feeding.

These mothers didn't try to force the nipple in, but got their babies to seek the nipple by brushing their cheeks with it. They fed the baby when she seemed to be hungry, and if they staved off the feeding they did it only briefly and did not let their baby get so hungry she was frantic. Some said their babies were pretty regular in their feeding habits, others said they were unpredictable. But whatever schedule the baby wanted, they went along with it.

The good feeders finished feeding as they had initiated it. They let the babies call the tune. When their babies gave them the message that they were finished eating, they stopped trying to feed them. They took their word for it. Oh, sure, they offered the nipple again, but it was apparent they were only checking to make sure they really understood what their babies were trying to tell them. When the babies were full, they often just ignored the nipple.

What was remarkable about all the mothers was the way they hung in there until they got things worked out with their babies. And some of the babies were REAL hard to read and to please. One little girl was so excitable that her mother had to sit with her for a long time and talk with her in a very soothing way before she finally settled down enough to eat well. Another started to breast-feed, and came immediately off the breast, yelling. His mother judged that her milk was flowing too fast, hand expressed a little, and he settled down very well. She figured right.

There was a big variation in the way the babies let their mothers know they had had enough to eat. Some nursed steadily and suddenly stopped and wouldn't take another swallow. Some started and stopped, started and stopped, until, finally, they got to the point where they only took a couple of swallows before a stop and their mothers quit feeding. Some just kept plugging away, but slower and slower, until they seemingly couldn't eat another bite, and reluctantly stopped nursing. Sometimes they drifted off to sleep with the nipple still in their mouth, and the milk drooling out of the corner.

Some Situations Were Not So Positive

There were some feeding situations that were not so positive, where it seemed that mothers had made little effort to work it out with their babies. Mothers controlled the feeding, and imposed certain amounts or certain schedules on their babies. These mothers were quick to assume they knew what was happening when their babies behaved in a certain way, and they didn't use any trial and error to check whether their assumptions were correct. For instance, when her baby had trouble eating, one mother announced, "He doesn't like his bottle." In essence, she was saying she wasn't going to look for a solution to the difficulties.

Some mothers were eager to get their babies on a schedule. To achieve that, they ignored their hunger and staved them off so long that they became over-hungry and upset. As a consequence, the babies had a difficult time settling down to nursing steadily, and seemed like they never really relaxed throughout the feeding. The mothers were frustrated with their behavior, and said they didn't feel very successful with their babies.

Some were impatient. They said they were feeding on demand, but they seemed so eager to be finished caring for their babies that they put them down whenever they paused or smiled or fussed during the feeding. The nipple holes were too big (perhaps because the mothers wanted to get the feedings over in a hurry), so the babies choked and gagged and paused in the feeding. When they paused, the mothers assumed they were full and terminated the feedings.

One mother appeared almost too willing to spend time with her baby. She was bottle feeding her baby, but very intrusive about it. She stopped the feeding every few minutes and wiped the baby's chin and checked the milk level. She straightened his clothes, and burped him four or five times during the course of the feeding. The feeding took forever, and it seemed they never really got a rhythm going.

One group of mothers overfed their babies, some to give them pleasure, and some to fill them up so they would sleep a long time. When it was for pleasure, both mother and baby appeared to enjoy prolonging the feeding process. The babies ate happily for a long time, even though the energy and excitement had gone out of the feeding, and they were sucking slower and slower.

The feedings I will describe next were so distorted that they should have gotten professional intervention. Mothers were uninvolved and babies were distressed. Neither party in the interactions were getting their emotional needs satisfied.

Some mothers overfed for stretching out feeding intervals, the babies spat out the nipple, struggled and tried to avert their heads. But the mothers were determined to get the food in, and they did. When they finally submitted, some babies did so passively, while others expressed their upset through the rigidity in their whole bodies. It was hard to watch those feedings, because babies were so upset and mothers were frustrated and so determined that they didn't even seem to see their babies.

Some mothers seemed uninterested in feeding, or in their babies in general. They didn't pay much attention to their babies during the feeding, held the bottle wrong, and let them sprawl out on their laps rather than giving them much support. Babies seemed listless, as though their mothers didn't interest them much, either.

In five striking cases Mary Ainsworth reported, the feeding was absolutely arbitrary in timing, pacing or both. In each case, the mother was having personal problems, such as depression or anxiety that made her detached and insensitive to the baby's signals. These mothers put their babies away for long periods and either tuned out the crying or failed to perceive it as a sign of hunger.

Feeding times were erratic, as were feeding styles. Sometimes the mothers forced their babies to eat long past the point where they indicated they were full, and sometimes they interpreted any pause as satiety and stopped feeding. Feeding was at the mother's own whim, and showed little reflection of the baby's wishes. Ainsworth commented in one case that a mother's determined stuffing of her baby "had to be seen to be believed."

I have been puzzled in working with cases of failure to thrive, because mothers have, in a very sincere fashion, reported a seemingly adequate food intake. Reading these observations, I can understand how someone this self-absorbed could really *not know* how much a baby had eaten.

Feeding In Broader Perspective

You can use feeding to connect with your baby, and to allow yourself to feel successful with her. You can use feeding to draw out a less-sociable baby, to quiet an agitated one, and to give pleasure to one who is not easily pleased. In the process of figuring out feeding, you will find out what makes her unique as a person. Working out ways to satisfy her and keep her comfortable with feeding will reflect on your whole relationship with her.

You probably noticed that the parents we talked about were not only getting food into their babies, they were teaching attitudes. The babies whose mothers were sympathetic, supportive and kind about feeding learned that the world is a great place, where they are going to be treated with attention and respect. The mothers who were domineering or controlling taught their babies that they had to fight to get what they wanted, or that they might just as well give up and go along with what they were given, or that nobody really cared how they felt about it anyway.

Pretty heavy lessons for such little ones. But feeding teaches those lessons because parents and babies spend most of their time during those early months in the feeding situation. Parents' attitudes and feelings about themselves and their children are acted out in the feeding situation.

What About Spoiling?

Don't let anybody tell you that you are spoiling your baby by being so solicitous. You can't really spoil a child until she is well into her toddlerhood. Until then, babies' upsets reflects their discomfort. It has nothing to do with struggles with you.

Babies who are picked up when they cry actually cry less than babies who are allowed to fuss longer before their needs are met. Picking a baby up is the very best way to comfort her, and is actually successful about 80% of the time[10]. Babies who are ignored either become cross and irritable to try to get through to you, or they withdraw[11]—either way isn't good for them or good for you.

It is easier to identify what a baby wants if you respond to her cry right away. That's when the cry has a different sound that gives you a clue to what the baby wants. After they fuss a while, all the cries start to sound like general misery[11].

Feeding And Growth

Working out a positive feeding relationship with your baby can make all the difference between whether your baby grows well or poorly. Children eat best when parents recognize and respond appropriately to their needs. When parents are either overactive or inattentive, babies eat poorly and they don't grow well[12].

Obesity

There is a chapter in this book about obesity, Helping All You Can to Keep Your Child From Being Fat (Chapter 14), and if you are concerned that your baby will grow up to be too fat, please read it now. There is no real reason to be concerned at this early age, but once you or your advisors start to worry that your baby will get too fat, it is an issue to be dealt with.

Let me tell you a fact, substantiated by considerable research, that is so hard to believe and so far removed from the usual perception that most people simply ignore it. There is no evidence that the fat baby will be the fat adult. Fat babies have no greater risk of growing up fat than thin babies[13].

Despite the fact that this has been common knowledge for years, many professionals and parents still withhold food from young, fat children. Nothing could be more destructive. It is THE most basic human need to get enough to eat. Starving a child to keep her slim is not only unnecessary and unproductive, it is brutal.

The best and potentially most successful way you can prevent your child from being obese is to cultivate a positive feeding relationship. When you let your baby be in control of the feeding and are sensitive and responsive to her cues, she will eat the amount she needs to grow properly. Because you are being supportive and not intrusive on her food regulation, she will grow up remembering how to eat according to her hunger, appetite and satiety. Then whatever body she turns out to have will be the body that is right for *her*. She might not be thin, but you will have helped her all you can.

Poor Growth

For a more complete treatment of the topic of poor growth, check The Child Who Grows Poorly (Chapter 13). I will simply summarize here.

Some babies are naturally slow about growing. They perk along, at or below the fifth percentile, giving everyone enormous concern. But they do all right, and eventually they grow up.

139

They cause so much concern because they look so much like other babies who *are* eating poorly and growing poorly, sometimes because they are sick.

About all you can do with these marginal eaters and growers is to work with the feeding relationship and try to make it as smooth and positive and infant-controlled as possible. If you try to force more food than your baby really wants to take, she may come to hate feeding and fight you rather than eating willingly. It can spoil your relationship with one another, because you'll be struggling over feeding so much.

Sometimes children are sick, and they have enormous problems taking in enough food to keep them going. Babies with heart defects, for instance, have to eat enough and grow enough to be ready for surgery. In some cases, these babies are fed by tube, even through tubes that are surgically implanted through the abdominal wall into the stomach. (These are called gastrostomy tubes.) They take whatever they can by mouth (and it is important for the normal development of feeding that they continue to do that), and get the rest of their meal through the tube. I have not worked with people who have had this experience, only talked with them, but it seems to me that it's better to go this route than to have struggles over feeding and spoil the feeding relationship.

Sometimes feeding goes so poorly and growth falls off so severely that babies are described as "failure to thrive." Studies of the feeding relationships in these cases show mothers who at times are overactive, jiggling the nipple, arranging the blankets, checking the formula level in the bottle. Other failure to thrive studies describe mothers who stop feeding at the first pause in feeding, when a baby coughs or rests or smiles. They see the pause as meaning their baby has had enough to eat, and rather than checking it out by again offering food, they simply quit feeding at that point[7].

You may have heard of those old orphanage studies where so many of the babies died, presumably from lack of love. Closer examination demonstrated that, while indeed they may not have gotten enough love, it took the form of feeders who had too much to do and were in such a hurry that they simply stopped the feeding and put the babies down when they first paused in feeding.

140

We've covered a great deal of information in this chapter. It may help you to sum up in a few lines—

• Keep your baby in control of the feeding.

• Try things out, see how they work, and if they don't work, try something else.

• Get some help figuring out your baby from someone you trust.

• If you've tried everything you both can think of, get professional help. It's that important.

References

1. Roger, R.P. and Smith, A.B.: Developing parental skills: An holistic, longitudinal process. Infant Mental Health Journal 7:103-111, 1986.

2. Greenberg, M. and Morris, N.: Engrossment: The newborn's impact upon the father. American Journal of Orthopsychiatry 44:520-531, 1974.

3. Macfarlane, A.: The Psychology of Childbirth. Cambridge, MA: Harvard University Press, 1977.

4. Kennel, J.H., et.al.: Maternal behavior one year after early and extended post-partum contact. Developmental Medicine and Child Neurology, 16:172-179, 1974.

5. Price, G.M.: Influencing maternal care through discussion of videotapes of maternal-infant feeding interaction. Unpublished dissertation, Boston University Graduate School, 1975.

6. Pollitt, E. and Wirtz, S.: Mother-infant feeding interaction and weight gain in the first month of life. Journal of the American Dietetic Association 78:596-601, 1981.

7. Wright, P., Fawcett, J., and Crow, R.: The development of differences in the feeding behavior of bottle and breast fed human infants from birth to two months. Behavioural Processes 5:1-20, l980.

8. Field, T.: Maternal stimulation during infant feeding. Developmental Psychology 13:539-540, l977.

9.   Price, G.M.: Sensitivity in mother-infant interactions: The AMIS scale. Infant Behavior and Development 6:353-360, 1983.

10.   Bell, S.M. and Ainsworth, M.D.S.: Infant crying and maternal responsiveness. Child Development 43:1171-1190, 1972.

11.   Ainsworth, M.D.S. and Bell, S.M.: Some contemporary patterns of mother-infant interaction in the feeding situation. IN Ambrose, Anthony: Stimulation in Early Infancy. New York: Academic Press, l969.

12.   Satter, E.M.: The feeding relationship. Journal of the American Dietetic Association 86:352-356, 1986.

13.   Shapiro, L.R., Crawford, P.B., Clark, M.J., Pearson, D.J., Raj, J. and Huenemann, R.L.: Obesity prognosis: a longitudinal study of children from the age of 6 months to 9 years. American Journal of Public Health 74:968-972, 1984.

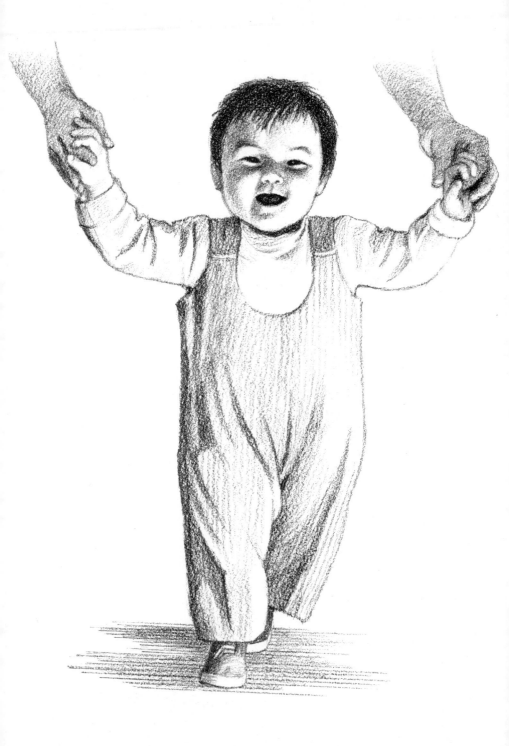

8

The Older Baby

During the second half of his first year, your baby will go through a transition in feeding: from all breast or bottle; to learning to eat semi-solids from a spoon; to feeding himself soft table food.

Once again, managing feeding during this time depends on a division of responsibility: You are responsible for what your child is offered to eat and the manner in which it is offered, and he is responsible for eating.

In this chapter, we will talk some about the food selection that goes into getting your baby started on solid foods and making the transition to table food. We'll talk more, however, about parenting your child through feeding: Feeding in an emotionally healthy way.

With feeding, and parenting, the developing child requires both patience and restraint. Being the bigger, stronger and more resourceful, you can take over and snatch the prerogative from your child at any moment. It may, in fact, seem like kindness itself for you to take the initiative and *do* things for your child. But children, even babies, don't want their parents to simply smooth the way and accomplish their tasks for them. They want

145

to do it *themselves*, whenever they can, because that's the way they grow and develop good feelings about themselves. On the other hand, they need your help.

If you and your baby are to be successful with feeding, you must be sensitive to him and let him take the lead. You have to pay attention to him, figure out what he can do and what works with him, and do it. You have to trust his reactions about what he wants and how he feels about food. In What is Normal Eating? (Chapter 5) I make the point that people feel about eating and react to eating in many different ways that are all normal and acceptable and functional. You will be safe going along with your child's eating behaviors, however odd.

The Six- To Twelve-Month-Old

Throughout the first year, your child is still an infant. He becomes more independent, in that he can sit up and crawl and maybe even walk. But he is still very much attached to you. He will cry like he did when he was smaller, but for not as long, and he will still benefit from your prompt attention[1]. He will play on the floor, but he will do it mostly at your feet. When he moves around the room, he will want to know where you are. At first he will keep an eye on you most of the time. Later on, he will wander out of sight, but will check back periodically to make sure you are still there—and interested.

To help your baby learn, you need to be available, patient and reassuring. You need to be interested in what he is doing, and supportive of it. You need to allow him the feeling that he is in control, that you are not simply going to impose something on him without his having any say in the matter.

The six- to twelve-month-old will show more initiative than before. He will want to go ahead on his own with things, like eating and playing and socializing. If you have been sensitive in responding to his crying when he was little, he will have learned a repertoire of ways to attract you to him[1]. He will talk, smile or gesture to capture your attention and will try new behaviors and watch you to see if you support him or not. You will make him feel good about himself and encourage his growth if you support his initiative, give him your attention, and at the same time hold back so he can demonstrate his abilities to you.

146

The way you respond to his initiatives is vitally important, because if he is to grow up feeling good about himself, he has to be successful in engaging other people and in keeping them involved with him. And you, his parents, are the most important people of all.

Parenting

If you handle feeding sensitively, you are helping your child to grow up to be a happy and healthy *person*. Much of the undivided attention you give your child is still going to be during feeding time, and the way you treat him then will have a big impact on him. The way you learn to treat him in feeding is also likely to rub off on the way you treat him in other areas, for example, introducing him to social situations and doing toilet training.

To get some clues about establishing positive feeding behaviors, let's look at tactics child psychologists use for improving parenting behaviors in general. Psychologists help parents to be sensitive and able to pick up on the baby's cues and signals and respond to them in a way that the baby finds satisfying. And the baby lets the parent know he takes pleasure in what the parent has done. They are in synchrony—they are getting along.

For instance, a parent and baby are in synchrony when a baby looks at the parent and makes a noise and perhaps even touches the parent's face or hand. The parent looks in the baby's eyes, and makes a similar noise. The baby smiles, and the parent smiles. They have connected with each other, and they both very obviously take pleasure in the connection.

But the parent and the baby are in *dys*synchrony when the baby tries to capture the parent's attention in much the same way and the parent doesn't respond. She might not look, or perhaps looks only at the baby's hand, and may even brush it away. The parent doesn't say anything in response to the baby's sound, or she might overwhelm the baby with a long string of words, or take over and impose lots of activity. If this happens often enough, the baby will show distress or even get depressed or get overactive, and the parent will feel frustrated and unsuccessful.

When a relationship isn't working, it often takes an outside observer to offer the parent suggestions about ways to operate so

147

the baby will respond better. T. Berry Brazelton demonstrated this kind of helping in his television program, "What Every Baby Knows." Adoptive parents of a Korean baby sought his help establishing synchrony with their child. "She doesn't like us," they worried, "she won't even look at us." Brazelton observed a bit, then told them that they were trying too hard to engage the little girl—being too talkative and too playful. Their daughter was feeling overwhelmed and withdrawing. When they settled back a bit and lowered their level of activity, she was able to approach and engage them, and things went better.

Karen Ostrov, a clinical psychologist, set out to do in a systematic fashion what Brazelton did with that family[2]. She did it on a broader scale in an early childhood intervention project, and she called it infant *psychotherapy*. Actually, she was doing *parent-child* psychotherapy, because what she was doing had an impact on the emotional health of both parent and baby.

Her technique of infant psychotherapy was simple. In a quiet and safe room, parents were instructed to get down on the floor with their baby and follow his activities without initiating or directing. They were not to start things or contribute ideas: Just watch, respond when approached, and show an interest. They were to stay within 12 to 18 inches of their baby, and make sure that both they and toys were available to him. Both parent and child were to be reasonably rested and alert and have the time free to devote to sharing time with each other.

The important idea was to let babies take the lead. Parents were to let babies initiate the activity, and were to respond in a restrained fashion, "with slightly less energy than the baby uses," so they didn't overwhelm them.

Babies, and relationships, blossomed when babies were allowed to take the lead. The technique of infant psychotherapy helped babies in at least four ways:

1. They got more of a feeling for themselves as individuals who were important to others;

2. They improved their ability to control their own behavior;

3. They were stimulated to explore even more; and

4. They got more of a feeling of competence.

148

The technique helped parents to know their babies better, to feel more relaxed and comfortable with them, and to enjoy them more.

Not all parents were able to operate in this supportive and engaged fashion. Some took over the activity, some remained unengaged with their babies, some competed rather than supported and some were overly protective of the baby or the setting[3].

Dr. Ostrov has two small children herself, now, and has some suggestions about how other parents can apply her infant psychotherapy work on a day-to-day basis. She suggests you take time to get down on the floor with your child, relax, and take an interest in what he does. You can use this method especially to reconnect with him after a time away.

And she says something else which is music to my ears. "The feeding relationship is a natural context for incorporating infant psychotherapy techniques. Parents can learn to do feeding in a way that is respectful of information coming from their child and follows his lead."

I couldn't have asked for a better opener for my section on feeding.

The Feeding Relationship

Remember the division of responsibility in feeding. You are responsible for what your child is offered to eat, but he is responsible for how much of it he eats, and even whether he eats. You are responsible for getting the food *there*. He is responsible for getting it *in*. Figure 8-1, "Division of Responsibility in Early Spoon Feeding," elaborates.

You can encourage your child's initiative and explorations in feeding by playing a supportive role. The infant needs your reassuring presence in order to feel free to explore with feeding.

If you hold him on your lap when you first introduce solids, he'll be braver. (Be sure to hold him up so his neck is straight and he is facing forward so he can swallow better.) Engage his participation by holding the spoon in front of him and waiting for him to open up before you try to feed it to him. Be ready to look into his eyes during the feeding process so you can share it with him.

149

Parents are responsible for what is presented to eat and the manner in which it is presented

• Choose food that is developmentally appropriate so he can control it in his mouth and swallow it as well as possible.

• Hold your baby on your lap to introduce solids. He'll be braver.

• Support him well in an upright position so he can explore his food.

• Have him sit up straight and face forward. He'll be able to swallow better and be less likely to choke.

• Talk to him in a quiet and encouraging manner while he eats. Don't entertain him or overwhelm him with attention, but do keep him company.

Children are responsible for how much and whether they eat

• Wait for him to pay attention to each spoonful before you try to feed it to him.

• Let him touch his food—in the dish, on the spoon. You wouldn't eat something if you didn't know anything about it, would you?

• Feed at his tempo. Don't try to get him to go faster or slower than he wants to.

• Allow him to feed himself with his fingers as soon as he shows an interest.

• Stop feeding when he indicates he has had enough.

Figure 8-1   Division of Responsibility in Early Spoon Feeding

Pay attention to him and respond to what he is doing, and let his actions determine what you will do next. You do that in a very concrete way by waiting to start solid foods until he is ready. He should be sitting up, able to open his mouth when he sees something coming, and able to move semi-solid food from the front of his tongue to the back. If you wait until he can do these things, he'll be more in charge of the process and more clear in giving you signals about what he wants to do.

You mustn't force in any way. That is taking over and running things to suit you. If you do that, he will likely just get quiet and stop letting you know what he wants.

You can gently support his efforts to use the spoon himself or to finger feed himself. If you do it for him because you can do it so much better and so much faster (and so much cleaner), you will take away his initiative and his opportunity to find out that he can get things to happen and that other people will support him when he does things his way.

Because your baby wants to do things for himself, it doesn't mean that he doesn't need you any more. The supportive role you play will help him to challenge himself and to stimulate his learning. Babies are more likely to go ahead on their own and do more, dare more and show new behaviors when they are lucky enough to have a supportive adult who is willing to follow and observe them, rather than trying to control them[4].

Good feeding is a sort of non-verbal, nicely flowing conversation. If you're talking with someone and they let you know they take an interest in what you say, that can make you feel real good. They can amplify what you were talking about and it is still fine. They can even introduce a new topic of conversation, and if it has something to do with the previous topic or if they've picked out something they think you'll be interested in, it is still OK.

But if during the course of the conversation, the other person abruptly changes the subject, that can take your breath away and usually brings the conversation to a screeching halt. Similarly, if you're talking with someone and, time after time, that person fails to acknowledge what you say or respond to it, or even worse, does the opposite of what you ask for, that can make you totally mad or totally discouraged. After awhile, you stop seeking out people like that.

The same thing happens in a non-verbal way in the feeding interaction. If you are feeding a baby and he is excited and wants to eat fast, you feed him fast, and probably even express back to him some of his pleasure and excitement in eating. You will be in synchrony. But if you hold back on the tempo and act displeased or upset at his excitement, you are not holding up

151

your end of the conversation, and both of you are going to feel disappointed and frustrated.

If he is hungry and you feed him until he gets full and then you take his word for it when he says he has had enough, you have had a positive interchange. But if he is eating along great guns and you suddenly stop for no apparent reason, you have broken a very basic rule of conversation. Your baby will feel upset by that, and if it happens too often, you are not going to be a very favorite conversation partner, and eating is not going to be a very favorite thing for you to do together.

The same thing happens if you ignore his signals that let you know he has had enough to eat. If you try to get him to eat more than he really wants, you are essentially ignoring everything he says and you will be shouting him down.

DO work on having nice feeding conversations with your baby. It is very important to your baby's emotional development, to your relationship, and to the way you feel about yourself as a parent. If you can develop a synchronous relationship, you will know your baby better and will feel more relaxed and comfortable. It is a basic human need to be effective with other people, particularly when that other person is your child.

If you are shy about getting to know your baby or fastidious about letting him take the lead (and make a mess) with feeding, you can get over it. If you have a hard time figuring out how your baby communicates, or if you have difficulty letting go of control and letting your baby take the lead, you can get help with it.

The Mechanics Of Feeding

The baby will move on to more sophisticated eating when he is ready. We're talking, of course, about eating from a spoon. Figure 8-2, "Introducing Solid Foods," summarizes when to add solid foods and why. The "why" includes the nutritional and developmental reasons why you add what you add, and when you add it[5].

You will know your baby is ready to start solid foods when he is able to sit up, open his mouth (or close it) when he sees something coming, and direct his hands where he wants them to go. Sitting puts him in position to look at the food and reach

152

Age	Feeding capability	Additional nutrient need	Food added
Birth-6 mo.	Roots for nipple Suckles	None beyond milk feeding and supplements	None
5-7 mo.	Begins sitting Follows food with eyes Opens up for spoon Lips close over spoon Begins to swallow	Iron	Iron fortified rice baby cereal
6-8 mo.	Tongue moves to side Controls position of food in mouth Controls swallow Munches: Up-and-down chew Hand-mouth pattern	Vitamins A & C Variety in diet	Vegetables and fruits: pureed or mashed
7-10 mo.	Bite matures Chews in rotary pattern Moves food from side to side in mouth Curves lips around cup Palmar grasp develops (Folds fingers over palm)	B Vitamins	Finger breads and cereals Lumpy fruits and vegetables Fruit juice from cup Milk from cup
8-12 mo.	Sociability increases Interest in solids increases Cup drinking improves Pincer grasp develops (Thumb and fingers work together)	Protein Trace elements	Soft and cooked table foods Ground or finely diced meats

Figure 8-2   Introducing Solid Foods

153

out and touch it. He will be able to turn his head toward and away from the spoon, to participate in the feeding and to let you know what he wants.

It is important not to rush the introduction of solid foods. Children don't need them until they become capable of eating them. You can't rush their capability by starting solids early. Studies have shown that parents and babies get into struggles over feeding when parents try to introduce solids too early[6].

The time from when you start solid foods until your child is eating from the table is called the *transition period*. During that brief time, your child learns to eat, starting with semi-solids that you feed from a spoon, and progressing to pieces of soft food that he picks up and gums. During that time, you help the learning process by picking out food that he can eat, but also food that challenges him to develop new eating skills.

Starting Solids

It is important to wait to start solids until your baby is ready. Children do better with feeding if they have some control over the process. The semi-reclining baby will have very little control over the spoon feeding process. The sitting baby can look at the spoon, feel the food with his fingers, get his fingers to his mouth and find out, "Hey, this is not a block! This stuff is good!" He can open his mouth and lean forward if he wants to eat; he can close his mouth and turn his head away if he is not interested. It is easy for a parent to pick up and understand feeding cues from a sitting-up baby who is eating solid food. It is much harder if you are starting out with one who is really too little, who is still lying back in his infant seat.

For your baby, learning to eat from a spoon is a pretty complicated business. First, when you are hungry and want nothing more than your nice, soft nipple, you have to learn to tolerate the spoon—that hard, cold, thing with the sharp edges. Then you have to figure out that that stuff in that strange object is for EATING. Very puzzling. Then you have to be willing to take a chance on it. After which you have to figure out how to get the stuff into your mouth. And down your throat. Without gagging.

The whole process is littered with pitfalls, especially if you have a parent who doesn't know what she is doing and is corre-

154

spondingly anxious and a little pushy, and who, every time you hesitate, thinks you are resisting and increases the pressure.

Keep in mind: Children want to grow up. They have built within them the nagging need to get better at everything they do. Eating is no exception. They have enough pressure within themselves to move things along; they don't need any more from us. What they need from us is support and encouragement and safety as they venture out into these strange unknowns.

To swallow effectively, a child has to gather the food together and propel it down his throat, past the opening to the wind pipe. If he doesn't swallow strongly enough, food will remain near the back of his tongue and make him gag, which pushes the food forward on the tongue. This gagging is a normal part of learning to eat, and won't frighten the child unless it frightens you or unless you get pushy and try to get him to be braver with eating than he really feels like being at the moment.

Up until about age four months, the gag reflex is very strong. After that time, it begins to get toned down by the mouthing of other things, like toys and fingers. That mouthing may be accompanied by a lot of gagging. I know a little girl who caused her parents great concern because she gagged herself with her fingers and even threw up a little. After a while that went away, as she became more able to judge how far to put her fingers into her mouth and as her gag reflex became less pronounced.

Before we go any farther with introducing solid foods, I want you to do a little experiment with your own eating. Get a cracker or a piece of apple or something that requires chewing. Now chew it, and notice what your bite and chew are like. What do your tongue and teeth do? How do you swallow?

Biting, chewing and swallowing are extraordinarily complex processes. First, you have to bite off the right amount. If you bite off too much you will have trouble handling it in your mouth and you might gag or choke. Then, you have to be able to retain the food in your mouth so you can chew it up before you swallow. (The young infant starting on solid foods does not retain food in his mouth; he just sends it right down.) Then, you have to control the position of food in your mouth with your tongue.

After you bit off the cracker, you probably used your tongue to move it from center front to between your teeth. And you further used your tongue to keep it between your teeth (likely moving it from side to side in your mouth) as you chewed it. Finally, the food was moved to the back of your tongue where you gathered it into a mass to be swallowed. (For later reference, also try chewing and swallowing when you are facing straight forward and holding your head up straight. Now try it with your head turned to the side—bent over forward—bent back.)

Whew! Do you see what I mean when I say there is a lot to be learned? You teach your child to swallow, chew and bite by gradually introducing him to a variety of foods. Lumpy solids follow smooth pureed solids—to get him to start to chew. If he has lumps in his mouth, he will be likely to use his tongue to move the lumps between his jaws rather than just sending them straight down.

If he doesn't move the lumps by himself, you get that chewing and tongue motion going by putting the lumpy food between his jaws. At first he'll mash the food between his jaws in an up and down motion, and later he'll learn to chew in a more grinding, rotary motion. This stage is really cute, because they work so hard at it. Often the baby's whole face gets into the act as he closes one eye and scowls, focusing his face toward the action.

About this time, you can start introducing juice from a cup. You can give a little formula or milk from the cup, too. Your child won't be very good at it at first, because he can't curve his lips around and make a seal on the rim. But as he gets older, he'll get better.

Engage your child's participation in the feeding process by offering him the lead whenever you can. Let your child go ahead with self feeding as soon as he shows the inclination and the ability—they may not appear at the same time. Some children finger feed before they chew, and vice versa. Let him finger feed himself pasty stuff, like mashed potatoes mixed with meat and vegetables, or hold his spoon hand to help him "do it himself." It's a time consuming and laborious process, but then, isn't everything at that age?

As your child's grasp develops, he will practice: picking up pieces of food and putting them in his mouth for himself; picking up a handful of mashed potatoes and putting it in his mouth; holding a cracker or piece of bread and biting off pieces.

156

That's just great. If he finger feeds himself (and you stay interested), he will feel in control and will be more confident about trying new things. Keep on being supportive even after you get all the way through the spoon-feeding phase and into the self feeding phase. When he starts eating from the table you will naturally occupy yourself by eating your own food. But you still help him to experiment by staying available and companionable.

He'll probably fill his mouth too full and gag some at this stage, because he has to develop judgment about how big a piece to bite off and how full to fill his mouth before he gets in trouble.

Gagging is very alarming for parents, but really just part of the process. Do stay available, but don't scream and snatch your child out of the high chair when he gags. Either he will be put off on learning to eat, or he will learn to gag or even throw up, just to give you an opportunity to go through your act.

Children are not diabolical, but they do learn to produce behaviors when their parents react or pay a lot of attention to them, even when it is negative attention. Actually, they are more likely to learn to work for *negative* attention when it is the only attention they get.

Table Food

The next stage is table food. Since the child has already been experimenting with finger foods and self feeding, the transition to table food is more of a social event than any change in type or preparation of food. He'll let you know he's ready for table food when he sees other family members eating and demands to join in. Be prepared for some fun and a mess, cover the floor with some plastic, cut, grind or mash up whatever you are having for dinner, and let him go at it with his fingers. A finger food is anything that hangs together long enough to get from the high chair tray to the mouth. Mashed potatoes are a finger food. A cut-up casserole is a finger food. Cooked carrots are certainly a finger food.

Weaning can be finished off at this time. It has really started when your child started on table food, or even earlier, when he started learning to drink from a cup. Nursing has been important to him, so it is important that you not wean too

157

abruptly. With the transition to table food, breast or bottle feedings can be dropped one by one after meals. If you don't say anything about it, your child likely won't miss it, because he'll be filled up on solid foods and drinking from a cup. Don't be worried about the fall-off in milk consumption at this stage. He'll start to drink more when he gets better at drinking from a cup.

Your child might eat a little or eat a lot. You can rely on him to regulate the amounts he eats. He might be consistent at accepting a variety of food, or go on food jags where he prefers first one thing and then another. As long as he is presented with appropriate and nutritious food, he will for the most part eat the types of food he needs.

He may feel passionately interested in food or only tolerant about eating. He can be curious and willing to experiment or act betrayed every time you introduce him to something new. He may have a powerful hunger drive, or react only mildly when he gets hungry. All these are normal reactions to eating, and your job as parent is not to change those reactions, but to go along with them and be supportive of your child's style in reacting to food.

Stop feeding when your child indicates he has had enough. If you try to force beyond that point you probably won't get anywhere, and you may turn him off on eating. He'll show you he is full by turning his head away from the spoon, by refusing to open up for it or by spitting the food back out again or pushing the dish away. Show him you trust him by stopping feeding at that point.

Observing Some Feedings

Now for the fun part. Let's take a look at some feeding interactions. Dr. Marguerite Stevenson, a professor in child development, did a series of videotapes with mothers feeding babies about eight months old. The goal of her study was to observe verbal communication between the mother and child, and she figured feeding was a pretty typical interaction to catch them in. I felt like she had done the tapes all for *me*. They were exactly what I wanted to see.

Feeding Going Well

When feeding was going well, both mothers and babies seemed to enjoy what they were doing. The effective mothers engaged their babies and showed both restraint and patience. Mothers sat their babies up straight in the high chairs and sat directly in front of them. They engaged their babies in the feeding process and let them take their time getting ready to eat.

There were some remarkable problem solvers. One little boy cried after every bite. He did not look angry or in pain or eager or anything else, but he did cry. His mother seemed not to think much about it, but just kept on feeding him. That seemed fine with him—he took it very readily. I wondered if his crying didn't come from his excitement about eating.

One little girl was absolutely independent and wanted nothing to do with her mother's feeding her. She grabbed the spoon out of her mother's hand and made it clear she intended to do it herself. And her mother let her. This eight-month-old also went at it with her hands, scooping up her food, which her mother had prepared to the thickness of mashed potatoes.

She ate with great gusto, making appreciative noises all the while. Her mother kept her company, talked with her a little, commented on the food, but didn't get over involved in the process. Her daughter let her know when she had had enough by picking up the dish and preparing to drop it on the floor. At that point the mother got involved—she caught it. The mother seemed amused by that: It was apparent she took pleasure in her daughter's independence and ability.

One baby sat in his high chair with some thick, lumpy stuff, feeding himself with both hands. He ate with great concentration and enjoyment, grunting occasionally at his mother. He had food from ear to ear, but was still getting quite a lot of it in.

It was apparent his mother was enjoying his pleasure in eating. She sat quietly and watched him and spoke to him softly from time to time about how good it was and how much he was enjoying it. If she had been at home, I think she would have been eating her own meal and keeping him company in much the same way.

Even though he enjoyed the food a lot, at a certain point he suddenly gave his dish a swipe and knocked it on the floor. It was no accident—every gesture he had made up to that point

159

was very dedicated to eating. It was a signal he'd had enough to eat. His mother laughed and picked it up and told him that next time they'd skip the dish like they do at home.

One mother was doling out the meal, a few pieces at a time. It seemed very positive, and like she wasn't being over-controlling. I speculated that she had found, as had one of my friends, that her child did better with feeding when she did it that way. When he had too much food in front of him, he just played with it.

One little girl was feeding herself wheat thins. She could bite off the right-sized piece, but she couldn't chew it and swallow it. It seemed they were just too hard to mush up in her mouth. She kept biting off little pieces, gumming them a while, and losing them on her chin. Periodically, she gagged and a piece flew out of her mouth. Her mother didn't get too excited about it. Then they tried some soft graham crackers, and she was able to munch those up with her jaws and swallow them.

Feeding Going Poorly

When feeding was going poorly, mothers were over managing and inattentive. They ignored or overwhelmed their babies' signals. They didn't engage with their babies or have any sort of give-and-take with them during the feeding process. And the babies showed the effects of that.

One mother was very charming, but she was entirely too overwhelming and distracting. She laughed and talked and clapped and sang, "I've been working on the railroad." Her baby was transfixed, but didn't have too much to offer for himself. He also didn't eat. His food wasn't very appropriate for a young baby. It was a cheese sandwich with whole wheat bread that looked pretty dry and crumbly. And that's just what he did: crumbled it.

One mother made it clear to her baby she was not going to let her feed herself. The little girl grabbed the spoon and put her fingers into the food, but the mother snatched the spoon back and restrained her daughter's hands so she couldn't touch the dish. Later in the feeding the mother put the bowl in her lap and restrained the little girl's hands with one hand while she fed with the other. The little girl got fed, but she didn't get to gain any pleasure in her own initiative and accomplishment.

160

One pair was feeding along very nicely when the mother stopped feeding for no apparent reason. Her baby was still eating with apparent eagerness and interest. But the mother just stopped. He looked a little stricken, but didn't put up much of a fuss. It made me wonder, so I reeled the tape back and looked at it again. This time through, what I had first thought was the baby's eagerness and interest looked more like haste and anxiety.

One mother did very well with the feeding—at first. She held the spoon out and waited for the baby to open her mouth before she gave it to her. The baby ate very happily, and showed a lot of interest in eating. They talked together, and seemed very companionable. But as they got near the end of the feeding, things started to disintegrate. There was a little food left in the jar and the mother seemed determined to get her daughter to finish it off. The little girl stopped opening her mouth and started to look around. The mother told her to "come on, eat this," and held it up to her.

At first the little girl reluctantly opened her mouth and showed by the expression on her face she didn't much care for it. The mother persisted, and eventually the little girl stopped even opening her mouth. Whereupon the mother started to force the spoon between her lips. The little girl objected. She shook her head from side to side, cried, and spit it back out again. The message could hardly have been more clear. But the mother persisted until the food was gone. I suspected that in this case the forcing was for the benefit of the camera. If the mother had been that domineering about feeding all the time, I don't think the little girl would have been as cooperative and comfortable as she was earlier in the feeding.

Another mother was offering smorgasbord. She had several different kinds of food that she offered to her baby. She held a spoonful out to him, and he clamped his lips shut and turned away. Then she tried another food—and another—with the same results. It seemed she was getting quite desperate as she went from one to the other. And he was getting a wicked little gleam in his eye as he exerted his control over the situation.

One young mother of an eight-month-old looked depressed. She sat slumped in her chair, and regarded her baby dully. He didn't even look at her, but sat with his arm hanging down on the side of the high chair, looking at the floor. She seemed to

161

regard the feeding as a difficult chore, and reached down and under him to force food into his mouth. From time to time he shook his head to refuse the food, and she said, disgustedly, "All right, then you're going to have some of this," straightened him in his high chair, and forced the bottle into his mouth. He shook his head and yelled, but she persisted, and finally he took a few swallows.

I could tell just by the way I *felt* when I watched those tapes that some of those relationships were working and some were not. In some cases it appeared to be a problem of technique and feeding expectations. In other cases the problems went deeper: the mothers seemed like they were having difficulties with both themselves and their babies. Some of those cases could have used some outside help.

All these parents were not just getting food into their children, they were teaching *attitudes*, and embedding patterns of emotional responses in them. Parents who were accepting and supportive of their children's initiatives were helping them to be open and expressive and trusting that they would be liked and treated well by other people. Parents who were insensitive to their children, and expressed it by being peremptory or unengaged, were teaching their children to be guarded and suspicious in their interactions with others.

The Rewards Of Good Feeding

As I pointed out at the beginning, this chapter has been about emotionally healthy parenting with food. The importance of giving your child a good emotional grounding cannot be overemphasized. It simply has everything to do with setting your child up to approach the world in a positive and confident way, establish relationships with others, and feel good about himself and other people.

A child who is secure in the knowledge that he can gain his parents' attention is in a good position to move out to explore and master his small world with the seeking-returning behavior of the toddler. Infants whose mothers treat them positively, as described in this chapter, end up more sociable and independent than babies whose mothers have been less sensitive and responsive to their needs. They are happy to be held, and equally happy to move off into independent exploration. Babies who are not given this positive attention tend to be ambivalent about contact by the end of the first year. They do not respond positively when held, but still protest when put down and do not turn readily to independent activity[1].

The infant during the second six months is mobile, but tends to stay near his parents. The toddler wanders farther afield, but has to go back to his parents from time to time to get some of the same reassurance and support he needed as a younger child.

In a pragmatic way, being sensitive and responsive to your baby's desires will pay off in the toddler period. As they approach a year of age, babies begin to be able to understand and obey simple commands—like No! and Come here! Babies whose mothers had been sensitive and responsive during the early months tended to comply with their mother's commands. Babies who had gotten rejection, intrusion and insensitivity from their mothers were less likely to do what their mothers asked them to. Babies learn to give back what they get. A mother who complies with her tiny infant's "requests" and "commands" will in turn find that her toddler will comply with hers[7].

References

1.   Bell, S.M. and Ainsworth, M.D.S.: Infant crying and maternal responsiveness. Child Development 43:1171-1190, 1972.

2.   Ostrov, K.: An approach to the study of infant-caregiver communication during infant-initiated activity sessions. Unpublished dissertation, Department of Education, Marquette University, Milwaukee, WI. 1980.

3.   Ostrov, K., Dowling, J., Wesner, D.O., Johnson, F.K.: Maternal styles in infant psychotherapy: Treatment and research implications. Infant Mental Health Journal 3:162-173, 1982

4.   Ainsworth, M.D.S. and Bell, S.M.: Some contemporary patterns of mother-infant interaction in the feeding situation. IN Ambrose, Anthony: Stimulation in Early Infancy. New York: Academic Press, 1969.

5.   Satter, E.M.: Introduction of solid foods to the infant diet. IN Child of Mine—Feeding with Love and Good Sense, pp 221-267. Bull Publishing, Palo Alto, CA. 1983/86.

6.   Beal, V.A.: On the acceptance of solid foods and other food patterns of infants and children. Pediatrics 28:448-456. 1957.

7.   Stayton, D.J., Hogan, R. and Ainsworth, M.D.S.: Infant obedience and maternal behavior: The origins of socialization reconsidered. Child Development 42:1057-1069, 1971.

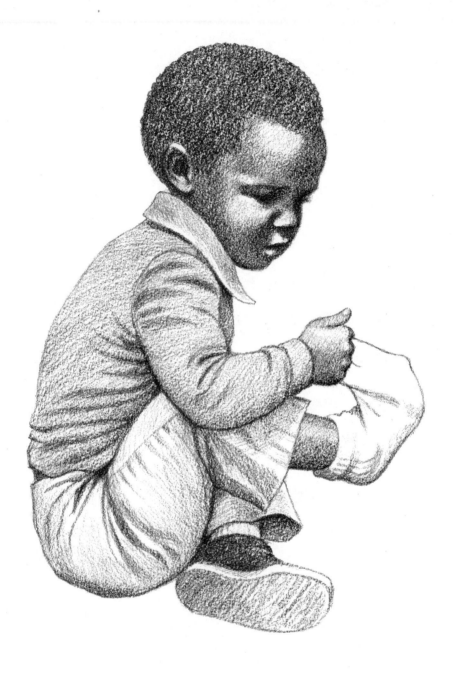

9

Is Your Toddler Jerking You Around At The Table?

Linda was still laughing when she arrived for breakfast. The night before, she had called her friend, Ellen. Ellen's husband answered. "She can't come to the phone right now. She and Michael (aged two) are having a fight."

Two hours later, Ellen called. "We were fighting about his dinner," she explained. "He has gotten so he likes dessert bars. Last night at dinner he handed his plate back to me, and said ' 'sert bar.' " I said, 'No, Michael, first you have to eat your dinner.' And he said, ' 'sert bar.' "

"I had read Ellyn's book (*Child of Mine*, naturally), and all the time we were going through this I could actually *see* the paragraph where she said to give them their dessert along with the rest of the meal, but I just couldn't bring myself to do it. So I told him he wasn't going to have his dessert bar, and if he wasn't going to eat, he could get down from the table."

"He got down, but he cried and sobbed the rest of the evening, and I felt so guilty and sorry for him. Finally it was bedtime, and I was afraid he wouldn't sleep. So I picked him up and

167

rocked him. I would think I got him to sleep, and start to get up to put him in his bed, and he would sit bolt upright and say, ' 'sert bar!' "

Ellen had found out what we all have: The way to learn is through trial and error. There are a lot of moves and counter moves in parenting a toddler. You have to respect her autonomy, but you also have to set limits. Sometimes you hit it right, sometimes you don't.

Understanding The Toddler

The toddler has moved from the intense intimacy of being a baby to exploring the separateness of being a child. She continues the process she began as an infant, that will continue throughout life, but is most accentuated in the toddler period: that of working out the balance between being separate and being connected with other people.

We generally think of the toddler period as starting when a child is about 15 to 18 months old, but babies acquire toddler-like behaviors long before that. They become mobile, they start to get into things, and, as early as 9 months of age, they can start to understand and obey their parents. A child becomes a full-blown toddler in her second year, when she gains a sense of her own capability, and gets around more and starts to have more of an opinion about what she wants to do.

A toddler is not an infant. If you treat her like a baby, you will fail her utterly. A toddler needs limits. The baby needed to establish trust, so you treated her with deference and understanding support. You tried to figure out what ailed her and fix it. That process was important, to allow her to feel secure and worthwhile and valued, and good about herself and about the world. If you have negotiated infancy in a positive way, your child will be well prepared for the inevitable struggles of the toddler period.

Actually, if you have negotiated infancy well, you may have *less* struggles with your toddler. Researchers at Johns Hopkins University[1] found that the idea of the terrible two's was largely a myth—most of the toddlers they observed were really quite cooperative. The toddlers who were the most obedient were the ones whose parents were compliant with *them*, and who *had*

168

been compliant throughout infancy. Mothers of the obedient children had been accepting, cooperative, and sensitive to them as babies. Mothers whose toddlers obeyed least well had been more rejecting, interfering and insensitive[2].

A toddler has endless mobility, energy and curiosity, and absolutely no judgment. It is as important to her to be treated like a separate person as it was when she was an infant. Now she is able to be a lot more assertive about it.

She says "no" a lot, because by saying no to you she can establish for herself that she is in control of what happens. A toddler will say no at the same time as she reaches for something.

A colleague told about her two-year-old daughter Rachel's ambivalence and struggle for autonomy. Carol had sung to Rachel since she was tiny. Six months ago, however, as bedtime approached, Rachel had begun saying to herself, "Yes, sing." But then, "No sing." Now when they settle down for bedtime and get ready to sing, the struggle is still there. Rachel as always, is at first delighted: "Sing! Sing!" Then she remembers. "No sing."

If Rachel is willing to give up her beloved singing in order to assert herself, what child wouldn't be willing to give up eating to accomplish the same goal?

At the same time that she is struggling with separation, your toddler is also struggling to learn self control. She is discovering that her whole small world and all the actions she can perform with her newly-mobile body are open to her. She is at once thrilled at the process, dedicated to exploring and manipulating everything, determined to do it her own way, frustrated at not being able to do everything she sets out to do, and profoundly afraid of being alone and losing contact with her parents.

The toddler is like the night watchman, checking the doors but not really wanting to find any of them open. She needs to be able to check the doors. To a certain point, you have to tolerate her aggression, but eventually she will go too far and get on your nerves and violate your civil rights and endanger herself and property. You will recognize it when you see it. And put a stop to it, preferably without making her feel that you don't like her. She has enough problems without your being mad at her too. She's not being naughty. Trial and error is the way *she* learns, too.

169

Parenting The Toddler

Your job in parenting your toddler is to offer her support for both sides of her ambivalent struggle between separation and security. You can help by teaching her to do things competently and independently, and by providing limits without taking away her self respect or individuality. She has to learn self control, but she has to do it without losing respect for herself.

It is a tight rope you're walking, between being over-restrictive and over-permissive, and it is a tight rope we will talk about again. If you go too far and are over-permissive, your child will not learn self control and won't feel as good about herself. If you go too far the other way and are over-controlling, your child won't get to experience the excitement and joy of learning a sense of *inner* control. She won't gain a sense of her independence and ability to choose her actions, and she still won't feel as good about herself.

We all learn. I got to meet Ellen the other day at a conference. I told her how much I enjoyed the story that Linda had shared with me about the dessert bars. Ellen laughed. "We're now letting him have his dessert bar along with the meal," she said. "And, sure enough, he eats it first and goes on and eats the rest of his meal."

Going Along, Helping

The trick for living with a toddler is to go along with what she wants unless it becomes downright harmful or dangerous or offensive. Toddlers do strange things, and they have their own reasons. When David, age 15 months, visited us recently with his father and brother, he took a liking to the door on the screened porch. He spent the better part of the two hours he was at our house opening and closing the screen door. We blocked the door's swing so he couldn't destroy it, and let him go at it. His father shuddered when I told him later I could no longer go through that door without thinking of David.

If you go along with toddlers, you can avoid a lot of unnecessary struggles. The other day, I stopped by at Ken Kopps, the little grocery store across the street from my office. In the front of the store were two kids—a girl about 12 and a boy about two.

170

They were having a disagreement about where to park the stroller.

"Here, here!" said the toddler, indicating an area over by the wall. "No, let's put it here," insisted the girl, pointing to an area by the grocery carts. (Actually, I thought he had the better idea.) "No, here!" demanded the toddler, pulling on the stroller and starting to get upset. "No, we're going to put it here!" insisted the girl, taking the stroller from him and planting it where she wanted it. They went back and forth a few more times, and finally she overruled him and walked back into the store. He followed her, crying and having a running tantrum.

The girl won, because she was bigger, but she paid a price for it. If she had been a little more grown up, she would have been able to go along with the toddler. She would have realized he wasn't hurting anything, and it was important to let him feel like she respected his judgment and like he had some control over what happened. But she was just a kid, and she had to assert herself, too. So they clashed.

You are not a kid, and you don't have to assert yourself. You can help your toddler through the process of detaching from you by enabling and teaching and encouraging her to do things competently and independently. You teach her what is acceptable and you limit disruptive, antisocial behavior. You do that by heading her off (as one study showed), nine times an hour when she is about to do something you don't want her to do. And you spend another average nine times an hour admiring or demonstrating something she wants your help with[1].

The encounters are brief, each lasting only a minute or two. They occur, on the average, every three minutes. It's all the interruptions that make it challenging to live with a toddler.

Setting Limits

But there will be times, no matter how accepting and flexible you are, when your toddler will go too far, and you will have to set limits. She will probably be angry with you, and may even have a tantrum, but that's all right. She doesn't have to like it—she just has to do what you say. Actually, her rage has a purpose. While you shouldn't deliberately provoke it, you needn't try too hard to avoid it. She, and you, both need to know you can stand up to even her strongest feelings.

171

Toddlers, like children of all ages, desperately need limits to make them feel safe and to free them up to learn to live in the world. If toddlers don't get limits, they become anxious and provocative and behave more and more desperately. They begin to look like the prototype "spoiled child."

As T. Berry Brazelton puts it in *Toddlers and Parents*[3], a spoiled child is one who is anxious about going too far, for children seem to know instinctively when they are doing that. The spoiled child constantly tests parents for limits which she knows are there somewhere, wanting them to come from the outside rather than having to find them for herself. When the child who is acting out is stopped, her response is one of relief.

Foster Cline, a psychiatrist who runs Evergreen Ranch for disturbed children in Colorado, says by 15 months a child has to have learned basic German Shepherd: Come, go, sit, stay, and no. It seems like good advice to me. The toddler period is the time to learn those basic disciplines, and a person who has not, is going to have a lot of trouble in life.

Hanging In There

A toddler is a challenging person to live with, but, like the purple cow, I'd rather see than be one. At times, she may be absolutely frustrated, excited and ambivalent. She acts "out of sorts," as the grandmothers used to say, and "like she doesn't know what to do with herself." Child development experts have a different name for it: Rapprochement. I like the way the grandmothers said it better.

At those times, you can't fix what ails a toddler, because what ails her is that she is trying to determine where her sphere of influence ends and yours begins, and to gain control of herself. Up until that time, she hasn't really been too conscious of boundaries.

The only way she can be sure about her boundaries is to make you the bang board against which she bounces her contrariness. You won't like it as well. It's not as much fun being a bang board as it is being a nice cuddly parent who is the cherished center of her universe.

The way you help is to hang in there and be friendly, and not overreact and not try too hard to make her feel better. It won't feel much like helping, because you won't see any immediate results. Your child will still be out of sorts. Eventually she will resolve the problem within herself—you can only wait. In many ways, living with rapprochement is a lot like living with colic.

The Parents' Relationship

Clearly, living with a toddler is challenging, and puts stress on parents. You have to be getting along with your spouse in order to do a good job with your toddler. You need the support, you need the help figuring out courses of action, and you need backing when you set limits. If your relationship is poor, you won't have the physical or emotional energy to manage this challenging time. And you'll undermine each other. If parents can't agree on what to do with a child, they fight with each other about it, and their child does exactly as she pleases.

Problems in feeding indirectly serve parents by keeping their minds off each other. Feeding difficulties that can't be resolved can generally be traced to wars between parents. If a child is refusing to progress from pureed food to table food, and one parent encourages more textured food and the other one says, "Leave her alone, she's just a baby," that child will likely not learn to eat more grown-up food.

Feeding The Toddler

To avoid unnecessary battles with your toddler about eating, observe a division of responsibility. Do your job as parent by maintaining indirect controls on feeding, like having set meals and snacks and limiting disruptive mealtime behaviors. But DON'T try to do your toddler's job of determining what and how much she eats. Figure 9-1, "Division of Responsibility in Feeding the Toddler," expands on the topic.

The eating situation gives the creative toddler many opportunities to test herself against her parents. The same two themes of learning skills and needing limits play themselves out in eating as in the rest of the toddler's life.

With feeding, it is time to get organized. The toddler no longer benefits from being fed on demand. She benefits from set

173

Parents are responsible for what is presented to eat and the manner in which it is presented

- Selecting and buying food
- Making and presenting meals
- Regulating timing of meals and snacks
- Presenting food in a form a child can handle
- Allowing eating methods a child can master
- Making family mealtimes pleasant
- Helping the child to participate in family meals
- Helping the child to attend to his eating
- Maintaining standards of behavior at the table

The parent is NOT responsible for

- How much a child eats
- Whether he eats
- How his body turns out

Figure 9-1   Division of Responsibility in Feeding the Toddler

meal times and scheduled food availability. It's time for a meals-and-snacks routine that imposes a reasonable routine on eating.

Continue to modify food (as appropriate) and the eating situation for your toddler, so she can be successful with eating. She still can't chew and swallow as well as an older child, and she will still be messy and have trouble manipulating her fork and spoon and glass. She still will feel more comfortable in a high chair or booster chair that holds her up at a reasonable height from the table. And she still will be very cautious about trying new foods, and will have to approach them in her own way and on her own schedule.

The toddler will react to any pressure on her eating as a

threat to her autonomy, and she would rather go hungry than be submissive. It will be difficult *not* to put pressure on your toddler's eating. Her appetite may seem to fall off considerably. Her growth rate will be slower during the second and third year than during the first. She will form definite food preferences, and won't be as ready to go along with your assumption that she will eat what you provide.

Whenever I ask for questions at workshops, parents raise the issues I'll deal with now. If it is any reassurance to you, all parents struggle with very much the same kind of quirky problems in feeding their toddlers.

Choose Your Battles.

Only fight battles you can win. Keep in mind that you can stop a toddler from doing what you don't want her to do, but you can't get her to do what you want her to do. You can get her to come to the table, but you can't make her eat.

Sooner or later, your child will say, in whatever language she happens to be speaking at the time, "I'm not eating." Usually that move comes very abruptly, as it did for me when Curtis, age two, climbed eagerly up in his high chair, apparently ready to do another thorough job of eating his dinner. However, this time he had another idea, and he couldn't wait to try it.

He sat back in his chair, crossed his arms, and announced, "I won't eat." Now, I don't know where he got the idea that his eating was my project. Maybe he just was running a little research trial to find out whose it was. I had my invitation to say back, "Oh, dear, you have to eat." But I looked at him, and I could see that little glint in his eye that I had come to recognize as meaning he was digging in for a contest.

I did some very quick thinking. It scared me that he might not eat, because I had seen how crabby he could be when he got hungry. I also realized he could get me to do lots of things, some of them rather awful, to get him to eat. Like beg. Or threaten. Or play games (here comes the choo-choo). Or bribe. All of it would make me look very silly and he probably still wouldn't eat.

So I said, "That's all right, you don't have to eat. Just sit here and keep us company while we eat." He looked absolutely crestfallen. It *seemed* like such a good game, and I just wouldn't

175

play. So he sat a minute, and then he said, "I want some of that." He ate it, and asked for something else, and so on until he had a full meal.

Now, at age 15, he still comes to the table at times and says, "I won't eat." He's heard me tell this story often enough so he is teasing. And I still say, "That's all right, you don't have to eat. Just keep us company."

Once you demonstrate to your child that you won't try to make her eat, she will likely go ahead and do it on her own. But you have to mean it—she'll know if you're just trying to trick her.

Have Regular Meals And Snacks.

Provide your toddler with three meals a day, and have planned snacks between times to bring the feeding intervals down to about every two or three hours. Her stomach is small and her energy needs are high, so she'll do better with frequent feedings.

I say *planned* snack to make the distinction from the "handout." The toddler's favorite trick is to get down from the table, having eaten little or nothing, then come around two minutes later wanting a cookie. If you dole out, your toddler will not learn that meals are for eating. It is dreadfully easy to dole out. They look so small and appealing and, especially if they are growing slowly, we worry that they're not going to be all right.

Don't give in. You'll have to show her what the limits are. Say no. Say, "Dinner is over. You are going to have to wait until snack time." Your toddler will cry and whine and make a nuisance of herself, but before too long, she'll get her snack, you'll both be happy, and she'll have learned that that ploy doesn't work.

The planned snack is the secret weapon of the beleaguered parent. You have to refuse the panhandling, or your toddler won't ever learn to eat her meals. But you'll need an out, because you won't be able to hold out until the next meal.

In the long run, she'll eat better if you're firm about adhering to a structure. You'll be in charge of what she eats, and not just doling it out in accordance with her special requests. With regular feedings, she'll have time to get hungry between times, and hunger increases her chances of trying new foods.

176

Having regular meals and snacks frees a child up from thinking about food all the time so she can get on with her other business. It also gives *you* some structure so you won't be tempted to use food to resolve the many emotional tangles you get into with your toddler.

You don't have to be hard-nosed about scheduling. Use snacks to remain flexible. If you have a hungry toddler and long meal intervals, you might have to give two snacks instead of one.

Make Mealtimes Pleasant

Make meals pleasant for your toddler by being companionable and by not putting pressure on food acceptance. Respect her tempo, and let her down when she indicates she has had enough. Equally, respect her slowness, and let her take her time with her eating. Talk and pay attention to her, but don't overwhelm her with attention.

Make meals pleasant for yourself, too. You don't have to put up with crying and whining, making a big fuss about eating generally or about particular foods, and making a *provocative* mess. (There will be a mess, but this kind is where the child seems to be trying to get your goat.) Most times, parents put up with misbehavior because they hope their child will eat a few more bites. That's like paying a very screwy form of blackmail. Whose food is it, anyway? Let her down when she loses interest in eating. There will be another snack or another meal, and she can eat then.

Your child needs to behave well enough to make her pleasant to be around, and you are the one who has to teach her that behavior. If you let her make a nuisance of herself at mealtime, the next step will be to feed her separately so you can have peace and quiet for your meal. Participating in family mealtimes is important, and isolating her to do her eating is too big a price to pay for your failure to set appropriate limits.

I think you'll find your tolerance of messes and noise increases when you have a toddler, and it should. But we all have our limits, and she will have to respect yours. You should also, to a certain extent, respect social convention. The world will not look kindly on a beastly toddler, although we both hope others will be tolerant of the usual range of small-child behavior.

177

Hang Loose About Food Acceptance

It should come as no surprise to you that university research has confirmed that toddlers are neophobic—they dislike new food. Studies have shown that the more familiar toddlers were with a food, the more they are inclined to like it. Simply looking at it increases their liking for a food, but tasting does it better. To get the children in the study to taste the foods, researchers had to reassure them that they could take the food back out of their mouths if they didn't like it[4].

The parents at a workshop gasped when I told them this. However, every toddler knows that putting something in your mouth is one thing, but getting it down your throat is QUITE another. My two-year old brunch guest the other day did just that with the quiche—he took a bite, mushed it around in his mouth long enough to taste it, then put it back on his place mat in a neat little pile. He did about the best we could hope for: He put it on HIS place mat.

The same researchers demonstrated that if you rewarded children for trying a new food, it interfered with their learning to like it. Children who were simply allowed to approach the food on their own were more likely to go back to it than those who had been rewarded to try it. (On the other hand, when food was used as a reward for doing something else, it increased the value of the food[5].)

Children react when they feel like they are being forced. It stands to reason that if you reward with dessert for eating broccoli, you will be teaching children to like the dessert more, the broccoli less.

Don't Short-order Cook

Your child comes to the table and says "What's that?" and you tell her and she says "I won't eat that," and you get up and make something else. That's short order cooking. Don't do it.

You won't be doing your child a favor by preparing mealtime substitutes. It gives her your job of planning the menu and fails to set appropriate limits. In the long run, it puts more pressure on her to eat, because it takes away not-eating as an option. And it is very counter-productive in terms of a child's food acceptance.

178

The ever-neophobic toddler takes a long time to get warmed up to try a new food. If you remove that food, she won't ever get around to it. You will give her the clearest message possible that you don't expect her to eat that. Leaving it there keeps eating it an option, and one of the times she sees it she will take you up on that option. It might be fourteen meals from now, but if all goes well, you will have lost interest in her number of refusals and gone back to enjoying your own meal.

Make one meal for everybody, put a variety of dishes on the table (always include bread—your toddler will generally accept that, even if she turns down everything else), and let her decide what to eat. She might decide not to eat her vegetables or her meat, and you mustn't blanche. She might, in fact, not eat much at all. She'll still be all right. She'll make up for it another meal or another day.

Be Realistic About Amounts

Toddlers don't eat very much, but when I have really analyzed their diets, it has almost always turned out that they are eating enough and eating the right foods. They don't *have* to eat so much to get what they need. Their portion size is only a fourth the size of an adult's, so they can get by on one or two tablespoons of vegetables or half an ounce of meat for a serving. If they eat more than that, it is all just a bonus.

Toddlers sometimes eat really tiny amounts of foods—when they are interested in other things, when they don't particularly like what they are offered, or when they just plain aren't hungry. Check Figures 4-4 and 4-5 in Chapter 4: "Range of Recommended Calorie Intakes at Different Ages for Boys and Men" and "...Girls and Women," respectively. You'll see that 1-3 year olds eat, on the average, 900 to 1800 calories a day. By the time you allow for day-to-day variation, some days your toddler won't eat very much at all, other days the amounts will seem more substantial.

If you present your toddler with a variety of foods—the favorites along with the not-so-favorites—she will eat what she needs. If you feel like you have to get her to eat enthusiastically all the time, you might end up going to the fast food place to get hamburgers every day, like one young mother I talked to, or, like

179

another, alienating the rest of the family by making meat loaf every night. In the short run it may seem like you are wasting food, to present things to your toddler, only to have them turned down. In the long run, however, you will waste less food, because your child will learn to eat what the rest of the family eats.

Get There First

You'll get to pick the food for a meal or a snack (and you really should—you're the parent), if you think it out ahead of time and present it before your child is ravenous. If she gets hungry first and gets her mind all made up what she wants to eat, you may have an unnecessary fight on your hands.

If you go ahead and do the meal planning, it will help you to moderate your child's food jags. If you ask, she'll tell you she wants her favorite food. If you don't ask, she will go ahead and take her chances like the rest of the family—sometimes you get lucky, sometimes you don't.

Present a variety of foods at meal time—a main dish, milk, fruit or vegetable, bread—then let your toddler pick and choose from what's available. Offer it all in a neutral fashion. Don't press things on her, or she'll play the toddler's favorite game of turning things down and watching you get desperate.

Keep Her Comfortable

The toddler can use a high chair or stool to get her at the right height to the table and to help her stay confined so she can keep her attention on eating. Make sure her feet are supported— dangling them is uncomfortable for toddlers just like for us. She benefits from child-sized silverware and from a glass or cup she can manage well.

Give her some emotional comfort, as well. Be pleasant to be around, and let her know you enjoy her. Spend some time with her. Your presence and example will give her all the encouragement she needs to try new foods. Be patient with her efforts, and overlook some of the things she does, like eating with her fingers. She needs to feel successful with eating, and your attitude will make all the difference to her.

180

Know Your Audience

People ask about the "one bite" requirement. You know, "you must take a bite of everything." Some children benefit from that, others will fight to the death before they do it. It's always better to suggest than command. That gives you an out when they turn you down. It gives them an out, too. As one young mother recalled the "three bite" rule in her growing-up household wasn't so bad unless they had pork and beans, and then it was *awful*.

All you are trying to accomplish with the "one bite" rule is to encourage her to taste it, so she can decide if she wants to eat it. You are not trying to get her to *eat* it. That is crossing the line into forcing, and the net result will be to decrease the likelihood that she will learn to like it. You'll be doing even better with this rule if you allow her the option of taking the bite back out again if she doesn't like it.

You, and your child, and the way you work things out between you are the ultimate authorities about feeding tactics in your household. You are going to have to make your feeding judgments based on what works with her. For instance, you are well aware that one of the major things I recommend is structured meals and snacks. But one young mother was telling me that her son begged a lot for a cracker between meals. She generally gave it to him, and observed that he didn't eat it—he just carried it around, and licked the salt a little bit. It kept him comfortable to have that cracker in his hand.

Know Your Nutrition

Parents worry on general principles if kids don't eat vegetables. It might help you to know that vitamin A is the main concern, and that kids can get that in other places besides their vegetables.

In the "Tools and Strategies" section in the Appendix is a list of Vitamin A sources in fruits and vegetables. If your child won't eat carrots, you can substitute cantaloupe or apricot nectar. But do it discreetly—you don't want her to get the idea that you are short order cooking for her.

181

Don't Be Too Free With Juice And Milk

Back in my pediatric nutrition clinic days, many parents of toddlers consulted with me about their toddler's poor eating at mealtimes. In figuring out the problem, the first thing I would take a look at was milk and juice consumption. (The second thing I looked at was amounts—generally parents were expecting their children to eat too much.)

More often than not, I would find toddlers were drinking way too much juice—sometimes as much as 24 ounces a day. The calories from the juice were filling them up, and they weren't hungry for their meals. When parents stopped the juice handouts between meals and began offering water for thirst instead, the kids' eating improved.

Often the juice of choice was apple juice. That's ironic, because parents felt like they were doing their child a nutritional favor to give her juice, and apple juice supplies very little, nutritionally. Some brands are fortified by the processor with vitamin C, but for the most part, apple juice doesn't have much to offer.

Milk can cause a similar problem. Sixteen to twenty-four ounces of milk a day is enough for a toddler. If she drinks too much milk, she won't be hungry for her meal. If she fills up on milk, you might have to impose a limit, and give her only one glass of milk and offer a glass of water to satisfy her thirst.

If your toddler is still on the bottle, it is because you missed your chance at weaning. Toward the end of the first year, when children get very interested in table food, they will gradually forget about bottle feeding, if you let them. During the second year the bottle can present problems, at meal time especially. If a toddler knows a bottle is waiting when she finishes eating, many times she holds out for the bottle and won't eat her meal. The same goes for the mealtime breast-feeding.

I can certainly understand why you would want to retain the closeness of nursing for a while longer. However, if you decide to continue with breast or bottle, keep it away from mealtime. Use it for snacks—maybe the mid-afternoon or late night snack.

Have milk at meals, and drink it yourself or at least limit yourself to water. Why should she drink her milk if she sees you having coke or apple juice? Here's one battle you set yourself up for. Offer milk or water, but don't force her to drink her milk or worry out loud because she isn't. Give her time to approach it on her own.

Don't Make Dessert A Reward

Don't promise your child a dessert if she eats her dinner. Put a moderate serving of dessert at each plate when you set the table, and let your child decide when to eat it.

Parents can't believe this until they try it, but children will eat the dessert first, discover they are still hungry, and go on to eat the rest of their meal. They haven't yet learned our strange idea that dessert marks the end of the meal. Presenting them right off the bat with dessert lets them decide how they are going to eat.

If you reward with dessert for eating dinner, she may over-eat twice: Once when she eats her dinner to get dessert, and once when she eats dessert when she is already full. Further-more, the dessert-after-you-eat-your-meal rule is hard to enforce. *Parents* value dessert, and it is hard for them to go ahead and have dessert when their child is still sitting and looking at her peas. They will likely try to get themselves off the hook by trying to force the peas, and then there is trouble.

Help Your Child Be Successful With Eating

Toddlers use their fingers and make a mess when they eat. They announce they are done by knocking the rest of the food on the floor—they are no longer interested, so they get rid of it. They aren't trying to annoy you—they are just very direct in their methods. Eventually, you'll get tired of it, or you'll observe she's trying to annoy you, and you'll put a stop to it. It's in the facial expression. Most times, saying "No," firmly, will do the trick. If she persists, put her down. Then ignore her when she has a tantrum.

Believe it or not, this is all part of allowing your toddler to be successful with her eating. She has to learn to eat, but she also has to learn to be pleasant at meals.

Present food in a way that she can handle it. Her muscles and coordination are still pretty immature, and she will need food that is easy to pick up and chew in order to manage it well.

183

Help her pay attention at meals by timing her snacks so she will be hungry (but not famished) when she gets to the table. Hungry children are very businesslike about their eating. It's when they start to get full that they become distractible and the other behaviors start to show up.

Allow eating methods she can handle. She'll use her fingers a lot and make a mess. She'll spill. That's normal for this period. If you get all caught up in requiring utensils and being neat she'll get self conscious or rebellious, and eating will lose out to the interaction between you.

You'll find yourself developing your eating skills, too. You'll be able to catch a glass as it tips to the table and be able to wipe up without losing your place in a conversation. Before the toddler period, it may never have occurred to you that no table is properly set unless it has a roll of paper towels for wiping up spills.

Your toddler continues to need some help to be successful with certain foods. She can't chew tough and fibrous food, like meat, and too-dry food seems to get stuck in her mouth.[6] You'll need to continue to do a little food modification. Figure 9-2, "Making Foods Easy to Eat for Toddlers," gives some suggestions.

Keep Her Safe

Children under age two have a higher risk of choking than older children. They aren't as experienced or as adept at chewing and swallowing, and things can get out of control in their mouths and slip down their throats without being chewed.

Most choking problems are readily preventable. Usually, children choke because they are being poorly supervised when they eat. Sometimes an older child gives them something they can't handle. Other times, they get into trouble when they are being allowed to run around and eat[7].

Choking is not the same thing as gagging. All children gag. It's their protection when they are learning to chew and swallow. When your child first starts chewing, she won't be too good at controlling the position of food in her mouth, and some will slip to the back of her tongue and activate the gag reflex. That will propel it right back out again. She won't get excited about this unless you do, and there is really no call for you to get excited.

184

- Cut foods into bite-sized pieces, cut meat up finely

- Make some foods soft and moist

- Serve foods near to room temperature

- Substitute ground beef patties for steaks or chops

- Serve salads without dressing as a finger food

- Make soups thin enough to drink or thick enough to spoon

- Give her a child-sized spoon and a small fork with dull prongs

- Give her unbreakable dishes

- Seat her at comfortable height to the table with feet supported

- Give her a plate or bowl with sides to push the food against

- Make food attractive and colorful, but don't bribe with gimmicks

Figure 9-2   Making Foods Easy to Eat for Toddlers

The problem arises when foods are too hard to chew, or slippery and smooth so they are hard to keep in position in the mouth. Something like a grape can slip back in a child's mouth and down her throat, and lodge at the entrance to her windpipe. *That's* choking, and that's dangerous.

Don't be hysterical and overprotective, but do take some precautions to prevent choking. Figure 9-3 "Preventing Choking," outlines some tactics you can use.

Obesity

You may be tempted to withhold food when you see how your toddler is built. She may be chubby and sway-backed and her stomach may stick out. That's simply a normal build for a toddler—try not to over-react.

It is still too early to worry that your fat toddler will

185

1.   Gradually build a child's feeding skills; let her work up slowly to more-difficult foods.

2.   For the child under age three, avoid foods that are hard to control in the mouth, chew and swallow, such as nuts, raw carrots, gum drops and jelly beans. Be cautious with these foods until your child can handle them.

3.   Modify some foods to reduce the risk of choking: Quarter hot dogs lengthwise, quarter grapes, cook carrots.

4.   Always be there during feeding. Don't let children supervise.

5.   Keep your child seated while she is eating. Most choking occurs when children eat on the run.

6.   Keep things calm at eating time. When children scream or laugh they catch their breath and they could inhale food.

Figure 9-3   Preventing Choking

remain fat when she grows up. Actually, age nine years is the youngest you can really begin to predict obesity in later life. If your child is fat, you don't need to be particularly worried about it. You *certainly* shouldn't try to restrict her food intake. Doing what you are already doing—maintaining a positive feeding relationship with a division of responsibility for feeding, is the best intervention for preventing obesity. Read more in Helping All You Can to Keep Your Child From Being Fat (Chapter 14).

There is one exception to the above generalization. Girls who gain weight rapidly between one and two years of age have a high risk of retaining that excess weight[8]. (With boys, the high-risk time, if you see a sudden weight gain, is between two and three years and four and six years.) If you see a sudden shift in your child's weight, try to determine what caused it. Has there been a major change in the way you feed her? Has there been any upset in the family as a whole? Are parents having a difficult time with each other? Have family relationships gotten organized around her eating in some way that makes her overeat?

These are important-enough concerns to warrant bringing in a professional to help you evaluate what is going on. It's hard to say what could be causing the problem. I have seen toddlers overeat because parents don't provide reliable meals and appropriate structure. I have seen parents inadvertently (or deliberately) encourage their children to eat more than they were hungry for, and I have seen them overfeed children during a time of stress to keep them quiet. I have often seen parents overuse food handouts in an attempt to quell toddler fractiousness.

At times, I have seen parents mismanage feeding and encourage overeating because of bad advice or simple misunderstanding of appropriate feeding. At other times, I have seen parents distort feeding because they weren't getting along with each other and, growing out of that, they haven't been able to parent their child in an effective fashion.

Distortions in family dynamics have to be considerable in order to disrupt a child's ability to regulate her food intake. In the face of a dysfunction of this magnitude, it is naive to impose food restriction (although that is the intervention most often chosen by medical professionals). The solution is to detect and change family dynamics that encourage the overeating, and to restore a positive feeding relationship.

Ignore Miscellaneous Kinky Behavior

Someone called me from the pediatrician's office with a mother's question. Her child was storing food in his cheeks when he left the table—should she be concerned? I wondered if the mother was trying to force her child to eat. (Toddlers sometimes will store food in their mouths as an alternative to eating it, to appease an over-pushy parent.) My caller said no, she didn't think so. In view of that, I said I didn't think there was any cause for concern, except possibly tooth decay. Furthermore, I didn't think it would grow into a problem unless the mother got all upset about it.

Since then, I have talked with lots of parents of toddlers who say their child leaves the table with food in their mouths. (What did I say earlier—putting food in your mouth is one thing, but swallowing is quite another?) The matter-of-fact ones ask them to swallow or they clean the food out with their finger. They don't want the child to choke, and they don't want

187

mushed-up food on the carpet. The worriers worry and make an issue of it and the child accentuates the behavior and then they have a problem that *is* worthy of concern.

Children are eager to please, and are always ready to produce a behavior that seems to get their parents excited. Other, more flamboyant behaviors include flinging food on the wall and throwing up at will. The latter is more difficult to be philosophical about. You'll probably need to check with your pediatrician to insure that there is nothing wrong. If your child is growing well and seems otherwise all right, try reacting very neutrally to it. Some children just regurgitate easily. If that doesn't do the trick, just say, very matter-of-factly, "I want you to stop doing that." If she doesn't stop, try a time out.

There is nothing that puts alarming or disgusting behaviors in their proper perspective any faster than treating them like any old, run-of-the-mill objectionable behavior. If you are matter-of-fact about it, she will likely learn to swallow instead of letting go. Ugh.

Living with a toddler is one of the most demanding—and entertaining—things you'll ever do. You'll learn to teach, to be home base, and to set limits. You'll begin to make demands on your toddler, and get so you can gauge those demands realistically. Your toddler will range out from you, and explore, and then come back to make sure you are still available. You'll develop your judgment about what is acceptable behavior and what is not, and sharpen your ability to set limits.

All these skills are essential parts of parenting throughout the growing up years. Children at all ages do best when parents set realistic requirements and give genuinely instructive messages.

References

1.　Minton, C., Kagan, J. and Levine, J.A.: Maternal control and obedience in the two-year-old. Child Development 42:1873-1894, 1971.

2.　Stayton, D.J., Hogan, R., and Ainsworth, M.D.S.: Infant obedience and maternal behavior: The origins of socialization reconsidered. Child Development 42:1057-1069, 1971.

3.	Brazelton, T.B.: Toddlers and Parents. . .A Declaration of Independence. New York: Delta, 1974.

4.	Birch, L.L. and Marlin, D.W.: I don't like it; I never tried it: Effects of exposure on two-year-old children's food preferences. Appetite 3:353-360, 1982.

5.	Birch, L.L., Marlin, D.W. and Rotter, J.: Eating as the "means" activity in a contingency: Effects on young children's food preference. Child Development 55(2):431-439. 1984.

6.	Lowenberg, M.E.: The development of food patterns in young children. IN Pipes, P.L. Nutrition in Infancy and Childhood. St. Louis: Times Mirror/Mosby, 1985.

7.	Harris, C.S., Baker, S.P. Smith, G.A. and Harris, R.M.: Childhood asphyxiation by food: A national analysis and overlook. Journal of the American Medical Association. 251-2231-2235, 1984.

8.	Shapiro, L.R., Crawford, P.B., Clark, M.J., Pearson, D.J., Raz, J. and Huenemann, R.L.: Obesity prognosis: a longitudinal study of children from the age of 6 months to 9 years. American Journal of Public Health 74:968-972, l984.

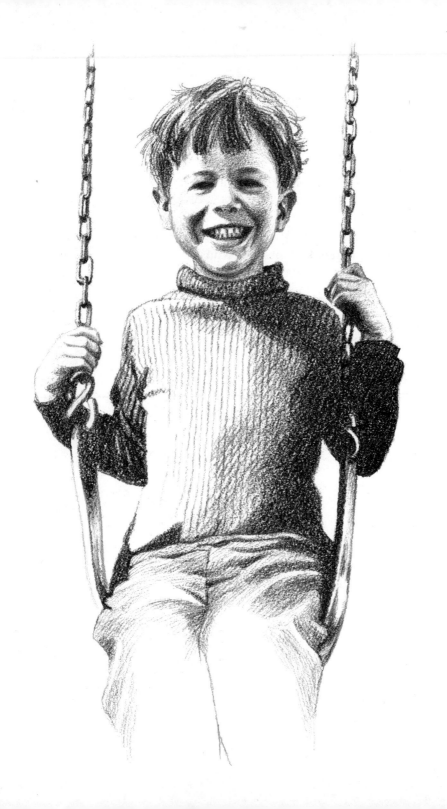

10

The Popular Preschooler

If he successfully negotiates the toddler period, the preschooler goes back to being a pleasant person who likes being in his own skin. He has demonstrated to himself and the rest of the world, in his struggles as a toddler, that he is an individual. His parents have demonstrated to him that he CAN be a separate person and that they will still help him (or stop him) when he needs it, and they will enjoy him as an individual, not just as a little foil who does everything they say.

Now his task is to grow up. He will increasingly take the initiative as he works at getting better at all he does. He learns, largely through trial and error, what is acceptable behavior and what is not, and to make some fine distinctions: acceptable behavior in one place or time isn't acceptable in another. He learns to express himself in appropriate ways and to work things out with other people. He learns to control his impulses and to wait or work for things. He develops his views about who he is and what he is, how much he is worth, and what he is capable of doing.

The preschooler is out to learn, and he is out to please you. He thinks you are the best thing ever. He will imitate what you do, listen when you tell him things, and require your help in demonstrating what is acceptable and what is unacceptable behavior. Your child will take the initiative in learning new things, because he is endlessly enthusiastic about growing up.

If you expect him to sit quietly, think logically, or act realistically, you are bound to be disappointed. But if you enjoy playfulness and surprises, you are going to have a great time with your preschooler.

You must continue to set limits and enforce rules, but those rules should have everything to do with the behavior of the child. In order to truly teach and to let him feel good about himself, you must neither criticize your child's character when he takes a wrong step nor respond in an arbitrary way that has more to do with your own whims or moods than with anything coming from your child.

Appropriate eating for a preschooler is sitting at the table with the rest of the family, being pleasant and being able to handle utensils and cup reasonably well. It is being able to accept most foods, try others, and politely refuse still others with the assumption that at some time he will want to eat whatever it is he has refused. The preschooler will develop his own ideas about eating, from day care, friends and the TV, and want to pick out snacks at the grocery store. But he will go along with his parents or day care provider if they tell him no.

Understanding The Preschooler

The preschooler is out to learn and improve in all areas of his life. Eating is no exception. Unlike the toddler, he is purposeful. He has a sense of what he can and can't do, and is willing to go along with his limitations. He has a feeling for what he can accomplish as well as for what is permissible. He is still, however, a child, and you will need to accommodate to his unique childishness.

Childishness

Even though he is a delightful and positive person, the preschooler is still a child and will have his own curious little ways of operating. There is no rush about giving up these little ways. Unless you make a big fuss about them, your child will outgrow them or get tired of them. Then he'll move on to other curious little ways! If you forget about molding this child of yours to be the next Miss Manners I think you will find his idiosyncrasies to be quite engaging. It helps to watch someone *else's* children.

I observed seven preschoolers in a day care center having their lunch of egg salad sandwiches and potato soup. The soup was a thin cream soup. All of the children started eating with spoons, but soon reverted to picking up their little bowls and drinking directly from them. The teacher, probably self conscious because I was there, made them put the bowls down and eat with spoons.

Most of them complied, but after two or three bites, gave up on it as a bad job. They stopped eating their soup, and turned to the sandwiches. One little girl, however, obviously *loved* the soup, and was not going to let anything get in the way of her enjoyment. She simply ignored the teacher, and continued to drink from her bowl. She asked for seconds. (As I sat and watched her enjoying her soup in her own special way, I discovered that there was something even MORE special about the way she ate: As she drank the soup, she was shelling the celery out of her mouth between her lower lip and the bowl!)

I *hope* the teacher was just having stage fright, because he was very nice in other ways. (I *have*, however, seen grownups be rigid and unreasonable with eating when they are really quite flexible and logical with other things.) He talked pleasantly with the children while they ate. He was careful to get rid of the tall thin glass because he knew that all the other kids, who had the short, squatty glasses, would be upset because they would think they were getting less.

And he left the sandwiches uncut and asked the children what shape they wanted. He knew from bitter experience that a preschooler is capable of loving a sandwich cut in triangles and may consider the same sandwich cut in squares to be totally inedible. Preschoolers aren't trying to bug anyone with those behaviors—they simply don't have the intellectual maturity to understand the basic similarities.

The preschooler's chewing and swallowing remain somewhat immature, so he still needs some toddler-type modifica-

193

tions in order to be successful with eating. Meat may continue to be a problem, and many children don't like plain meat until they get older. If they run into a piece of dry meat, they may chew it a while and then sneak the cud out their mouth and under the edge of the plate.

Preschoolers Are Purposeful

Preschoolers generally are quite purposeful. I was reminded of that on the same grand tour in which I visited the day care center. I was out looking for preschoolers in their native habitat to get some ideas about how they operate with eating. To find them, the first thing I thought of was a day care center. The second thing I thought of was McDonalds.

At McDonalds I struck it rich. There were a number of children, and a number of interesting things going on with eating. I have since discovered that wherever there are children and there is food, something engaging is *bound* to happen.

Two preschoolers were just sitting in the booth while their mother got their lunch. It was a nice day, and some other children, who had gotten there first, had already finished and were running back and forth from their table to the outdoor playground.

The two latecomers watched them while they waited. But after they got their food, they paid absolutely no attention to the two running around. They ate their hamburgers and french fries steadily and with total absorption. After eating for a while, they began to slow down a bit and look around, still eating. Finally, they put their food down and sidled out of the booth and ran off to play. As long as they were hungry, they attended strictly to their eating. When they got full, they lost interest in it completely.

Learning And Improving

Preschoolers make a point of learning from other people. They observe, they role play, and they start to accumulate and process information. They begin to think out ahead of time what they want to do, and make provision for it, and are able to put off something they want to do and realize that it *will* happen. The toddler couldn't do any of those things. That's why the preschooler is easier to live with.

194

He gets better at chewing and swallowing. He gets neater and more consistent at using his utensils to eat and at drinking from a cup without spilling, even though he doesn't have the fine muscle control that will let him pour milk or cut meat. He still has short fat fingers that make it hard for him to manipulate things. If he is given modest help, he can achieve. He takes pride in his eating abilities and likes eating with the rest of the family.

Your preschooler is capable of observing what you eat, and being influenced by that. Don't forget that you are being perceived as this all-knowing person, and if you eat green beans, it must be the thing to do. You don't have to say another word. All you have to do is enjoy your green beans. Observing that, your child will make the assumption that he, too, will eat green beans. If not today, then someday. It is just a matter of time.

I have made the point MANY times that you shouldn't put pressure on your child to eat. The pressure is already there, in your child's built-in desire and drive to grow and in your demonstrating what it means to be grown up. Your child will imitate what you do. One of the preschooler's favorite games is role playing to find out what it's like to be a grownup.

Parenting The Preschooler

Kids need to learn what the world expects, and the only way they can do that is from your reactions and from the reactions of other grownups around them.

During the preschool phase, you will evolve the parenting style you will likely use throughout your child's growing up years. It is worth spending some time considering your approach to parenting: It can make an enormous difference to your child.

Children do best with eating, as with every other thing, when they are exposed to love AND limits. Diane Baumrind, a child development specialist at University of California, Berkeley, observed 110 3- and 4-year old children in nursery school to see how well they operated with other people[1]. She then observed them with their parents at home and in the nursery school to see what kind of parenting environment the kids had grown up in.

Some parents set limits and enforced rules, but were also

195

willing to listen receptively to children's requests and questions and support them in surveying and mastering their world. They made use of power and reason, rather than guilt or fear, to enforce rules. If children disobeyed them, parents used a further show of force, but did it calmly and kept control of the situation.

Children raised in this fashion were self-reliant, self-controlled, explorative, and content. They were successful, happy with themselves, and generous with others.

Some parents were overly strict. They were arbitrary in the way they handed down directives, and didn't explain reasons for their actions or allow their child to express himself or disagree with them. They disciplined harshly or frightened their children to get compliance. Their children were relatively discontent, withdrawn and distrustful. They weren't as curious, independent, or achievement-oriented. They were likely to be obedient but unhappy.

Some parents were overly lenient. They didn't expect their child to eat, sleep or contribute in any sort of a regular way. They allowed babyish behavior, and they didn't enforce the expectations they had communicated to their children. They had a difficult time distinguishing between appropriate and inappropriate behavior in their child. They simply went along with the child's demands until their patience was exhausted and then punished him, sometimes very harshly.

Children of these permissive parents learned little from their disciplinary techniques. They were likely to be aggressive and lack self control, and were often openly disobedient or disrespectful.

Baumrind called these three styles *authoritative, authoritarian* and *permissive*, respectively. Other studies of children at other ages focussing on issues ranging from latch key after school situations to adjustment to divorce have used these same categories (although sometimes different names) in describing parenting styles. And they have reached the same conclusions: To do well, children need appropriate guidance and limits. As a textbook on child development pointed out[2], "authoritative parenting...is most likely to produce a happy child rather than a distrustful puppet or an uncontrolled little devil."

The advantages are so many, one wonders why we don't all parent in an authoritative fashion. It won't surprise you that I have some ideas about that. Authoritative parenting takes more time, energy, judgment and nerve than either being peremptory or being permissive. If you are lacking in any of those areas, it is hard to pull it off.

Of course, we can't overlook the child's part in inducing a certain parenting style. If your particular child is easy to instill self control and self reliance in, you may turn out to be more relaxed and flexible than you would be otherwise. On the other hand, a hostile, unfriendly child may make you more authoritarian than you really want to be. (Or you may have made him hostile and unfriendly in the first place by being so authoritarian. As we family therapists say, sometimes it is hard to tell where the punctuation is—where the vicious cycle starts.) A child who has so darned much initiative that he wears you out, may cause you to be permissive from simple exhaustion.

For whatever reason, if you are going too far to either extreme, you would be wise to do whatever is necessary to get yourself back toward the middle. It will take time and energy and maybe even some painful self-examination to change, but it will pay off in the long run. With child raising, we simply can't dispute the old adage that an ounce of prevention is worth a pound of cure.

Even though your preschool child becomes more independent of you, the way you treat him will have an enormous impact on him. Although parents' attitudes toward their children are important throughout childhood, they are especially so during the preschool years, partly because the child's self-concept is in the early stages of formation at this time. But it is also because of the way your preschooler thinks and feels about you. Your preschooler thinks you are just great and that you know all the answers. It follows directly from that that your attitude toward him is the gospel truth.

If you think he is just great in return, you are off to a fine start. Keep in mind that your preschooler doesn't have to do everything right or be a well-behaved little angel in order for you to feel like he is just great. Neither do you have to ignore bad behavior and pretend to yourself that he can do no wrong. He's just great because he IS, that's all. If you are having a hard time feeling that way, you had better get some help with it.

You can be helpful with a child's growth only if you are trusting and curious about him as his personality and behavior develops. With a positive attitude, you can correct him matter-

197

of-factly, and say, "No, you can't do that," and even enforce it with a time out if he ignores what you say. With a negative attitude, you say, "How *could* you do that! What *is* the matter with you?" And for the parent who uses love and guilt for leverage, "How can you do this to me? I am so disappointed." There's *nothing* the matter with him—he's just being a kid. Or *was*, until his grownup started chewing on him. Ever heard of the self-fulfilling prophecy?

To do a good job of parenting, you have to support the preschooler's initiative in appropriate ways. You provide tasks that are do-able and challenging. You notice when he accomplishes something. You let him take the lead, whenever possible, in conducting his affairs. You don't need a rule book to let you know when you are being appropriately supportive. Normal sensitivity and a little trial and error will show you the way. Your child will glow, and act proud of himself, and show similar warmth toward you. He will strive for further achievement, just for the joy of it, not to get your praise.

On the other end of the spectrum, there are thousands of ways of taking his initiative away—you can ignore his achievements, or criticize his efforts, or insist on taking over and doing it your way, or over-baby him when he hits a little snag. You may be misfiring by always having a better way of doing something or by waxing so enthusiastic that he gets suspicious that you don't really mean it. And he'll act hurt or discouraged or disgusted, and either turn away or get naughty.

It is a serious issue to trample on your child's feelings. We all do it at times, and if you're sensitive to it, you can apologize and change your behavior. But if it just goes on and on, your child will either withdraw or get angry, and you won't get many more chances to be supportive. And he'll end up not feeling very good about himself.

Having had this short course in parenting, you and I both need a little reassurance. Authorities writing on child abuse, Ruth and Henry Kempe[3], see a continuum of parent care, from the highly pathological at one end to the "only possible claimant to perfection as a mother, the Madonna" at the other. "But let us not forget," they caution, "Mary also had the perfect child." The Kempes estimate that between 20 and 30 percent of all parents have considerable difficulty caring for their child adequately. Figure 10-1, "Range of Parenting Styles," tells the story.

198

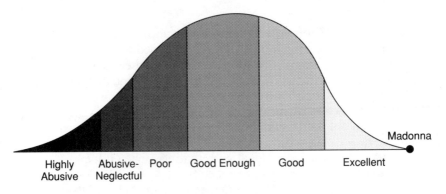

Highly Abusive   Abusive- Neglectful   Poor   Good Enough   Good   Excellent   Madonna

Figure 10-1   Range of Parenting Styles

Most of us are at least "good enough," and relatively few parents are completely bad. The "good enough" parent provides reasonably well for a child's physical and emotional needs, sets limits, and provides support and opportunity for achievement.

Parenting With Food

The themes of growth and responsibility and love and limits play themselves out with eating, the same as with every other aspect of your preschooler's life. If you lay out clear and realistic expectations with eating, he will work toward achieving those expectations. If you put certain foods on the table, he will work toward mastering those foods. He will learn, for the most part, to eat and enjoy them.

The goals regarding eating are to help him increase food acceptance, and to learn to conduct himself appropriately when he eats in a variety of social situations. The guidelines from the previous chapter, Is Your Toddler Jerking You Around at the Table, apply to the preschooler, as well. If you haven't read it recently, go back and review some of the ideas about food and eating management that we talked about there.

Have Structured Meals And Snacks

We have repeatedly discussed this previously, but it's important enough to lay it out again. Make meals, provide struc-

199

tured snacks, and limit grazing behavior (including juices and caloric beverages) between times. Present the food to the children, and let them do the rest. Don't try to force them to eat.

Having family meals doesn't just happen. As one mother confided, "Things are so miserable when we try to eat as a family, my husband and I have started eating alone." I pried a little, and it turned out her husband was insisting the kids finish their meals, so they didn't come around later panhandling for food. I commented that the time to deal with that was when it happened, and to refuse snacks until snack time.

"I know I make my kids eat for self-defense," said another. "If my four-year-old doesn't eat his dinner, he wakes me up at five a.m. to feed him." I pointed out that you can refuse snacks as well at four a.m. as at four p.m., and that she'll have to do that if her child is to learn to take responsibility for his eating.

You have to let kids have a feedback loop. The only way they will really learn to regulate their own eating is if they are allowed to experience the consequences of their behavior. If they don't eat dinner, they will find out that they will get hungry long before the next feeding time and that next time they had better take eating more seriously. If you are overbearing and insist they eat dinner, or permissive and dole out a snack when they come around begging, they won't find out anything about taking responsibility for managing their own eating.

Avoid Pressure On Food Acceptance

Your preschooler will not be as neophobic as he was when he was a toddler. For one thing, there won't be as many things that are new to him. If he does encounter something strange, you can talk about it with him, and that will give him the courage to try it. He'll no longer make the assumption that if the taste is novel, it is bad.

It still is important not to apply pressure on the preschooler to accept new foods or to eat his vegetables—any kind of pressure. Cooperative as they are, preschoolers still like foods less if they are given rewards for eating them[4]. Probably they reason, "If I have to get something in order to eat this, it must not be so good." (They also learn to value a food more if it is used as a reward for doing other things. Since adults tend to reward with what *they* value, and they think *children* value, the traditional child's preference for cookies is easy to explain.)

200

Preschoolers' food preferences reflect those of their parents as well as those of other people in their lives. Their parents can be especially helpful in demonstrating eating a new food[5]. But preschoolers learn to eat new foods from other children as well as from their parents. Children in preschool or day care situations learn to eat foods that they have turned down before[6].

Depend on other people to expose your child to foods you don't have around—the more familiar he is with a variety of foods, the more comfortable he'll feel in the world. You might, however, get some surprises. I will never forget the disgruntled expression on the face of my friend, the gourmet cook, the day her children came home and excitedly told her they had discovered a great new food: boxed macaroni and cheese dinner!

Mealtime Behavior

Lay out clear expectations for mealtime behavior. Your preschooler needs to know ahead of time that if he behaves badly at the table, he'll have to leave.

It's all a matter of degree—and attitude. He won't be the neatest person around, and you can overlook a lot of messiness if he is genuinely applying himself to his food. He'll still be inept at using a knife, but he'll manage a fork and spoon pretty well. He will still use his fingers a lot for pushing the peas onto the spoon and picking up the pieces of meat. He will likely have a difficult time sitting still, although he won't *really* start to move around on his chair until he's about six.

Those are simple kid behaviors. Bad behaviors go further, and include an attitudinal shift: Your preschooler will be twitting you. Bad behaviors include whining or complaining about the food, begging for foods that are not on the table, or eating in disgusting ways. If he can't behave properly, ask him to leave the table, don't let him take anything with him (or come back for dessert), and don't let him eat until the next planned snack time.

While this may seem like alarming advice to you, it is essentially the same maneuver that you used with the toddler in refusing him food handouts when he got down without having eaten. With this immediate and clear response, children get the message very quickly that they have to behave at the table.

Asking him to leave the table doesn't have to be punitive. It is just a matter-of-fact way of protecting your own mealtime

201

from disruptive behavior. It is also a way you teach him that eating with the family is important, and that you expect him to participate in making it pleasant.

If you let him persist with undesirable eating behavior, you give him the very clear message that you don't think he is capable of taking responsibility for his eating. You can *tell* him otherwise one million times, but what you *do* will still have more of an impact.

Make Maturity Demands

Cultivate the attitude that, sooner or later, your child will learn to eat almost everything. Keep presenting a variety of food, and offering it. Expect that your preschooler will be polite if he turns it down. That will keep the issue of learning to eat new foods before your child, and he will keep working to eat almost everything. But, when he does, it will be his idea, not yours.

You shouldn't put pressure on your child to eat, but neither should you baby your child and take away his motivation to grow up. If you need to, you can say, "When you get a little older you will eat that." But you don't even have to state that expectation out loud. It is assumed by both of you. We've talked before, at length, about not putting pressure on your child to eat. I think we all need to realize that the simple process of growing up puts pressure on your child, and most of it comes from within him. He *wants* to grow up. He *wants* to do the things he sees others around him doing.

I watched a movie on feeding toddlers[7], where the day care provider capitalized very skillfully on her charge's drive to grow. A little boy was examining the cheese he had for lunch.

"What is this?"

"Cheese," answered his provider, knowing full well he knew exactly what it was.

"Do I have to eat it?"

"No, you don't," she replied in a matter-of-fact voice, but making no move to remove the cheese.

So, there it sat, and there he sat, left to his own devices in figuring out what he was going to do about his cheese. He looked at the other kids, who were happily eating their cheese, and looked at the provider, who was happily eating her cheese. He thought about it a few seconds, then ate it.

202

Nobody applauded or even said, enthusiastically, "That's wonderful, I'm glad you ate it." Their approval was implicit—they simply assumed he'd be able to handle it.

Kids are wonderful. You can just *see* the wheels going around in their heads. And so was that care provider. She did just the right thing to set free that child's need to explore and master.

Trust Their Desire To Grow

Children in the most difficult situations can draw on that need to help themselves grow. I realized that when I was talking with Dr. Thomas Linscheid, a Clinical Psychologist in Cleveland who works with children with what he calls Type II Failure to Thrive. These are children who have major problems with their eating and who may be growing poorly because of them.

These kids might have had something wrong with them when they were little, like a heart defect, that kept them from eating all they needed to, so they were tube fed instead. Then, when the defect was corrected surgically, they were older and had never learned how to eat. And they didn't WANT to learn how to eat. Well, they wanted to, because they could see that people around them were eating and that they were odd because they didn't, but they were desperately afraid to.

In order to learn to eat, these older children had to learn everything they had missed as infants and toddlers. They had to learn to tolerate food in their mouth, to chew and to swallow. Because they had been away from those experiences for so long, it was profoundly aversive to them, and they had a terrible time getting past their aversion.

They were afraid of choking. They hadn't had the experience of swallowing, and they were afraid the food would get stuck in their throat and they wouldn't be able to breathe. Of course, they wouldn't have been able to say that in so many words, but the experience was there, and the reaction was there. One little boy in Omaha who was trying to learn to eat after his heart surgery got so reactive to food that he threw up when it was brought into the room.

Dr. Linscheid considers it very important that children learn to eat. And of *course* it is important—they have to learn to fit into the world. He takes the process seriously enough to set

203

up a very careful program to teach eating[8]. He puts the children in the hospital, cuts back on the tube feeding so they are hungry, and presents them with very carefully-chosen eating tasks.

At first the task is simple. He asks them to sit with the food in front of them. He progresses slowly, through touching to smelling to finally putting some of the food in their mouth. Without having to swallow it.

At every step of the process he is matter-of-fact about laying down his expectations. He explains what he wants the child to do and why he wants him to do it. Then he sits with the child while he gets ready to comply. Dr. Linscheid says the children's anxiety is tremendous. They cry and delay. Since he is being firm and dispassionate about his demands, the children soon learn that the struggle is with themselves. And they do struggle. Eventually they summon their courage and do what is asked of them, and they are very proud.

Now, I am not asking you to be an eating therapist for your child. It is a tremendously skilled procedure that requires carefully calibrated tasks to challenge the children without overwhelming them. I am using this story as a vivid example of just how powerful that drive is that children have within them to grow up and to respond to the matter-of-fact examples and expectations of grownups around them.

Teach Your Child How To Behave

The preschool child needs to behave acceptably with eating. He needs clear and realistic expectations about mealtime behaviors so he knows what standard to strive for. Kids thrive on challenging themselves. They don't appreciate it when you fail to set goals of achievement for them. They feel lost and not as good about themselves.

Children need limits. They feel lost and afraid when they can't count on their adults to let them know when they have gone too far. Lack of limits, in fact, is so distressing for children that you must realize that permissiveness is truly a form of neglect.

I became aware that setting eating behavior standards was a particularly hard point to put across with eating when I spoke the other day to a parenting support group. The topic, of course, was feeding children. I went through my usual rap about division of responsibility in feeding, and that went down all right. And I talked about letting the child be responsible for what and how much he eats, and they did all right with that. But when I got to the part about encouraging parents to take charge of what the child should be offered to eat and when the child should be allowed to eat, people began to avoid my eyes. Suspecting something was afoot, I opened the topic up for discussion.

People had a lot of reservations about taking situational control with their children's eating. One commented, "I don't think they should have to sit at the table for a long time. I had to do that when I was little, and it was awful. If I try that with my child, he has such a fit that I don't enjoy my meal." It hadn't occurred to her that she could let him down when he finished his meal.

Another said, "My four-year-old gets so busy playing, and it is so much trouble to get her to come in for meals, that I just don't bother. And besides, mealtime is more pleasant when she isn't around."

Even the group leader, who ran a parenting class and had said earlier in the evening that she thought children needed clear limits, waffled when it came to setting clear limits and putting demands on her child about eating. She said she did make meals, but she did not expect her four-year-old to come to the table and to participate in the meal. She let him come if he wanted to and even let him take something from the table and eat it elsewhere, but she did not expect that he sit there while he ate.

I pointed out to her, and to the group as a whole, that the same principles of laying out appropriate expectations and setting reasonable limits apply to eating as to any other area of parenting. They had all grown up with *un*reasonable expectations and *un*realistic limits, and they had never made the shift in their thinking.

Negative experiences with eating in childhood do make us want to back off from the topic entirely. But being totally permissive about the issue can be as destructive as being domineering. We're talking here about teaching children to be grown up. Children who are simply allowed to do as they please with eating don't learn anything about behaving as more-mature individuals and participating appropriately in the social activity of eating.

Maybe the most powerful argument of all is a pragmatic one: Being permissive simply doesn't work. When children are allowed to wander around and eat when and where they will, they make a nuisance of themselves. Even though your intention is to "feed without guilt," sooner or later you'll get upset about the mess they make or the food they select and scatter around. One day it will get to you, and you will react by taking over their arena. "You can't have the cookie," you'll yell for no apparent logical reason, or "You can't have anything to eat right now—I just cleaned up the kitchen."

Avoid Forcing

Laying out achievable expectations about eating and setting reasonable limits on mealtime behavior is not the same thing as forcing children to eat. As we said earlier, the preschooler *wants* to get better at all that he does. Learning to come to the table and manage himself there is no exception.

Sometimes I have to help a family sort things out before they can free a preschooler up to do that. In all of the problem cases I have ever worked with, and in all of the ones I have discussed in this book, the first step in resolving the struggles around eating was establishing a clear division of responsibility in eating.

A young couple came to see me recently for advice on solving their problems with their four year old's eating. They worried about her limited food selection, and they also worried about her bad behavior at mealtime. They ate and liked a variety of nutritious food, and they found themselves cajoling her to eat. And she was playing it for all she was worth. "How many bites of broccoli before I get my cookie?" she would ask. "Do I have to eat those carrots?" And her poor parents would tell her, and she would whine.

When she behaved like that, they said they remembered the 16-year-old they had met traveling in England with his parents. He would only eat steak, and every night his parents searched out a different steak house to appease his limited palate.

The daughter had gotten to be very unpleasant to have at the dinner table. In fact, she often had a big snack around five o'clock, and then the mother felt relieved because she felt like her daughter's eating had been taken care of. I said it seemed to me the little girl was old enough to take care of her own eating. One of the ways she might decide to take care of it was to choose not to eat at dinner.

But it should *not* be her choice to eat early and eat whatever she wanted and stay away from the table. She had to adhere to the schedule her parents set for meals and snacks. She didn't have to eat, but she *did* have to come to the dinner table, and she had to be pleasant while she was there.

Put the cookie by her place, I said. And say to her, "It's up to you. You can eat it whenever you want." And pertaining to the carrots, "It's up to you. It's your dinner."

They were pleased to have a way to deal with her rudeness around food. She could learn to say "No, thank you", instead of "Aagh, that smells awful." And if she couldn't, she could miss the meal. Experiencing the consequences of her misbehavior was very important for her, because she was becoming very unpleasant to have around at mealtime. And the mother (and probably the daughter) was starting to worry that her daughter would be equally obnoxious around food when she ate at the neighbor's house.

They chuckled gleefully, anticipating the shocked expression on her face when they changed the way they operated with her eating. I hastened to tell them that they had to sit down with her and explain the new rules and the reasons for the rules. But they couldn't expect that to take care of the problem—she would still test them, and they would still have to follow through with consequences before she knew they meant what they said.

They left feeling much more optimistic than when they had come in. Suddenly, in seeing that they didn't have to get their daughter to eat, that it was *really* up to her, they freed themselves up to deal with her eating behaviors. Once they do that, I am sure they will find her food acceptance improves.

Obesity

We can't really predict adult obesity from childhood obesity until a child gets to be at least nine years old. Children have natural increases in their weight, which they later lose spontaneously. However, if a boy *suddenly* puts on a lot of weight between ages two to three years or between ages four to six years, there is an increased risk that that weight excess will be retained[9] when he gets older.

As I will explain in Helping All You Can to Keep Your Child from Being Fat (Chapter 14), you can help prevent obesity by maintaining a positive feeding relationship, by using indirect controls on eating and by giving your child freedom to move around and be physically active. The preschooler is a busy and energetic person, and you need to develop a tolerance for reasonable movement and commotion so he can get the exercise he needs to grow properly.

Generally, if a child's weight changes drastically, there is something wrong. Before you take any action, consult a pediatrician to see if you can sort out the cause. Ask to see a dietitian— not to get a diet, but to find out if there are any changes or excesses in your eating. It could be emotional, so an evaluation with a child psychologist or, even better, a family therapist might be in order. Do this, particularly, if you have recently had some major changes in your family and you all have been under stress.

If the weight gain is stress-related, perhaps you can get some help relieving stress and decrease the pressure on the child's eating. Whether you find the weight gain is stress-related or whether it is not, the eating intervention is the same. Maintain a positive feeding relationship, observing a division of responsibility in feeding. If you do that, your child will grow up regulating his food intake based as accurately as possible on his internal cues of hunger, appetite and satiety.

Even if a child is too fat, you should not try to do his job of regulating the amount he eats, nor should you put pressure on him to eat less. A preschooler is much too young to be put on a diet. It could disrupt physical and emotional growth.

It is upsetting for children to feel like they are going to go hungry and, in the long run, could make the problem worse. Children who are put on diets by their elders become preoccupied with food and learn to sneak around to get enough to eat. In the long run, they could eat more, not less.

Television

I would be remiss if I didn't introduce the topic of television in the Preschooler chapter. Above all, don't allow television at mealtime. It profoundly interferes with family social time, and with children's eating. After you get mealtime television under control, you can worry about the other negatives.

By the time they graduate from high school, kids on the average watch 15,000 hours of TV. They spend 13,000 hours in the classroom. During those hours of TV watching, they will be exposed to 350,000 commercials, 55% of which are for edibles, 65% of which are for heavily sugared products[10].

A Harvard University researcher found that children who spend more time in front of the TV set are fatter[11]. The connection may be inactivity, increased reminders to eat, or a depressing effect on basal metabolic rate from the hypnotic effect of the TV.

Too much TV is certainly to be avoided. But even moderate amounts can play havoc with trips to the grocery store. Your child will want what he sees on TV, and you'll have to decide. A lot of those food products will be things you never heard of before. You and your child will be learning about food together.

Perhaps you can use that to make positive use of TV advertising. Why not talk with your child about what will make a food worth buying, and do some investigating? You probably will disagree on some of your criteria—children think heavily sugared cereals are just fine, their parents do not. The parents get to win. However, you also can bend—sugared cereals could be all right occasionally, as are toaster pastries and some of the other weird and wondrous fabricated foods that are coming on the market. Many parents define sugared cereals and toaster pastries as dessert. (In my opinion, they really are). The important part is explaining to your child the basis for your choices.

Give me real food, any day. On the other hand, I eat some of that strange stuff from time to time myself, and some of it isn't so bad!

Your child will end his preschool years when he goes off to school. He will turn his focus outward, to friends, to teachers, to projects away from home. You'll begin to understand what the sage meant when he said, "Parenting is putting yourself out of a job."

If all has gone well these last five years, he'll be ready, and so will you, even if you do shed a tear or two about it. He'll have a good feeling about himself, and be able to manage what he needs to make it in his small world.

References

1. Baumrind, Diane. Current patterns of parental authority. Developmental Psychology 4: 1-103. 1971

2. Berger, K.S.: The Developing Person. New York, Worth, 1980.

3. Kempe, R.S. and Kempe, C.H. Child Abuse. Harvard University Press, Cambridge, MA, 1978.

4. Birch, L.L., Marlin, D.W. and Rotter, J. Eating as the "means" activity in a contingency: Effects on young children's food preference. Child Development 55:431-439, 1984.

5. Birch, L.L.: The relationship between children's food preferences and those of their parents. Journal of Nutrition Education 12:14-18, 1980.

6. Birch, L.L.: Effect of peer models' food choices and eating behavior on preschoolers' food preferences. Child Development 51:14-18, 1980.

7. Cotterman, S. No Better Gift: Nutrition for Preschoolers. Society for Nutrition Education, Oakland, CA, 1984.

8. Linscheid, T.R.: Disturbances of eating and feeding. IN Drotar, Dennis. New Directions in Failure to Thrive; Proceedings of a Conference. New York, Plenum, 1986.

9. Shapiro, L.R., Crawford, P.B., Clark, M.J., Pearson, D.J., Raz, J. and Huenemann, R.L.: Obesity prognosis: A longitudinal study of children from the age of 6 months to 9 years. American Journal of Public Health 74:968-972, 1984.

10. Rothenberg, M.B. The role of television in shaping attitudes of children. Journal of the American Academy of Child Psychiatry 22:86-87, 1983.

11. Dietz, W.H. and Gortmaker, S.L.: Do we fatten our children at the television set? Obesity and television viewing in children and adolescents. Pediatrics 75:807-812, 1985.

210

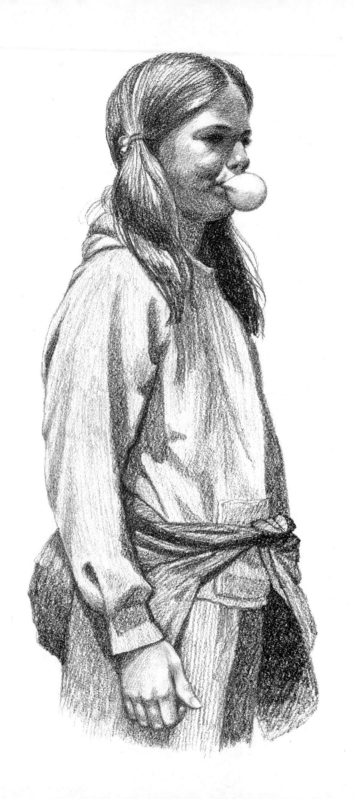

11

The Industrious
Schoolager

The connections between parenting and feeding during middle childhood are less clear and concrete than they were earlier. This is particularly true when parenting is going well and children are growing in a satisfying way.

Parents do their job in maintaining structure and providing support with feeding, children take appropriate responsibility, and feeding and eating just happens. As problems come up, like, "Can I stop at the store for a candy bar after school?" children and parents solve them with little upset, like, "It's up to you, it's your money. Just eat it early so you are hungry for your dinner."

However, when feeding problems arise, the connections become abundantly clear. The way parents operate overall is absolutely related to the way they operate with feeding. The parenting principles we talked about in the previous chapter, The Popular Preschooler, quite simply permeate everything you do

213

with your child. Children *at every age* do better when they get acceptance *and* clear limits.

Some time ago, I worked with a young family whose nine-year-old daughter was obese. They were extremely concerned about her weight, because they saw it as a total impediment to a happy life. At the time I met them, they had been attempting to intervene by holding down on the amount of food they would let her have. They dished up her plate in the kitchen, and told her she could not have second helpings.

That upset her, and the minute she saw her plate, or even before, she would start yelling and demanding more food. They would tell her no, and plead with her to stop being so naughty, and try to explain how her eating less was going to make her thin so she could be happy. She would continue to storm, and finally they would give in to her and tell her how naughty and unmanageable she was being and they would feel like she was an enormous amount of trouble and, secretly (they thought), they didn't like her very much. But of course she knew they felt that way about her—children do.

They would tell her she couldn't have snacks, and she would go in the refrigerator and get ice cream. They would catch her and tell her she couldn't have it, and she would cry and fuss and they would again plead with her, or try to placate her with an apple, or threaten her that she couldn't go to the zoo on Saturday if she didn't mind. But eventually they would give in and tell her that if she kept that up she would surely be fat and it would be her own fault.

Many of their parenting tactics put more pressure on her eating. They would reward with food, and explain difficulties she was having with her friends by blaming her weight ("If they are calling you too fat, we'll just get you thin, and then it won't be a problem.") They allowed her to wolf down her food, and labelled her "uncontrollable," because they couldn't control her.

I have worked with very similar scenarios that feature finicky children, children with diabetes, children who won't live up to the family standards about healthful eating—the list goes on and on. In every case, the problem was not only the child's eating—the problem was the parent's attitude about the child and the manner in which parenting was done. In every case, before the problems with feeding could be corrected, the parenting had to be corrected.

The School-age Child

The ages six through eleven, roughly, are the school-age years. This period can be subdivided into *early* and *late* stages.

Early School-age

The early school-age child is much like an older and more-competent preschooler. She is positive and curious and shows a great deal of initiative. She attacks a task for the pure joy of being on the move and trying out what the world has to offer. Unlike the toddler, and like the preschooler, the early school-age child is positive in her energy. If all goes well for her, she no longer shows the toddler's need to protest her independence. She *knows* she is separate, and she is out to learn—from parents, from teachers, and from other kids[1].

She is an energetic person who is busy learning and doing, and is engrossed in trying out what the world has to offer. Her surplus of energy allows her to forget setbacks, and to approach what seems desirable, even if it seems uncertain.

For the early school-age child, the emphasis is on *initiative* as she begins to develop social, physical and school skills. She engages in new situations simply for the pleasure of it. In the process, she gains an increased sense of herself, and improves her judgment about what is acceptable behavior in the many situations she encounters.

She differs from the late school-age child in the playful and enthusiastic way she approaches a task and her capability (or relative lack of it) in carrying it through to completion. For instance, in setting herself the task of straightening up her room, she may become engrossed in playing with her toys in part of the room and forget all about what she set out to do. Because her enthusiasms carry her in a variety of directions, she may need help in remembering the task at hand.

A child up to age six or seven has basic limitations in the way she thinks. She is *prelogical*. She can't understand that amount is conserved when shape changes, she can't understand gradual change, as in getting gradually older, and she can't classify things, like shapes. She is egocentric: She can't understand that someone else may have a different point of view than she does. She is less interested in how things work than in how it

215

affects her: She may believe that a toy has wheels so it will move when she pushes it. And she may believe she can cause things to happen by the way she feels: That her mother became ill because she was angry at her.

Preschoolers and early school-age children work hard at identifying—primarily with their same-sex parent, but also with both parents. The child this age explores her body, and relishes the feelings she generates with her explorations. She observes and imitates her mother to find out what it means to be female. She may be very rigid about her definition of feminine roles, and may insist that she, not her boy friend, be the one to do the cooking in her play house. Children this age persist in stereo-typed views of male and female roles, even if their parents avoid the stereotypes.

She absorbs her conscience and social and physical skills from both parents. If her process of identification goes well, she will feel secure and free to move into the outside world without always having her parents physically present.

Most times, she will feel good about herself, and compe-tent. At other times, however, she will feel less good, and dis-couraged as she becomes aware of the discrepancy between her own abilities and those of other children, especially older children.

The 5- to 7-year-old stands at the cross roads between initi-ative and guilt. If she is provided with suitable opportunities, and firmly (and tactfully) steered away from what is not suita-ble, she can come out of this period with a positive view of her-self with her delighted enjoyment and manipulation of what the world has to offer. If, however, she is repeatedly allowed to blun-der into situations that will hurt or defeat her, and then is sub-jected to criticism for her lack of judgment, she can come out of this stage feeling guilty about her curiosity and her desire to explore.

Late School-age

From about age 7 or 8 on, the child begins to harness her initiative, and begins to carry her exploration through to some sort of a conclusion or product. She becomes more diligent and systematic about pursuing a task, and is interested in its useful purpose or creating something of value. She is more persistent, and no longer gets as easily distracted by the possibilities for play in a situation. She also becomes able to evaluate her performance when she completes a task.

The school-age child values being independent of parents. She takes pride in doing the work her parents set out for her, but she prefers to do it when she is not closely supervised. She relishes a feeling of independence, but won't like it if parents cut loose of all controls or fail to recognize her achievements.

During the later elementary school years, the child needs to *achieve* to establish her worth to herself and to other people. She imitates parents, teachers and other adults she sees as being successful. Inside the family, she makes whatever contribution the family asks. If all goes well for her, she strives to please the adults in her world, and it is important to her to get recognition for her achievements. It is only when things go badly, and she is thwarted again and again in her efforts to please, that she gives up and stops caring what parents and other adults think of her.

Parents sometimes fail to recognize how important they continue to be to the late school-age child, because it is during this time she enters into a society of children. Another of her major priorities becomes achieving whatever tasks the child culture values. It is a time of having best friends, and cliques, and having things go well and being so engrossed in it all, and having things go poorly and being devastated. It is a time of games that have rules that are *followed*, and often debated and hammered out. The games deal with real-life issues, like playing on teams, and "in and out" and "tag" and "fox and goose." They delight in scaring themselves with night games like "ghost in the graveyard" and by telling scary stories.

Late school-age children become more accomplished at thinking, learning, remembering and communicating because their mental processes become less self-centered and more logical. They can tell when something is bigger or smaller than another thing, can sort objects into categories, and have an understanding of time and distance.

The joke-telling of children this age demands these thinking skills. (Telling jokes is beyond most preschool children.) They

have to know how things really *are* in order to find the humor in
a situation:

> How many balls of string does it take to reach around the
> world? (One, but it had better be a big one.)

They also have to understand words enough to play on them:

> Why didn't the woman leave the house even when a bear
> was chasing her? (Because she didn't want to be seen with a
> bare behind.)

The child ages 7 or 8 to 11 or 12 works to achieve self control, and uses techniques to help herself. She may set herself the
task of practicing the cello for fifteen minutes after school before
she has her snack, or of kicking the soccer ball for an hour every
day. After a few days, her resolve may waver, but the fact that
she makes plans at all demonstrates she is thinking about ways
to manage.
  Children use these self control techniques to wait for something they want. In one experiment, preschoolers and school-age
children were offered marshmallows: One if they wanted to eat
it right away, two if they waited for five minutes. At least half of
the preschoolers went ahead and ate. Almost all the older children waited. To help them with their waiting, they used little
mental exercises, like thinking about something else entirely,
or telling themselves the marshmallow was poison for the next
five minutes[2].
  Many late school-age children think they know more than
adults. You'll perhaps be relieved to know that this trait, which
so many parents find so obnoxious, is common enough to have a
name: cognitive conceit. If your child beats you at checkers, she
may take that as proof that she is brilliant and you are stupid.
Books popular with this age group feature clever and creative
children who help each other outwit bumbling adults—consider
Peter Pan (the children don't need parents), Nancy Drew, The
Hardy Boys, or the very popular Judy Blume books, in which
adults are peripheral and naive.
  While sexual issues are pretty much relegated to the back
burner during this time, school-age children do think about
appearance and looking good to the opposite sex. They talk
about boyfriends and girlfriends, but they really mean who

looks at whom or who talks to whom in the lunch line. Boys and girls fight, tease and harass each other—you can tell if a boy and girl are interested in each other because they *fight*.

Boys and girls break down into sex segregated groups, and it's a rare girl who will play soccer with the boys or a rare boy who will talk to the girls as they stand at the edge of the playground. Children do successfully break these rules but, to do it, they have to know how to stand up to teasing.

Children grow relatively slowly at this age, which gives them time to develop their skills and coordination. They vary greatly in their height and body shape, and are very aware of their individual differences.

The middle childhood years are rather uneventful, because a child grows (physically, intellectually and emotionally) steadily and has no big hurdles to overcome. The school years are sandwiched between the stress of the toddler and the struggles of the adolescent. But these years can make or break what has gone before.

Despite all older children's opinions to the contrary, parents continue to have an important role to play. As you move though the school years, you are less and less the star of your child's life. Friends have become the stars. You may embarrass your child if you treat her like your child, by doing things like kissing her in public or expressing concern about her. But you can, and must, work behind the scenes. In fact, you *will* work behind the scenes, and your work will benefit your child or fail to benefit her.

Parenting The School-age Child

As I prepared to write this chapter, I talked with a colleague, Dr. Erica Serlin, a child psychologist who has wonderful ability to understand the world from a kid's point of view and a knack for helping parents to do the same.

After we talked for an hour, about middle childhood—children and parents—I asked her to summarize in a sentence or two her advice about parenting a school-age child. She thought a moment, then said it seemed to her that the issue with children and parents, the same as what has gone before and what will come afterward, is *autonomy*: supporting the child in growing into a separate and independent person. Let me quote her.

"The key is to respect your child's autonomy, but don't give her so much rope that she hangs herself. You always have to balance license with security and guidance. That balance shifts as the child gains experience and capability."

First, foremost, and undergirding everything else, you help by respecting your child as an individual, by listening and appreciating what she says, and by supporting her in working things out for herself. For this child, as you have at every age up to this time, you hold back and let her take the lead. And you support that lead in appropriate ways.

The same qualities of parenting that were important at earlier stages are important now—warmth, encouragement, and authoritative guidelines without authoritarian control. Listening to the child's opinions and ideas about what she should and shouldn't be allowed to do, and explaining rules and reasons for punishment are especially important. As her ability develops to think logically about specific events, she needs to know about your logic. Instead of doing things for her, you must provide guidance and support while allowing her to think for herself.

Setting Limits

School-age children are quite capable of testing their limits. There are times she'll be angry with you, and put a lot of pressure on you. It's important for you to stand your ground, and not be intimidated by her outrage.

Some parents try to avoid a confrontation, and undermine themselves in the process, by placating and arguing and trying to persuade. If you are one of them, and can't stand up to your child, you'd better look around for causes. Maybe you are being too arbitrary and taking a stand you later find you don't want to follow through on. Maybe you can't stand emotional intensity, and you back off when the heat goes on. And maybe, under it all, you need to be needed. Promoting your child's independence is not what you *really* want. So you retreat, and say, "She is such a problem—I just don't know what to do with her!"

In all cases, the problem is that *you* don't have any real sense of limits for your child. That is serious. She won't be able to tolerate a lack of limits. She will push until she knows what the limits are—or become very frightened because she realizes there are *no* limits. Your child's respect for you hinges on her realization that you can set limits, and it will break down if you fail in this area.

If she knows you can set limits, it will free her up to learn about her world. Then, she'll need you to provide her with tasks that match her abilities, with instruction that will allow her to be successful in doing things, and with recognition when she does what she sets out to do.

Presenting Tasks

Presenting her with achievable, worthwhile tasks will take some thought. One of the prices of our changing and mobile society is that we have fewer and fewer traditions to fall back on in instructing our children. In many cultures, adults rely on children between ages 6 and 11 to perform important work: They herd cattle, or make ropes, or put in crops. There are traditions that say at what age children are ready to assume these responsibilities, and traditional ways of recognizing children when they do.

When I grew up on the farm in South Dakota, children were expected to begin gathering eggs at about age seven, helping with the milking at age 10, and with driving the tractor to do simple jobs at about the same time. Adults recognized us when we began doing these things. But most important was the tacit approval—now people relied on us to do part of the work.

It takes some planning to develop these traditions in our present families. You'll need to think through age-appropriate tasks and make sure the tasks make a real contribution. Then you'll have to develop methods that a child can use to get the job done. If you want your child to help prepare dinner, you'll need to do some menu planning to figure out what she is capable of preparing, and give her some basic lessons so she knows how to cook, and think through the timing of things. I still have a number of recipes in my file written in child language: "Take the big stainless steel pan and fill it half full of water. Put it on the big burner and turn it up to 10. . ."

The process takes time, and for a while it will probably be easier to do it yourself. The early payoff, however, is in your child's joy and pride of accomplishment. The later payoff is some genuine help in getting the household chores accomplished.

Too often, parents instruct by giving their child a task, leaving her to her own devices in figuring out how to do it, and criticizing her mistakes. That *is* a way of learning, but it is a painful and laborious way, with very little good feeling at the end.

Give positive praise when she does a reasonable job for someone her age. In *Between Parent and Teenager*, Haim Ginot[3] made quite a point of concrete praise that is specific to the situation. He recommended that a parent say, "The kitchen looks wonderful! I really like the way you cleaned it up. You even rinsed out the sink"—not, "What a good boy you are!" Ginot said if you give specific praise, children will draw their own conclusions about themselves: "What a fine fellow I am for doing such a good job."

Even praising requires you to use good judgment and sensitivity to your child's responses. If you praise too effusively, it is like saying, "I didn't think you could do it!" It also overshadows your child's inner sense of achievement, and could encourage her to work for *your* praise, not *her* own sense of pleasure and accomplishment.

You also need to maintain realistic standards, and not settle for a shoddy job. Or, at least, not praise for it. If she turns in only part of the task, praise the part of the task done well, and encourage her to finish up in the same manner.

Giving Support

The school-age child wants to solve her own problems. Kids this age have *bad* problems. I am not being facetious. Their friends mean a *great* deal to them, and when things go badly with friends, they are *very* unhappy. Sooner or later, your child will come home, and say, "Nobody is playing with me any more. Jennie and Kate are just playing with each other and they don't want me." It is a rare parent who doesn't have memories of just such an instance, and of all the hurt and painful feelings that go along with it.

The way you react can make all the difference. The best response is one that respects your child's feelings. "That must make you feel pretty bad." Then you may hear more about it. After she's told you all she wants to, ask, "What do you think you are going to do about it?" Her answers might surprise you.

She might remember that other kids have had the same problem, and think about how they have solved it. Or she might decide she is going to start playing with someone else. Or she might decide that she is going to have to play what Jennie and Kate want to play instead of insisting they play her games.

There are lots of *un*helpful ways of responding to this situation, and they are almost all based on your taking over the problem.

Nobody likes to see their child being hurt, and your first impulse will be to try to make it go away. You can insult her feelings, "Oh, that's just silly to get so upset about that. Tomorrow, you'll forget all about it." You can insult her friends, and insult her for caring about them, "Oh, who cares about them anyway? They're not very nice girls." You can encourage her to withdraw, and not try to work things out with other people, "Well, you and I will just play a game and you won't need them." Or critical, "Well, what are you doing that they don't want to play with you?"

Friends *are* important, and making it with other kids is *all* important. You need to manage your own feelings so you can recognize hers, accept her feelings and help her screw up her courage to go back out there and work it out with them. Sometimes that may require you to try to figure out what your child is doing that is calling out this response in other kids, and work with her in changing it.

Children often have an idea of what they are doing that is creating their difficulty. However, it's important to approach that topic tactfully, and to wait until you have gone through all the other steps to do it. Otherwise you'll just be critical and taking over, and neither one will help your child.

For the most part, it is best if you don't get directly involved. Whenever you fix things, your child misses an opportunity to grow.

Feeding The School-age Child

The themes of the school-age child play themselves out in eating, as well as in every other area of her life. She will be as curious and enthusiastic about her eating as she is about everything else. As she gets older, she will work toward competence with food and eating, again, the same as with everything else.

223

During the school-age years, you begin to reap the benefits (or the bitter harvest) of all that has gone before with feeding. If you have supported your child's individuality in feeding and growth, and provided firm and consistent structure, she will arrive at her elementary school years with a positive attitude and the ability to take care of her food needs in a matter-of-fact fashion at the same time that she explores and continues to grow in that area.

She will assume that there will be a family meal, that she will be at it, and that she will be pleasant while she is there. She will be reasonably adept at joining in mealtime sociability and pretty good at using eating utensils. She will eat in a business-like and reasonably orderly fashion, she will accept most foods she is offered, and will know how to turn down the rest, politely. And she will value working at and improving all these skills, the same as she does every other facet of her life.

If your child is not able to do these things, you may have to go all the way back to toddler limit-setting to right the situation. And ignoring a seven-year-old who is having a tantrum is a lot harder and more aggravating than ignoring a two-year-old doing the same thing.

With eating, you encourage a child's initiative by increasingly letting her pick her own snacks. The younger school-age child will still depend on you to be there to help prepare the snack and to keep her company while she eats. The older school-age child will want to do more of the planning and preparations herself, but will still appreciate knowing you're there, and benefit when you make yourself available for conversation during snack time. Even if your child is pretty independent with snacking, you set limits by letting her know *when* you expect her to eat her snacks and by maintaining meals.

Feeding still demands a division of responsibility between you and your child: You/what, she/how much. You are still the primary food planner and the gatekeeper on what foods come, in quantity, into the house.

Responsibility for meals will start to shift. As you approach the later end of this period, you may share with your child in the preparation of breakfast as she gets her own cereal and toast in the morning. You provide structure by seeing that the food is there, and, very importantly, by eating breakfast yourself and by taking a few minutes in the morning to connect with your child and her schedule. You'll be involved in planning, and maybe packing, lunch. Dinners can still be a family meal, and should be. But she will take over with getting her snacks, and she will regulate the eating she does away from home.

Meals

I hope you are having family meals. I hope it a lot, and I admire you if you are doing it. I know it is hard, with busy family schedules and all the demands put on you. But if you're not having meals, do try to start during these school-age years.

School-age children are still small and dependent enough to be worried if you don't look out for them. They may not show it, but they do worry if there aren't meals, or if the meal times are erratic. They wonder if they are going to be fed, and their concern makes it hard for them to move on to their other tasks.

You have to make time for your child during this stage if she is to make time for you later on. Soon she will be a teenager, and the ritual of meals can help carry you through all that will involve. It will give you a chance to see her and give you all an anchor when she is struggling for independence and identity as much as she will be then. But it will be too late to start the ritual then, when you need it. You have to start early.

Children who eat meals do better nutritionally than children who merely snack, and the nutrients they miss out on are vitamins A and C: vegetables and fruit[4]. Children who eat meals are better at liking and managing a variety of food. They know how to conduct themselves in polite company, and they take pride in their eating skills.

School-age children are more restful to have at the table than children who have gone before. They are more coordinated, and you'll have less spills and messes. You may even begin to leave the roll of paper towels in the kitchen.

They don't exactly sit *still*, however, especially when they are six. For some reason, six-year-olds have more skill than anyone else at moving around on a chair and moving a chair around on a floor. Constantly. A sense of humor, and the patience to wait until it passes, seem to be the only solutions to this entertaining problem.

Be realistic in your expectations. Children under age ten still use their fingers quite a lot in ways that adults don't, like

225

pushing peas onto a spoon and picking up pieces of meat. They still have some trouble chewing and swallowing tough or dry or fibrous foods, like steak or chops.

Part of the problem might be that they don't have the jaw strength to chew up the meat (although their ability to manage bubble gum belies this theory). Another part is that up until about age eight their swallow is immature. They swallow with their cheeks, as if they were sucking from a straw, not using their tongues, like you and I do.

Children this age still have a limited number of foods they readily accept. Do not despair. The number of accepted foods will gradually increase as they get older. The numbers will increase—that is, provided you don't make a big issue about it. Then they will not increase. In fact, they will probably decrease.

It is important that your child comes to the table hungry. By the time she gets to middle childhood, she will be able to learn how to control her hunger and wait for the meal to be ready. She can develop strategies to help her with that, like going away from where food is being prepared, or by thinking about something other than how hungry she is. It's important for her to learn that skill, because if she's hungry when she approaches a meal, the food will taste better to her and she'll be more inclined to eat, and enjoy, foods that are not her favorites.

But even if mealtime is pleasant, out playing with the other kids is where she would rather be. Especially in the summer, your child might rush through her meal so she can get back out to play. Try asking her to stay at the table and socialize for a certain length of time—maybe 20 minutes— whether she eats or not. (That will also provide you with a comeback when she tells you she's not hungry and she doesn't want her dinner.) Of course, the next move is yours. If you ask for sociability, you have to *give* sociability, and make the table a pleasant place to be.

Do not criticize. Recognize positive eating, and wait for the rest to happen. If parents criticize (even about non-food behavior) and mealtimes are tense, it will show up in a child's eating. Studies have shown that children eat less and do not do as well nutritionally when they are catching a lot of criticism from their parents—on any topic, not just on eating[4].

While nagging and criticism don't work for improving mealtime behaviors, consequences do. If you are setting reasonable expectations, and your child is being unpleasant at the table, ask her to leave, and don't let her have anything to eat until the next regularly scheduled feeding time. Let her know ahead of time about the mealtime expectations, and what will happen if she doesn't comply. If you are prompt about handing out consequences, she'll know you mean business. If you protect the quality of *your* mealtime, in the long run she'll value her meals more, and take responsibility for governing her own behavior while she is there.

The family needs to be functioning well in order for feeding to be going well. That means that parents have to be doing well with each other. If there is a lot of tension and dissatisfaction between parents, they don't do as well with providing food and modeling appropriate eating behaviors, and children don't eat as well[5]. Also, in studies where parents were very permissive about eating, the nutritional quality of children's diets decreased[6].

Older children start to have their opinions about what they like to eat, and you'll find yourself getting advice and suggestions and even criticism about the food you prepare. Here is where you start to teach tact. It is also where you start to teach meal planning and cooking.

Why not take advantage of some of that industry and world experience to get some help with the chores? Your child this age can help with planning menus and food preparation. You can make it something fun that you can do together, and in the process teach her to cook. And *him*, too, for that matter. Boys benefit as much as girls from accumulating food-preparation skills.

Single Parenting

When you are the only adult in the household, it is tempting to cook to please the kids. That is a mistake. A perfectly understandable one, but a mistake, none the less.

When there are two adults in the household, you tend to cook for yourselves, and each other, and give secondary attention to the kids' preferences. That's the way it should be. They are, after all, the kids, and their job is to fit into *your* household, not vice versa. (Obviously, this whole philosophy can be taken to the extremes of neglect and even child abuse. But taken appropriately, it can be pretty relieving to a child to be allowed to be, simply, a child.)

227

As the only adult, it still is most important that you cook to please yourself. Give yourself the same care and concern with meal planning and preparation that you would if you were cooking for two adults. And let the kids pick and choose from what is available. They need that approach to learn to eat a variety of food and to conduct themselves appropriately at mealtime.

I think you'll find if you don't get started catering to their wishes, it won't be an issue. They will just think that that is the way it is done. If you've been catering to them, you might have to sit down and have a talk with them before you swing things back the other way again.

I am well aware of the reasons for cooking to please the children: over the short run, the kids eat better and there is less wasted food. It is easier to avoid hassles over mealtime behavior if they like what you cook. And so on. But as a single parent, you still have to set limits and teach appropriate behavior. You can deal with all those difficulties, and in the long run, it will be better for you all if you make yourself, not them, the priority when it comes to planning meals.

Snacks

Increasingly your child will have opportunities to eat in places besides home. She'll begin to make choices about her money, and often want to buy snacks with it. And sometimes snacks are things you may not approve of, like candy or snack cakes or potato chips.

All that interest in snack food is coming from the all-important peer culture. It doesn't work to get hard-nosed about forbidding snacks you don't approve of, because it puts your child in a bind: Does she go along with you and be a "baby" in the other kids' eyes, or does she defy you and risk your wrath and give up on getting any help from you? Your child this age is going to have enough of a challenge figuring out how to get along with her friends and how to be successful without selling herself out. She doesn't need showdowns with you.

Between you, you should be able to figure something out. You can let her know you don't want her spoiling her dinner with snacks, and suggest a time limit on how late she can have a snack and still be hungry for dinner. You can remind her that she's eating too many candy bars—and suggest alternatives that are more nutritious, but still acceptable in kids' eyes.

There are real options, even with candy—some kinds are more nutritious than others. (There are some suggestions in "Choosing Nutritious Snacks," in the "Tools and Strategies" section at the end of the book.) She'll be learning about nutrition in school, and you can encourage her to think about what she has learned when she makes her choices.

Experimenting With Eating

They all laughed at me when we went to the office picnic and my then ten-year-old-son ate six snow cones. "The dietitian's son," they chortled, "and he eats like that." I don't know if his being my son had anything to do with it, but I do know that that kind of behavior is pretty typical of the school-age child.

Elementary school children are learning about food regulation. Part of that is eating too much, and even stuffing, on foods that are ordinarily available in limited amounts. From that they learn that some is good, but enormous quantities are not necessarily any better. They learn what their limits are, and they make some fine adjustments in their ability to regulate their food intake.

Fluctuations In Appetite

Like younger and older children, sometimes the school-age child eats a little, sometimes a lot. Fatigue, excitement, and vigorous activity can all interfere with food intake. For instance, your child will start to play sports, and you'll find that a game right before a meal will interfere greatly with her appetite.

Ask her to come to the table, even if she isn't hungry. She may eat a little. But it may also take her an hour or two to get hungry after she quiets down. Continue to schedule a regular snack for this older child, and let her have as much to eat as she wants at snack time. If your child regularly snacks instead of eating her meals, however, you may have to talk about it with her and put some limits on snacking.

Finickiness

Very finicky children start to have trouble when they begin to eat in public. It's hard to know how other kids will react to

229

finickiness—they might think it's cool or they might think it's babyish, which is the WORST thing of all. However they react, it will become a problem to your child, and she will need some help with it.

If you are matter-of-fact and respectful about your child's finickiness (or of anything else about her), you are halfway there. And so is she. She won't be touchy when kids tease her about it, and they will lay off. (It may seem like school-age children are little savages who pick on each other about any weakness. Some of them are. But if you look at that behavior in another way, children can be little psychotherapists who help each other change, or help each other develop a thick skin about their idiosyncrasies. If your child feels comfortable about herself, she won't let the teasing get her goat.)

She'll also, maybe with your help, think of ways to be discreet and tactful in handling her food preferences, rather than being awkward and calling a lot of attention to herself. And maybe she will be able to hear your suggestion that she try a little bit of the foods she doesn't like, and over a long time she might get so she can eat them.

You may think I am soft on finickiness. I'm not, if it is the kind of contrived finickiness where a child is just jerking you around at the table, getting you to short order cook for her just for the joy of dominating the situation. Or where you are over babying her with food because you need to be needed. But I *am* soft on finickiness if it means taking a child's word for it if she says she really doesn't like something.

Some people seem to start out in the world with an exquisitely developed sense of taste (and caution), and it is very painful for them to try to eat something they don't like. That is more of a handicap for the child than an aggravation for her parent. She needs help with learning to live with that kind of a sensitivity, not criticism for having it. Maybe she'll even parlay it into something wonderful, like becoming a great restaurateur.

You keep a child from being capriciously or manipulatively finicky by presenting food to her in a neutral fashion so she can approach it and find out about it at her own speed. Give her the same consideration in planning menus that you do the rest of the family—put on a variety of food, don't offer substitutes, and let her pick and choose from what is available. Left to her own devices, she will most likely gradually increase the variety of food she eats. But don't hover, or you will be hovering for a long time.

As I said earlier, you work behind the scenes, but sometimes you have to help more directly. One of my friends called for advice the other day about helping her seven-year-old son, Tom, with a school lunch situation. Tom has quite a long list of foods he doesn't like and she has been respecting his preferences. Some days they order school lunch, some days they pack a lunch. It was working until the lunch room supervisors become aware of his pickiness, and took it upon themselves to make him change. They started to put a lot of pressure on him to eat his food, and even refused to let him go outside until he finished.

There is nothing worse for a seven-year-old. Those supervisors were separating him out and treating him like a *baby*, reducing him in his friends' eyes and depriving him of their company. Wisely, the mother recognized he needed help and saw that he got it. Together, they talked to the principal and finally to the supervisors, and they reached an agreement. Tom would taste his food, and that was enough. The supervisors were to take his word for it when he said he had tasted everything.

School Lunch

School lunch can be good, or bad, or come out some place in the middle. If you are fortunate (or if you have worked hard to achieve it), your school will have a high quality program that serves tasty, attractive food. Good school lunch programs have pleasant settings with short lines, ample time to eat, and accepting and supportive supervisors. Poor school lunch programs don't have the amenities, but federal regulations assure that they at least have nutritious food.

Even if it's good, your child will have complaints about school lunch food—it's one of those kid-culture traditions. And she'll have outrageous rumors, like, "Did you hear they use kangaroo meat for their hamburgers?" (When it starts out "Did you hear" I always perk up my ears. The food rumor I like the best is, "Did you hear about the guy who opened a can of peaches and found a thumb?")

"Ugh!" "Gross!"

But, I digress.

Good nutrition is the real objective, and the reason to

231

encourage your child to participate and to moderate your own criticism, even if the program isn't very good. I'm not suggesting you try to talk your child out of her dissatisfaction. Acknowledge that the food isn't always the best, but make the point that it *is* nutritious and it *does* give her a chance to try some foods that she might not otherwise. School lunch menus have to conform to certain nutritional standards. Home packed meals, on the average, are less nutritious and have less variety.

Children can be exposed to new foods at school lunch, and the more foods they learn to handle, the more comfortable they will be in the world. Even learning to live with less-than-delicious food has something to offer. She won't always be home with your good cooking. If she learns to eat institutional food in grade school, she'll be all set to go off to college and live in the dorm—or to military service—or to a hospital. I have seen too many adults in hospitals who haven't been able to do that. They have behaved very badly when they have been confronted with food that doesn't meet their standards.

During the early years, you might ask her to take school lunch a certain number of days a week. Later on, you can let her decide how to handle it. If you have been talking about it, she will know what the issues are, and she'll be able to make up her own mind.

Don't Be Too Protective

It doesn't do your child any favors to baby her with food. I know some people who were worried about taking their children to Europe because they were afraid they couldn't eat the food there. Those are the fruits of a lifetime of being over concerned and over solicitous about children's food acceptance.

There is room in feeding for benign neglect. I previewed a movie on feeding young children with a friend of mine the other day. After a while she said, "For heavens' sakes! Did you hang over your children like that when they ate?" I allowed as how I hadn't—I was always too busy eating my own meal. The parents were being very attentive, watching and admiring every bite the children ate.

I thought of that interchange a few days later when our family went to Ginza of Tokyo for dinner. We had Japanese onion soup and salad with ginger dressing and hibachi chicken with sesame and mushrooms, and the vegetables on the side were mushrooms and summer squash and bean sprouts. And we all ate and enjoyed it enormously and commented on the food.

When we finished, a woman across the table from us said, "My, your children eat well." I was quite startled, because it hadn't occurred to me to think about it. I was enjoying my meal, and if they didn't like it they knew what they could do about it.

(If they don't like something, they don't eat very much. They don't make a fuss about it and neither do I. They seem very relaxed about under eating and seem to know that they will make up for it at meal time or snack time. Since we haven't made a big deal about their eating or not eating, it doesn't worry them or put pressure on them when they encounter food they don't like.)

Dieting

The dieting craze has reached into grade school. A study done in the San Francisco Bay area showed that almost half of the nine-year-old girls and close to 80% of the 10- and 11-year-old girls studied were dieting to lose weight[7].

You don't have to go along passively with this. You can use some of the same techniques you have used before—find out what your child is thinking and how she's feeling, give her a reality check, let her know *your* view of the situation, and maintain the same guidelines on eating as before. Ideally, you will be pretty relaxed and accepting of your body, and hers as well.

Children toward the end of the school-age period begin to look in the mirror a lot, and wonder what mother nature will do for them. Your encouraging her to hang in there, and wait to see how her body turns out will be a real help.

Children almost all gain fat as they approach puberty. Some get quite chubby. Don't over react to that, and encourage her not to over react, either. That is a common and normal part of her growth process. She has a very good chance of losing her extra fat as she goes into her growth spurt.

Don't put pressure on her weight, and don't let anyone else do it either. If your child is plumping up, warn the medical people ahead of time that they are NOT to say anything about it to her when she goes in for her camp physical.

233

To a great extent, the way your child gets along in the world will be determined by your parenting. You teach her attitudes about herself and other people, you set up the home environment where she can learn to work things out with her brothers and sisters, you model relationships with other people, you set limits that are reasonably in line with those of other parents', and you provide backup and support when she has difficulty.

I can't overemphasize the importance of letting your child take the lead during middle childhood. There are grave consequences if you try to take over. In the process you will interfere with her self-development and pleasure in learning new skills and responsibilities. If you over-manage, a child may become withdrawn and too compliant. She may decide, "OK, if you're going to take charge, I'll just let you. I won't take any responsibility." Or she may become openly defiant, and fight you every step of the way.

Children may go along, and not say much, but inside of them they are very angry at what you are doing, and hurt that you treat them in such a disrespectful fashion. They will find a way to make you pay dearly for your actions: by becoming exactly the kind of person you assume they are. Unfortunately, that way makes them pay most dearly of all.

If you operate in a peremptory fashion, chances are you won't have too many problems when your child is young. Preschoolers and school-age children, for the most part, respect their parents' authority and try to please. But when your child becomes a teenager, the feathers will hit the fan. Then all the pent-up feelings and frustration will come bursting out along with adolescent rebelliousness, and you will have a *real* problem on your hands.

References

1. Erikson, E.H.: Childhood and Society. W.W. Norton, New York, 1950.

2. Berger, K.S.: The Developing Person. Worth, New York, 1980.

3. Ginot, H.G. Between Parent and Teenager. Avon, New York, 1969.

234

4.   Pipes, P.L. Nutrition in Infancy and Childhood, Times Mirror/Mosby, St. Louis, 1985.

5.   Kinter, M., Boss, P.G. and Johnson, N.: The relationship between dysfunctional family environments and family member food intake. Journal of Marriage and the Family 43:633-641, 1981.

6.   Eppright, E.S. Eating behavior of preschool children. Journal of Nutrition Education 1:16, 1969.

7.   Mellin, L. Disordered eating characteristics in preadolescent girls. Presentation, The American Dietetic Association Annual Meeting, 1986.

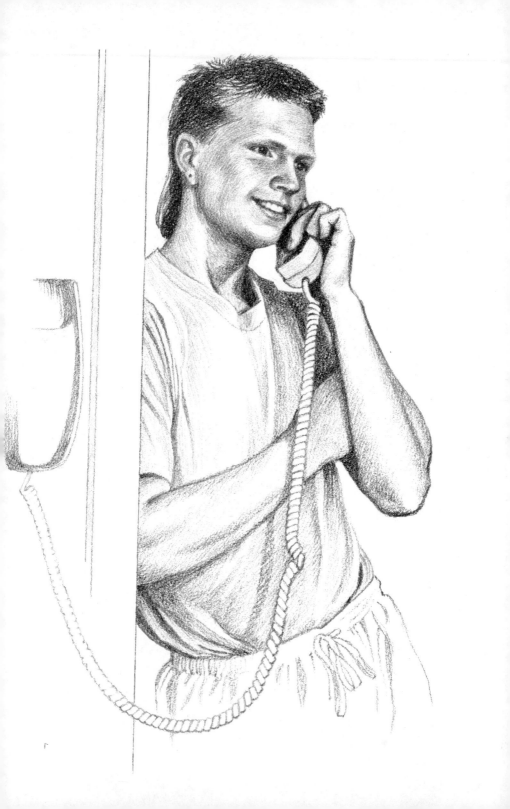

12

The Individualistic Teenager

Someone said that an adolescent is a toddler with hormones and wheels. It feels like that at times—the difference being that when you go toe-to-toe and lay down the law with an adolescent, you have to look UP to look him straight in the eye. Someone *else* said the only way to deal with adolescents is to bury them when they are 12 and dig them up when they are 21. Which, unfortunately, is an all-to-common view of the hopelessness of dealing with kids this age.

Teenagers are not as bad as they say. Teenagers are even good. Even delightful, at times. Maybe beauty is in the eye of the beholder. *I* think teenagers are delightful. They have so much energy and humor and such a stimulating view of things. In fact, as my children get older, I keep adjusting my estimate upward of what is the very nicest age a child can be.

But we must be realistic. Stress levels in both parents and children are the highest during adolescence[1]. Marital satisfaction, which starts to dip with the birth of the first child, declines even further during adolescence, although it doesn't dip as far if parents feel they are being generally successful with their child. It isn't until the nest empties out that marital satisfaction again improves[2].

237

Even with these negative reviews, like the stories about the terrible twos, the stories about adolescents are much exaggerated. The stories got started, of course, by adults who expected adolescents to be little grownups and who wanted to have the final say on how the younger generation should conduct their affairs. The stories got supported by early researchers and psychotherapists whose clients were the ones people were most likely to notice: the adolescents who were disrespectful, disturbed and delinquent. They saw the problem cases. It's no wonder they saw the teen years as a time of *storm and stress*[3].

These descriptions hung on until twenty years ago, when studies began of large groups of ordinary teenagers. Those studies showed that, taken as a whole, adolescents are *not* in turmoil, *not* deeply disturbed, *not* at the mercy of their impulses, *not* resistant to parental values, *not* politically active, and *not* rebellious[4].

Some teenagers are, and some aren't, having trouble. One study that followed boys throughout their teen years[5] showed that about a fifth of the boys experienced *tumultuous* growth—the turbulent, crisis-filled maturation that we all hear about. Another fifth experienced *continuous* growth—"a smoothness of purpose and self-assurance" and a "mutual respect, trust and affection" between them and their parents.

A third of the boys experienced *surgent* growth. They were reasonably well adjusted and coped with the tasks of adolescence quite well, but they also went through times when they were angry and retreated from growing up. But they came out of retreat, and moved on again, working on coping with the increased demands their bodies and their cultures placed on them. (The rest of the boys were put in a "mixed" group and showed combinations of patterns.)

The Adolescent

The basic themes of adolescence are *autonomy* and *identity*. The adolescent grows rapidly toward being an adult physically, emotionally and functionally. Early in adolescence, the major sub-theme is *autonomy*, as a child focuses on peers and learning to make it in a teenage world. Later in adolescence, the sub-theme is *identity*: taking on a more adult identity and learning the skills that are necessary to make it in the adult world.

Early Adolescence

Early on, roughly ages 12 through 16, everything about the adolescent is subject to change. His body develops very rapidly, and it quite simply disorganizes everything about him. His hormone levels shoot up, and along with that comes insistent sexual feelings. As his body changes, he has to cope with a new size and shape and distressing side effects, like transitory breast formation and pimples.

Typically, his hands and feet get longer before his arms and legs do, and his torso is the last part to grow. His nose, lips and ears usually grow before his head does. A fourteen-year-old boy may worry that his nose is the only part of him that is getting any bigger. Little wonder that it is rather terrifying to have to wait and see how it will all turn out.

His world changes. He may go off to a new middle school or a new junior high, where all the rules of socializing are different, from the way you treat a teacher to what you do on the playground at recess. If there even is a recess.

Between 11 and 13 or 14, adolescents start not feeling as good about themselves. They become more self conscious, their good (and bad) feelings about themselves come and go, and their overall self esteem goes down significantly. But by about fifteen, most measures of self confidence start to improve, and between 16 and 18, kids start feeling even better about themselves than they did in middle childhood[6].

Physical changes put enormous pressure on the adolescent, especially the one who is out of sync with the other kids. Girls who mature early and boys who mature late are likely to be particularly distressed by their physical development, or lack of it. Children who are relatively fat, or thin in what they consider an unattractive way, feel the same.

Early-maturing girls might be perceived as boy-crazy and snobbish by their classmates as their sexual maturation and interests carry them beyond the level of the other girls. But later, as the others catch up, the early ones are able to share their worldly wisdom and help their friends learn about bras and their periods.

For boys, however, it is a different problem, and one that can hang on beyond the adolescent years. The boy who matures late may feel less capable than his friends, self conscious, and

239

out of the social main stream. It's important to help this child find ways of feeling successful, or those limitations on his self esteem can last for life. Indeed, there are many reasons for the late-maturing boy to feel successful: he is likely to be more playful, creative and flexible, all certainly attractive qualities[7].

The early adolescent has matured considerably in his thinking from his preschool and elementary school years. He is able to be logical and imaginative, and he can tell the difference between what is hypothetical and what is real.

But his thinking also has some limitations. One of them is egocentrism. He thinks he is unique among people. While he recognizes the fact that others have similar experiences, he believes there is something about his particular experience that sets it apart from all others. It is egocentrism that makes the adolescent believe that his parents can't possibly know what it feels like to be in love. The same process convinces him that, while other kids may have car accidents, it can't possibly happen to him.

The young adolescent acts as if he is on stage and the whole rest of the world is his audience. He thinks that everyone else is paying as close attention to him as he pays to himself. The adolescent also has personal fables—he spins fantasies of great fame or fortune. He has the unique ability both to imagine many logical possibilities and also to deny reality when it interferes with his hopes and fantasies.

As a child gets older, he overcomes these limitations in thinking. In the meantime, though, he has to be protected against some of the dangers that these limitations offer. He may be convinced, for instance, that he alone can ride his bike at night without having need for a reflector. He may think his parents are totally crazy to insist on it, and will be angry when they do. He will just have to feel that way, and later, when he develops more mature judgment, he can make the decision for himself.

In early adolescence, some teachers feel like they are really up against it. Others enjoy the adolescent's willingness to speak out and be intrigued by social, political and moral issues. (Some, like the rest of us, feel both ways.) In the adolescent view, the *really* important issues of life revolve around what goes on in school. The pressures of peer culture carry the day. Kids worry about appearance, personality, their strengths and weaknesses, and their relationships with their parents and the other kids.

240

They feel that they think about sex too much, and some worry that they are sex crazy. The boys can get an erection at any moment, and they worry that they will have a visible erection at the swimming pool or when they are standing in front of the class. Girls worry that they will let their sexual interest show too much—or too little.

Everybody worries about their sexual appearance—girls are concerned about the size and shape of their breasts, boys worry about their height and muscles and the size of their genitals. Greetings from friends in the high school annual during the freshman year are totally raunchy—"Are you going to get laid this summer? Haw, haw, haw." For most of them, it's all talk, but some of the kids do become sexually active at ages 13 or 14 or even earlier.

Late Adolescence

In late high school, the annuals are considerably tamer, as sex becomes a more *real* possibility and at the same time kids begin thinking of the future, if only with tongue in cheek: "I wish you luck in the five B's of life: bikes, broads, beans, beer and brats*." They start to think seriously about their sexual morals, as they are starting to pair off and establish longer-term relationships with the opposite sex.

The high school upper classman wants to fit himself into the world, while at the same time he establishes a sense of himself as a unique person. In the process of "finding themselves," adolescents must establish a sexual, moral, political, and vocational identity that is stable and mature. If things go well, the adolescent will accept some of his parents' values and goals but reject others.

Older adolescents begin breaking away from home, and moving toward their future. They struggle with how to be close with people without being bound to them, and how to let go without rejecting them. That is a struggle that can continue throughout life.

---

*Brats: Not a pejorative name for children, but a German sausage popular in Wisconsin.

241

Why Parents Don't Like The Teen Years

Both early and late, adolescents have some characteristics that may make them less attractive to their parents than they were earlier. They may have mood swings that shift from euphoric to despondent. It may be difficult for them to make decisions, and they can become extremely frustrated when they are confronted with a choice.

They may shift between autonomy and dependence, one day insisting on being out in the world and doing things their own way, the next day coming back and wanting to be guided. More often than not, however, the advice won't be taken—nothing seems to suit.

Is this starting to sound a lot like the rapprochement of the toddler period? Very much the same process is taking place: The adolescent is trying to cope emotionally with the dilemma of being separate—but being attached, of being let go—but not abandoned.

Adolescents are extremely sensitive to criticism—any but the most tactful of suggestions is likely to provoke a hurt reaction. At the same time, *they* are very critical. They have to assert their own selves and ideas, and the first step in that process is to *tear down* what has gone before. The next step is to build their own.

Adolescents are more of a challenge to raise because they challenge *us*. You'll delight in your teenagers' energy and curiosity and sense of humor, and despair in his ability to find all the weaknesses in your character and inconsistencies in your reasoning. He will pin you to the wall if you are being illogical and challenge you absolutely if you are being arbitrary. He will *hate* you if you are being a jerk, but at the same time desperately want you to keep on trying to work it out with him.

Despite all the struggles, most young people have considerable respect for their parents as individuals[8]. They wish their parents and they agreed more about some of their issues, but generally their disagreements are on finer points rather than overall persuasions. For instance, the adolescent and his parents might disagree on whether he shall attend or cut study hall, but he will be likely to do well in school if his parents value an education.

For some adolescents and parents, the time is simply

242

awful. It isn't that adolescents suddenly turn on their parents and become different people when they hit thirteen. In families that produce troubled adolescents, problems of interaction have always been there, they just become apparent during this stage.

Parents have to be doing well with each other in order for them to do well with parenting their adolescent. Parents have to talk things out, and back each other up in dealing with the challenges adolescents present. If they don't talk, or don't agree, they can't be helpful. As at earlier ages, if parents undermine each other, the child will simply do as he wants (or do the best he can).

The adolescent can easily become a scapegoat. His trials and challenges make him a ready target, and any tensions in the parents' relationship can easily be displaced on to him. His habit of challenging his parents' ideas makes that even more likely.

Little children believe everything about their parents is right. School age children preserve many of the same ideas, and are so busy with their friends they don't bug their parents. Much. But adolescents have the insight and world experience to see their parents in a wider view, and if parents behave in such a way that gives kids no choice but to either accept their parents' values or reject them, the situation can get very grim.

I have been amused at times, but more often saddened, to see kids who have seemingly gotten along well during their growing-up years, begin to act out in some pretty alarming ways when they have become teenagers. They start out by flaunting hours and school responsibilities and family limits. If parents don't react in a helpful way at that level, they increase the pressure. They get into drugs and alcohol and sex and start doing things to assert themselves that really hurt them a lot. And they look very lonely.

The other kids who concern me are the ones who are oh, so good, who turn out just like their very controlling and careful and moralistic parents. These seem like just as much of a loss to me. I see the liveliness and sparkle of their middle childhood start to fade and they turn into guarded people who are very careful about doing the right thing.

While the rebellion looks more alarming, both are very costly in human terms. Whether an adolescent spends his time reacting against adult authority or submitting himself to it and

243

striving to please, he won't be asserting himself and growing up to be his own person. He will fail himself in some essential parts of his development.

Parenting The Adolescent

The theme for parenting during adolescence is, "Oh, no, *now* what am I going to do?" Your teenager will present you with difficult and terrifying issues—drinking, sex, drugs, driving. None of these dilemmas had easy answers for us when we were growing up, and our kids, if anything, have even more pressures. Teachers surveyed thirty years ago about their classroom concerns said their biggest problems were smoking in the rest rooms, running in the halls and gum chewing. Teachers surveyed currently said their concerns were drugs and alcohol, school dropouts, and teen suicide.

The real theme for parenting during adolescence is *teaching responsibility*. By now, you are beginning to understand what I meant back in The Popular Preschooler (Chapter 10) when I said effective parenting is putting yourself out of a job. Once he hits adolescence, your child is approaching the time when he'll have to be ready to go on his own. When he leaves home, he'll have no limits except for the ones he sets for himself. But he hasn't left home yet. There is still work to do.

Adolescents think they should have every freedom, be given every privilege, and can handle any situation. Parents don't. The solution to the dispute is letting the child gradually earn his privileges as he demonstrates he can handle them.

Adolescents want to drive, they want to set their own hours, they want the freedom to decide where they will go and with whom. They want to go to school mixers and rock concerts and movies and the shopping malls with their friends. To be allowed to do those things, they have to demonstrate they can handle themselves in the relative freedom of unstructured situations.

For instance, a teenager who wants to go hang out at the shopping mall is going to have to demonstrate that he considers it important to be courteous to the other people there, that he can respect property, and that he can separate himself from anyone who is up to no good, like shoplifting. If he wants to go to rock concerts, he'll have to demonstrate that he is capable of staying away from the drugs and alcohol there.

Driving carries with it a whole host of attitudes and responsibilities. He has to be able to resist drugs and alcohol. He has to be willing to accept authority and not get angry with other drivers who do dumb things. He has to be able to contain his impulses and plan ahead and not get in dangerous situations that are avoidable. He has to be willing and able to put gas in the car (or provide work to pay for gas) and take care of simple problems, like flat tires and stalled engines.

He has to demonstrate he'll respect your property, and take good care of the car when he's driving it. If he demonstrates those capabilities, you provide the opportunity to share the family car.

The key is *talking*. Share your thinking and your feelings with your adolescent about how he operates. Let him know about your concerns. Find out from him how he sees himself operating, and check your own thinking to find out if your concerns are justified. Let him know what you want from him and why.

If you do all that, his options will be clear to him, and he'll be able to make up his own mind. You will be able to avoid either being neglectful, and just letting him find his own way, or being arbitrary, and ordering him around.

Parenting in this way is the adolescent variant of the authoritative parenting we talked about earlier. This kind of parenting includes a real sensitivity to the child's feelings and needs, and a respect for him as a person, as well as a willingness to set firm, realistic and intelligible limits.

Dr. Melinda Bailey, a clinical psychologist who has had much experience with adolescents and has a great appreciation for them, summarized for me what she saw as the essential issues in parenting the adolescent. Her answer, in different words, came out sounding remarkably like what Dr. Serlin said about the school-age child in the last chapter. "Being a good parent to the adolescent is continuing to be present and taking an active interest without being overly critical or intrusive. It is vital to continue to establish appropriate boundaries and to offer guidance and support."

During the teen years, you continue to teach and guide your child, building on the foundation of instruction and interaction that has gone before. The way you *treat* your child is the most powerful part of the instruction, as it has been at all previous times. Your attitude of respect and interest and your willingness to play a supportive, rather than a controlling role, will have an enormous impact on the way you and your child feel about each other.

You will also powerfully teach and guide with your own behavior. Your adolescent can start to visualize himself moving in your kind of world. You teach with direct instruction—It's vital to be *truly* instructive, and not just critical. Finally, you teach and guide by setting limits. It's here you teach your child to limit his impulses in deference to other people and to hazards in the world around him. You have to set limits, in order for your child to gain an inner sense of his ability to get along with other people.

You teach your adolescent about feelings in much the same way that you teach about behavior. If you regard feelings as important, and consider feelings in the same matter-of-fact way that you consider everything else about a situation, your adolescent will too. And he will benefit in more ways than anyone can count. He'll learn to express his feelings openly, and in tactful and respectful ways.

He'll be able to hear and respect others when they share their feelings. And together, they'll be able to work out solutions that are satisfactory to both, and in the process gain greater respect and trust.

Being able to deal openly with feelings has, quite simply, everything to do with being comfortable in the world and getting emotional needs met.

When the growing-up process goes reasonably smoothly, it is hardly noticeable. Adolescents take pretty readily to their responsibilities and take pride in managing well (and so do parents). They often take the lead in mastering more grown-up skills and handling the challenges of their world.

It's when the process *doesn't* go well that you have to be aware of it and have to develop more clear expectations. A kid who is defiant, or arrogant, or sneaky will do things his own way no matter how anybody else feels about it. There are some real consequences for operating that way. In the long run, his undesirable methods will catch up with him and he won't be very successful in life, and it won't be very satisfying for him to

246

work things out with other people. In the short run, you can see to it that he doesn't get the privileges he wants until he comes up with more positive ways of operating.

Earning privileges demands willingness to talk about what's coming up, to work out arrangements with you, and to adhere to whatever limits you have set. If all has gone well during the early years, those attitudes and behaviors will be in place. If they are not, you're going to have to work on them. During adolescence, especially early adolescence, you have your last chance to change negative patterns before they harden into adult characteristics. If you let your child get around you to get what he wants, rather than working things out with you, he will use the same attitudes and behaviors to get around his wife and get around his boss.

I have watched lots of families, both professionally and personally, struggle with issues in adolescence. Some handle them well and some don't. Families err at both ends of the continuum. Some are arbitrary and lay down the law and don't talk. They set a restriction they can't abide by, and then they have to back down or let the consequences drift. Others prefer not to know what kids are doing and ignore them and in the process tacitly condone almost anything. Eventually the child goes too far and then they scream and yell and insult him (there's a teenage word for it—*rag*), and don't do anything. The middle ground is the kind of parenting we have talked about in these last three chapters: authoritative parenting.

Authoritative parenting takes sensitivity, effort, thought and courage. In the short run, it takes more time than operating at the ends of the continuum. During adolescence, you begin to get compensated for your time. Authoritative parenting has the best chance of producing an emotionally healthy, pleasant, and responsible child.

Authoritarian or permissive parenting has a much greater likelihood of producing a more troublesome child. Children of authoritarian parents are angry, and either passive and compliant or aggressive and defiant. Children of permissive parents are undisciplined and inconsiderate. Neither set of children will be as appealing to others, or as willing or capable of taking responsibility for themselves.

Raising an adolescent today is a whole new ball game. Nobody has really raised anybody before in a world like ours. It is enormously difficult, and you can't do it alone.

247

You'll benefit from help—across the whole range from anticipating and managing routine challenges to turning around the really difficult situation. Finding that help provides opportunity for you to get to know some fine people who have caring concern for you and your child. Friends, older kids who are willing to talk, teachers and the school administration, pastors and youth workers and professionals in agencies are all people who will enrich your life and give you guidance and the emotional support you need as you provide for your child.

If you get stuck, get professional help. You're stuck if you keep having the same fights over and over again, if your child seems unhappy, won't talk, doesn't have friends and isn't having any fun at school. You're stuck if he doesn't seem to care about how you feel about him and what he's doing. You're stuck if he repeatedly does things that are dangerous, like drinking or doing drugs or staying out nights without your permission.

If you need professional help, *get it*. If you don't, your child will pay the price. And so will you—it will be terribly painful for you to see him having such a difficult time.

Letting Go

Dr. Bailey, whom I mentioned earlier in this chapter, does therapy with many children who are in the later stages of adolescence. She has observed that in many cases parents of these older children begin to forget how important they still are. She says the junior and senior in high school and the person a couple of years out of high school seem so competent and put so much priority on their own affairs, it's easy to get the impression that parenting doesn't matter any more. And she points out that part of this forgetting is because of what we as parents are going through.

We are getting ready to let go, ourselves. As our stint of active parenting comes to an end, we begin to turn our time and attention more and more to our own, individual activities and away from our children. Our similar, yet contrasting, needs present a basic dilemma. We are moving out and letting go of the involvement of childhood at the same time that our children are. Somehow we must resolve that dilemma so we can continue to nurture our children appropriately, at the same time that we provide for our own social, emotional and vocational needs.

248

Children, even seventeen- to twenty-year-old children, can feel abandoned if you forget to watch out for their needs during their late adolescent years. It's a very delicate process. You have to be involved without intruding, and establish the few boundaries that still need to be established at the same time that you offer guidance and support.

You need to frequently take time to put yourself in your child's shoes and imagine, or try to remember, what he is going through. He might need help figuring out how to go to the prom or how to write a resume' or how to invest his money or how to pick out a college. He may not ask. But *you* can ask, and you can talk about it together. The important thing is that you continue to be actively involved. You shouldn't just wait until things go wrong to offer your services.

But don't take over and do it for him, and don't insist he do it your way. You'll spoil it.

Once again, we are talking about promoting autonomy—the ability to be responsible for self. Autonomy is being able to be self governing, as Webster put it. More than anything, responsibility for self is an *attitude*. You and your child have to know in your *bones* that it is his life, and that ultimately he has to make the decisions about it. The adolescent who takes responsibility for himself wears a seat belt when he drives because he knows the risks and consequences and chooses to be on the safe side. The adolescent who does not take responsibility for himself wears one only when his parents are in the car because they make him.

Making your child responsible for himself is not being punitive or neglectful. Being neglectful is sending a child out into the world still reacting against you rather than acting on his own behalf. You get to the point as parent where you can turn responsibility over to him in a kind and nurturing way when you know you have done all you can. You have taught him what he needs to know, or have seen that someone else has, you have made all the necessary provisions, you have laid it out to him what the issues are, and you have let him know that the rest is up to him.

It's ironic, but as parents recognize a child's authority more, he comes back around and recognizes theirs. Between the ages of 14 and 19, most young people consult with their parents more often than they did earlier[9].

249

Parenting With Food

As with everything else, the adolescent eats pretty much in his own world—much of it beyond our control. As with everything else, the adolescent is developing skills so he can become capable of handling his eating, and what he does can be alarming.

Teens can push the nutritional quality of their diet to the limit. They snack on high-calorie, low-nutrient foods, eat out with friends at fast food establishments and choose pop for meals instead of milk, miss meals with the family, skip breakfast, go on diets, try to make weight for sports.

Nutritional Experimentation

Their tastes in food border on the outrageous. Curtis, my 15½-year-old, is taking drivers' ed right now, so every Monday and Wednesday night we take him over to the business college for a two-hour class. Sometimes, instead of driving the three miles back home again, I settle down in the break room to do some reading. Not only does that trap me away from chores and other more self-indulgent diversions, but it puts me in the position of being a *spy*. I watch the kids when they come in for their break.

What they choose for snacks is enough to make your teeth fall out. How does a candy bar and a can of pop sound? How about an ice cream bar and a can of pop? How about an ice cream bar and a candy bar? It doesn't even *sound* good.

Primarily in the early teens, kids pig out with their eating. They buy great quantities of non-nutritious foods and have parties and even boast about how much they can eat and drink. That kind of eating is not the same thing as the binge-eating behavior of the bulimic. It is simply the natural exploration of kids who are trying to assess their own limits. They try out what it feels like to be unsupervised with their eating and to go to excess and don't like it and decide there are better ways of operating.

Adolescents *do* take nutritional risks. You can't stop them. Kids hanging out with other kids are on their own, and they will, for the most part, eat what everyone else eats.

250

Nutritional Considerations

During their rapid growth phase, adolescents have higher requirements for nutrients than at any time since their infancy. But teenagers also have a big calorie requirement, and that is what saves their diet, in many cases, from nutritional impoverishment.

There is a gap between the calories teenagers need to get in their basic nutritional requirements and the calories they need to provide their energy needs. Teenagers can eat anywhere from 500 to 1800 calories of nutritionally worthless food a day, and still get the nutrients they need if the rest of the food they eat is reasonably well-balanced. In "Tools and Strategies," the figure, "Calorie Requirements Compared with Basic Needs" illustrates (for people of different ages) the gap between the calories necessary to cover for basic nutritional needs and the average total calories. You see that for children throughout the teen years, the gap is considerable. It's only when you get into the adult and later-adult years that the gap narrows.

Even though they have volume on their side, adolescents still should give some minimal attention to their diets to get the protein, minerals and vitamins they need. The nutrients most likely to be deficient in the diets of teenage girls are iron, calcium, magnesium and vitamin B_6. Teenage girls on weight-reduction diets have the poorest quality diets of any group[10].

The diets of teenage boys appear to be somewhat better, although when their intakes fall short of their requirements, they are deficient in the same nutrients as girls. For boys as well as girls, iron-deficiency anemia is a common problem.

For the average teenager, it has been shown that eating one of the day's meals away from home significantly decreases the intake of calcium, iron, vitamin C and thiamin. Of those studied, 19% of teenage girls and 11% of teenage boys missed breakfast, and 56% of teenagers ate four or more times in the day[11]. Essentially, the foods that are low or missing in teen diets are fruits and vegetables, whole grains and milk: the foods they have the best chance of getting at family meals.

Nevertheless, teens are not that far from nutritional excellence. If they meet the requirements of the basic four food plan on a fairly regular basis, and give some attention to getting in the foods that nutritional studies say they are likely to miss, they can continue to get a very high-quality diet.

Some teens eat a marginal or below-optimum diet. Teens who are under stress are the ones whose diets are most likely to be poor. Emotional stress decreases the chances that a child will be at family meals and that he will go to the trouble of choosing nutritious foods.

Pregnant teenagers and ones with injuries and illnesses have particular problems getting the extra nutrients they need. Teenagers who diet to look good or who restrict their total calorie intake to make weight for sports will, too. If kids cut down on calories, protein nutrition will suffer. There is no way you can have adequate protein nutrition if the total calories in the diet are too low.

What's A Parent To Do?

So what's a parent to do? A great deal—and almost nothing. Most of what you should do is almost done. You have developed in your child the food habits he will carry with him for the rest of his life. Even if he does veer away from them through his teen years, the habits will be there, ready to take over when his life gets more stable again. That's a start.

You can continue to have meals, and continue to expect your child be at them. He won't be there, a lot of time, but the expectation is important, and having him assume he needs to let you know where he will eat is also important. The message is clear: If you don't make use of the structure I provide for you, you need to provide it for yourself. Your child may complain about this, but secretly in his heart of hearts he will be glad that you look out for him.

Meals will provide you with a reliable social time with your child when he is so very busy with his adolescent life. Reliable rituals that keep a family in touch are almost all centered around eating: dinners, Sunday breakfast, holidays, picnics.

You can get good food into the house for snacks. In "Tools and Strategies," the figure "Nutritious Snacks" gives a list of snack suggestions. Take a look at it—maybe you'll get some ideas.

When you have teenagers, you will have to develop a policy about whether or not you will feed friends snacks. This is not a commitment to be undertaken lightly. Teenagers, boys OR girls, are expensive to feed. Boys eat anything in large amounts. Girls

252

are more selective, but they eat *expensive* food, like cottage cheese and fruit. It's nice if you can provide, but don't feel like you have to. Teens really need clear expectations and they need to learn to respect the feelings of others—they don't necessarily need handouts at every home they go to.

That's about all you'll have direct control over. The rest is up to your child. He'll be in charge of lunch and one or two snacks a day, maybe even breakfast, and dinner some of the time. Combine that with the kind of foods we all know teens like, and there is a VERY big margin for error.

Giving Nutritional Guidance

What does your child need to know in order to manage this part of his life? Is he capable of doing it? You're going to have to talk to him to find out. You may discover he knows a lot. Chances are he has studied nutrition in school since he was little. Chances are he hasn't really thought much about applying it to himself, because you have been taking care of it.

You can talk about what he takes for school lunch, and encourage him to get in his milk and a fruit or vegetable. Later on, when he starts missing dinners, it will be harder. But he can still get a can of fruit or vegetable juice to have along with a sandwich, or take salad bar at the fast food place.

You might have him take a look at the nutritious snack list. The figure, "Fun Foods that Make Nutritional Sense" list, in "Tools and Strategies," is another list that might be helpful. It demonstrates how to get good nutrition from the teenager's favorite foods. I originally developed it when I was counseling pregnant teenage girls.

The "Milk Group Portion Sizes" list is important for all teens, but especially for teenage girls who might start cutting down on their milk in hopes of losing a little weight. It's important that they continue to get their calcium so they can build their bones when they are young. Once they get to be our age it's too late. As far as bones are concerned, after age 35, it's all down hill.

Unless you make a big issue about it, teens will be concerned about their nutrition and taking care of their bodies. Teens like information better if they find it themselves, so encourage cooking classes and nutrition and health classes.

253

Don't get defensive when they question your shopping and cooking—they can be helpful in choosing family foods and expanding the choices available.

Once you are satisfied that he understands his basic requirements and knows some strategies for getting those requirements attended to, your job is over. He'll provide better for himself if he takes responsibility for his eating than if you follow him around and try to supervise it for him.

Don't criticize the way he eats. That will give him a script for rebellion. If you get in a struggle over the way he eats, his nutritional status will suffer. Teenagers who are criticized about their eating skip more meals and have worse diets than those whose families are more supportive and accepting[11].

It might be that the nutritional quality of his diet isn't as bad as you fear. Despite our worst fears, most teens consume a good-enough quality diet.

As adolescents, children's eating continues to develop. Their table manners improve, and as teenagers they accept a wider variety of foods than they did when they were smaller, and they continue to experiment. They experiment, that is, provided you don't put pressure on them. It has to be *their* thing, not yours.

Finally, you need to be philosophical about the fact that, no matter how much food there is in the house, they will still complain that there is nothing to eat.

Eating For Sports

The best training diet is one that is adequate in all essential nutrients, including water, and including sufficient calories to maintain the level of extra exertion that is involved.

The concerns that arise in sports nutrition come from the kinds of distortions that kids impose on their diets in the name of increasing fitness: Weight loss regimens to decrease body fat percentage, protein dosing to increase body weight or musculature, vitamin supplementation based on a variety of theories. At times, these extreme methods are endorsed by coaches. But none of it does much good, and all of it carries some hazard.

Moderate changes in diet, as long as basic nutritional adequacy is maintained, are probably not a big cause for concern.

254

However, if your child is imposing severe measures on himself to change his body, chances are it isn't doing him any good. In the long run, it will probably detract from his performance.

The problem is getting your adolescent, who is so committed to making the team and doing well once he gets there, to be moderate about his eating. It's a ticklish topic, because if you question the coach and try to move in, you will be asking your adolescent to choose between you. It's better to work indirectly, if you can. Certainly, express your concern and let your adolescent know what you see that is worrying you. Tell him you want him to take some steps to find out the facts. But let him know that, ultimately, he is going to have to be the one to decide.

If he is agreeable, you can send him to an outside professional to help him. A dietitian who is knowledgeable in sports nutrition can be an enormous help. She can give good information, and help your child figure out a healthful eating program and set some reasonable goals for weight management. He'll get some valuable information, and it will get you out of the role of trying to be the voice of reason.

Weight Reduction Dieting

Eventually, your child, especially your girl child, is pretty likely to get to the point where she wants to go on a weight reduction diet. And once they get through the rapid growth of puberty, weight reduction efforts may be a reasonable possibility. But it's an important step, and not one that should be undertaken lightly.

I will talk in the obesity chapter about the dangers of weight reduction efforts. They can lower body metabolism, increase pressure to eat, and cause rebound eating that in the long run makes people fatter, not thinner. This is your child's one big first effort to see if he can lose weight, and it's important that he not screw it up.

Again, if he decides to proceed, encourage him to go to a professional. A registered dietitian will be able to advise him about making modest eating and exercise changes that, consistently applied over time, have the greatest chance of being successful without causing reactive weight gain.

But keep it his thing. Read Helping All You Can To Keep Your Child From Being Fat (Chapter 14) to get some ideas about

255

being supportive, but don't take over. You're not going to be there forever, and you shouldn't try to stimulate him to do anything with your help that he can't sustain without it.

Eating Disorders

An eating disorder, as I will explain in Chapter 15, is made up of two components: a distortion in eating, and an underlying emotional struggle. The emotional struggle is one that involves the whole family. Anorexia, bulimia and obesity of emotional origin are all diseases of adolescence. The eating disorder is the product of lifelong distortions in the way parents and children deal with eating—and with other issues in their lives.

Typically, children with severe emotionally-based problems with their eating have not been encouraged to develop autonomy, so they arrive at the teen years with a poor sense of themselves and their own capabilities. They simply don't feel equal to the adolescent challenges of making friends and, eventually, emancipating themselves from their parents and getting out in the world. They see getting thin as the way to help them accomplish both goals. In the process, they get engrossed in a struggle with their bodies, and that struggle distracts them from the other, more real, and more frightening issues that are confronting them.

Eating disorders most often appear in girls. No one is quite sure why that is. It may be because societal pressure for thinness is greater on girls. Also, families may feed girls differently from boys. Studies of obese children show their parents to be more controlling and critical of girls, more indulgent of boys[12]. And girls may simply choose a more passive way of acting out than boys do. They stop eating rather than staying out nights or being truant from school.

Read Eating Disorders (Chapter 15) to get a more complete discussion of the causes and treatment of eating disorders.

The struggles of the eating disordered teenager help point up the considerable accomplishments of the adequately-functioning adolescent. In respecting your child as an individual and encouraging his autonomy from birth onwards, you have been enabling him to take his place in the world. When the time comes, it will be hard to see him go. But you'll be proud. You'll be proud of him for being ready to handle what he encounters, and proud of yourself, too.

References

1. Small, Stephen. Personal communication based on unpublished research. June, 1987.

2. Menaghan, E.: Marital stress and family transitions: A panel analysis. Journal of Marriage and the Family 47:371-386, 1983.

3. Berger, K.S.: The Developing Person. NY, Worth, 1980.

4. Adelson, J. Adolescence and the generalization gap. Psychology Today 12(9):33-37. 1979.

5. Offer, D., and Offer, J.B.: From Teenage to Young Manhood...A Psychological Study. New York: Basic Books, 1975.

6. Simmons, R.G., Rosenberg, F., and Rosenberg, M.: Disturbance in the self-image at adolescence. American Sociological Review 38:553-568, 1973.

7. Jones, M.C. and Bayley, N.: Physical maturing among boys as related to behavior. Journal of Educational Psychology, 41:129-148, 1950.

8. Sorenson, R.C.: Adolescent Sexuality in Contemporary America: Personal Values and Sexual Behavior, ages thirteen to nineteen. New York: World. 1973.

9. Kandel, D. and Lesser, G.S. Parent-adolescent relationships and adolescent independence in the United States and Denmark. Journal of Marriage and the Family. 31:348-358. 1969.

10. Christian, J. and Greger, J. Nutrition for Living. Menlo Park, CA: Benjamin Cummings, 1985.

11. Pipes, P.L.: Nutrition in Infancy and Childhood. St. Louis: Times Mirror/Mosby. 1985.

12. Costanzo, P.R. and Woody, E.Z.: Domain-specific parenting styles and their impact on the child's development of particular deviance: The example of obesity proneness. Journal of Social and Clinical Psychology 3: 425-445, 1985.

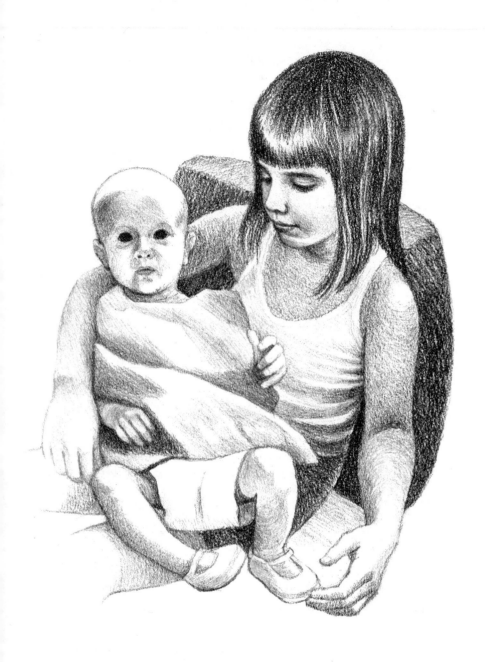

13

The Child Who Grows Poorly

Feeding problems are extremely common. The best esti-
mates suggest that approximately 25% of the pediatric population has some complication with feeding. In specialized centers
treating developmentally disabled children, the incidence is even
higher—estimated at about 33%. Keep in mind these statistics
are based on cases in which parents seek professional help.
There are many who don't[1].

Poor growth is often related to difficulties in feeding. Of
1,120 infants with growth failure reviewed by one researcher,
29% were found to have no medical reason for their poor
growth, and an additional 13% were categorized as having
feeding problems[1].

The feeding relationship should be routinely examined
whenever a child is growing poorly. If distortions in feeding are
not the cause of poor growth, they are almost certain to be
the effect. In either case, the distortions must be corrected if
a child is to grow as well as possible. Unfortunately, that
seldom happens.

259

Treatment—The Optimum

Once detected, the next problem is finding treatment. Expertise in the area of eating and eating problems is relatively new. Furthermore, there seems to be a real mystique about childhood feeding problems—most professionals are reluctant to treat them. These may be the very same people who, with respect to other types of problems, are willing to read and learn as they go along.

That mystique is largely unnecessary; skillful professionals can learn about feeding. Approach your doctor or pediatric nurse. They are accustomed to seeking out services for their patients. They might have to encourage a mental health worker and dietitian they trust to learn about feeding and give you some help. It needs to be a team effort—it takes expertise in both areas to resolve difficult feeding problems. (I do both parts, but I have training and experience in both disciplines.)

The treatment methods I have described in this chapter, as well as the basic information about feeding, will give an adequate start to anyone who works with you on your child's feeding problems. In many cases the problem will yield to simply getting the pressure off feeding and giving some attention to properly supporting the child in the eating situation. The methods at least provide a first step in teasing apart the problem, to find out if the child will recover in her food acceptance once parents quit putting pressure on feeding.

At times, the eating problem will yield to behavioral modification techniques that treat only the eating and leave the other interactional problems alone. (Often parents may find they are inadvertently provoking or reinforcing the behavior they most object to.) While this type of treatment is available in only a few areas, it *has* been written up[2], and it has been shown to be effective when applied by a mental health worker operating as part of a team with a registered dietitian. Those professionals have the basic skills to move readily into working with your child's eating problems. But you may have to provide the initial push to get them started.

Some treatment teams hospitalize the child and use careful behavioral programs to teach desirable behaviors and get rid of undesirable ones. Inpatient treatment is a logical step for children who are really sensitized to eating or who seem fragile, either medically or nutritionally. I will talk about some of these treatment approaches in the next chapter.

Many cases of marked childhood eating problems require looking at the problem in the context of the way the whole family operates. At times, children's eating problems are so bound up in family emotional and social functioning that I have called the cases *childhood eating disorders*[3]. To resolve these problems, the family as a whole needs counseling to detect and change what is going wrong in the way they interact with each other. It may start with the child, but it always gets back to the parents. Parents have to be getting along with each other before they can do a good job with their child. Most battles with a child over eating are really battles between the parents.

Treatment—The Reality

In most cases, when a child is growing poorly, she gets evaluated medically and nutritionally. She has a physical examination and lab tests. Sometimes, lots of lab tests. A dietitian may question the parents about what the child has eaten in the previous day, and may do an analysis of several days' written record of her food intake. All of that is desirable, and even essential. However, finding out what the child has eaten doesn't give any information about the interaction between parent and child around feeding, and that interaction may be what is causing the growth problem.

Poor growth can be constitutional, or it can be caused by disease or by eating problems. It is always difficult to sort out the cause. When the feeding relationship is ignored, it is even harder. To illustrate the difficulty, let me tell you about Richie.

Richie was breast fed, and as you can see by his growth chart, Figure 13-1, he grew well for his first two months.

Then his weight started to fall steeply off the growth curve. No evaluation was done on the breast-feeding, and at his four-month checkup his mother was told to start solid foods to supplement her breast milk supply. She tried, but Richie took solids only reluctantly. At six months, his growth had continued to fall, and she was told to give even more solid foods. On neither occasion did she receive instructions on which solid foods to use to increase the calories in his diet.

261

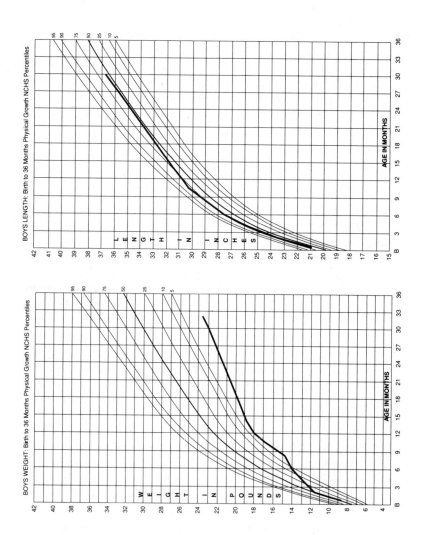

Figure 13-1   Richie's Growth Chart

His weight kept going down, and finally at eight months a dietitian was asked to do a nutritional evaluation of his food intake and advise his mother on food selection. She observed that Richie was depending pretty heavily on solid foods to get his calories, and that a high proportion of those solid foods was made up of relatively low-calorie fruits and vegetables.

The dietitian suggested the mother begin to supplement breast-feeding with formula, cut down on the fruits and vegetables in his diet, and instead offer him the higher calorie baby cereal mixed with formula. The dietitian didn't attempt to evaluate the feeding relationship, but she was a good observer. She saw that Richie was a very wiry child, not at all cuddly, and that his mother didn't seem to like that. She had to hang on to him tightly or he would throw himself out of her arms.

Throughout his early months, Richie had had one cold and ear infection after another. When he was sick, his appetite would fall off. When he got better, he'd eat well for a while, but then he would get sick again. At 14 months, his growth still hadn't improved and, since he was having so much lung congestion, the doctor decided to have him tested for cystic fibrosis.

The parents were extremely alarmed, because they knew just how serious that could be. In their alarm, they increased their efforts to get Richie to eat, and feeding deteriorated even further. His mother said she was getting quite desperate as she tried first one food and then another to see if he would accept it. And Richie was getting a wicked little gleam in his eye as he got his mother to perform for him.

It turned out that he didn't have cystic fibrosis, but the feeding struggle continued. I saw the family when Richie was 16 months old. By then, the parents felt they were having to force in every mouthful Richie took, and he was getting increasingly reluctant to come to the table and increasingly upset while he was there.

We reviewed what had gone on during Richie's early months, and the parents remembered being under an enormous amount of stress. The father was working extremely hard, and the mother felt isolated and unsupported in her efforts to care for Richie. Some of Richie's lack of cuddliness could have been coming from *her* inability to cuddle. When she tried to let her husband know how she was feeling, he refused to listen, and reminded her there was nothing he could do to change the demands on him. He was having trouble keeping his family first in his list of priorities, and his wife was feeling abandoned. Since, that time, however, they had begun having some counseling, and things were going better between them.

Since they were doing better with each other, they were in a position to do better with Richie. I encouraged them to stop forcing Richie to eat, and simply to present his food to him in a matter-of-fact way. We talked about tactics for feeding the toddler, including modifying food so he could be more successful eating it. I encouraged them to make sure Richie was getting enough fat in his diet, and emphasized giving him whole milk rather than the 2% milk they had gone to when they took him off formula.

They were relieved to get the advice, and at a couple of follow up appointments they told of having regular meals and snacks, and letting Richie pick and choose from what was available. They were doing better and feeling more confident in handling his toddler-type eating behavior. After a few days of eating very little, he was starting to show more interest in food.

When Richie came in at 17 months for a checkup, he was breathing strangely. The doctor made an immediate diagnosis: he was having an asthma attack. Asthma may been part of his problem for some time.

Richie continues to grow in his own slow way, he is not enthusiastic about eating, and at last sighting he was a tall and very slender boy. (Both his parents are also tall and very slender.)

Almost from the first, Richie's feeding was mishandled. When things get off on the wrong foot with feeding, the problem can persist for a long time. Parents don't build up trust in either themselves or their child to handle feeding appropriately, and each stage that comes along can make the struggle worse.

It would have been helpful to his mother, and not at all intrusive, if someone had sat down with her and evaluated her breast-feeding and helped her improve it. Instead, she got some sketchy and bad advice, and went on to feed in a way that was increasingly ineffective.

As a routine part of a breast-feeding evaluation, she could have been told that mothers often have problems with milk supply because they are under too much stress, and encouraged to share what was going on with her emotionally. Despite her hus-

264

band's protests, something can almost always be done about high-pressure situations like the one they had been in when Richie was little.

If breast-feeding couldn't improve, she should have been told to give a formula supplement instead of solid foods. At age four months, Richie needed the calories and nutrients in more breast milk or formula, and he needed a satisfying nipple feeding experience.

The solid-food tactic was intended to help preserve the breast-feeding, but in that instance it wasn't a good one. Formula supplementation would not necessarily have interfered with the breast-feeding. But even if it had, Richie's need for satisfying feeding and adequate growth should have taken precedence over his mother's need to breast-feed.

Richie didn't need solid foods, he didn't need the spoon, and he wasn't ready for it. By the time he was old enough to take some pleasure in eating solid food, the experience was already tainted for him by their earlier struggles. Feeding continued to be unpleasant for both of them.

Richie's case was a complex one, made more complex than it had to be by the way breast-feeding was mishandled and by the fact that a whole body of information was missing—what was going on with the feeding relationship. Looking at that might have prevented some problems. It certainly would have saved him and his parents a lot of struggles, and improved the quality of their relationship. And that's a lot.

Distinguishing Poor Growth From Slow-but-normal Growth

Your doctor is the best person to advise you about your child's growth. Anything I say I mean as a supplement to that information, to help you with your own thinking about your child's growth.

It is always difficult to distinguish the child who grows naturally for her, but slowly, from the child who grows more slowly than she should. Children who perk along at or below the fifth percentile on the growth charts are a concern for us all. However, there is nothing *wrong* with growing at a slower rate.

265

The charts are set up, after all, to define the variations in normal growth. Children who on the bottom line are just as normal as kids who are in the middle or at the top, and there are still 5% of children who are below the fifth percentile, and still grow normally. To have us question a child's growth pattern, she has to be considerably below the fifth percentile or show an erratic growth pattern.

Ultimately, genetics provides the greatest influence on your child's growth. Chances are very good that your child's size and shape will be influenced most by her mother's shape or her father's shape, or by a combination of the two. Her constitutional endowment for height and weight will start to show up in the second half of the first year, when she may gradually either go up or down to different percentile levels for height and weight on the growth chart.

It is the shift in growth that raises questions about whether a child is doing as well as she should. Generally, a modest shift in growth over several months is nothing to worry about. It is the major shift that goes on for several months, or the abrupt shift over a shorter time that gives a greater cause for concern.

If a child seems to be not doing well emotionally, it provides an additional sign that growth is not all it should be. If she is withdrawn and depressed or over-active, it is likely that something happening in the family is bothering her, and it should be examined.

When growth is puzzling, it is important to look for causes. The cause might be illness, inappropriate food or the feeding relationship. The three are also interactional—a problem in one area can lead to difficulties in another.

Naturally Slow Growth

It is difficult to have a child who grows slowly. It is nerve-wracking for you, because she will seem fragile. Actually, a small, slim child's food intake is just as stable as a larger child's. Her feelings of hunger and satiety are just as strong, and she is just as capable of letting you know how much she is hungry for.

Because a child eats small amounts, at times parents get the idea that she isn't interested in eating. Quite the opposite is true. Even children who don't eat much are very interested when they are hungry, and if feeding is smooth and not disrupted, they generally eat in a businesslike fashion. It is only when they start to get full, or the feeding gets interrupted, that they lose interest and can't be persuaded to take any more. It's at that point that parents get upset and form their impression that she isn't interested in eating.

Actually, what they are seeing is normal satiety. Anybody loses interest in food when they are full or they get jostled around. You are just more aware of it with someone who is so small.

In many cases, however, parents' concern about growth leads them to be *too* helpful with feeding, and therein lies the rub. They get a little pushy with feeding, and their baby doesn't like it. She resists, or gets confused, and eats a little less. The parent gets more concerned and pushes a little harder, the child eats even less, and feeding deteriorates into a struggle —eventually it starts to look like she *won't* eat unless she is pushed into it.

That's what happened with Bethany. As you can see by her growth chart, Figure 13-2, Bethany was tiny when she was born, and stayed tiny during her early months.

In fact, she got tinier. From the beginning, her parents struggled with her about feeding, and throughout her young life the feeding struggles got worse and worse. By the time she was 15 months old, their fights over eating were so vehement that her parents worried the neighbors would think they were beating her. Her father held her head and tried to force food between her lips. And she screamed and fought back. Food regulation can't get much more emphatic than that.

When she was 15 months old, Bethany's parents were advised to back off on the forcing, and the situation improved somewhat. She grew a little better, and as her mother put it, "Her eating is still the pits, but at least we're not fighting about it all the time."

There is probably not much you can do if your child appears to be a naturally slow grower. If she is like most babies, she won't eat any more than she wants to. Even if the amounts she eats seem tiny to you, and are tiny compared to what other children eat, they are right for her. If you try to persuade her to eat more than she is hungry for, she is likely to be very firm indeed about it, and if you try harder to persuade, she will become even firmer.

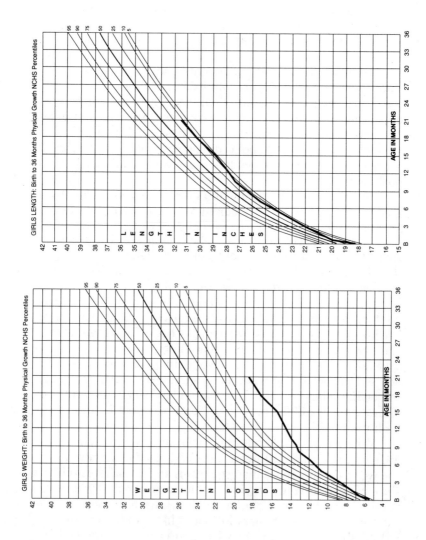

Figure 13-2 Bethany's Growth Chart

I told you in Quit When the Job is Done (Chapter 2) about little Alice Black, our miniature child who regulated decidedly on about 14 ounces of formula a day. Despite her parents' gentle persuasion and our nutritional trickery, Alice did not eat more than she wanted. She had her own agenda about how she would grow, and WE adhered to IT.

Almost everybody tries too hard to feed babies who seem like they are fragile. A number of studies have been done on children who were either growing poorly or had been labeled as being "at nutritional risk" because of their smallness. These studies showed that parents were more active with babies who seemed vulnerable. And the increased activity interfered with, rather than encouraged, food intake[4].

Instead of waiting for the baby's feeding cues and following her lead in feeding, too-active parents take charge. They push the nipple into the baby's mouth (rather than waiting for her to open up), jiggle the nipple in her mouth whenever she pauses (rather than waiting for her to go back to sucking), use any means at their disposal to get her to take the rest of formula in the bottle (rather than taking her word that she is full and stopping feeding), and impose a feeding schedule (rather than feeding her on demand).

It is natural to try to help out when someone seems to be having a hard time with eating. Ironically, these studies showed that these all-too-natural attempts backfired. When parents got too forceful or too active in feeding, babies ate less, rather than more. Babies did best with feeding when parents worked to calm them, helped them to stay organized and alert enough to persist in eating, and conducted the feeding in a smooth and uninterrupted fashion.

When babies get a lot of interruptions in feeding, they don't do as well. It could be that they just get tired out with all the extraneous activity. It could also be that they get too much stimulation, and they withdraw from it. Newborn babies must keep themselves composed at the same time as they take an interest in what goes on around them. It is hard for them, because they emerge from the relative quiet of the womb to encounter a new world of sights, smells, sounds, touches and tastes. They have to remain calm in spite of it all. It over-stimulates them when a parent comes on too strong, and they react by becoming agitated or withdrawing. Either can disrupt feeding.

Once in a while a child will allow herself to be overfed. There is no doubt that overfeeding is effective in producing growth. But there is a price to pay, and you only have to observe overfeeding to realize what that price is. A child who is being overfed will submit, but look withdrawn and passive, or she will express her unhappiness with her whole body. That child will grow up with bad feelings about feeding and about herself.

The Sick Child

I'll talk in Feeding the Child with Special Needs (Chapter 16) about feeding sick children. To summarize here, I want to warn you that a sick child, or a child who grows poorly for whatever reason, is very likely to stimulate you to do counter-productive things with feeding. Parents regularly cross the lines of division of responsibility in feeding children who are sick. It is understandable, if a child's health depends on her taking enough food or the right kind of food, for a parent to get over-concerned and try to manage the child's eating for her.

It doesn't work any better to be over-managing with a sick child than with a well child. Their sense of themselves and their need to be in control of this very important part of their lives is just as strong—or even stronger. (When children are undergoing medical treatment, eating may be the only thing in their lives that they can control.) They will react emphatically when parents try to take over in their area. If parents are over-concerned about feeding, children can get manipulative, and the bad feelings on both sides can worsen an already very trying situation.

My advice for feeding a sick child is the same as for feeding a well child: Maintain the division of responsibility in feeding, maintain structure, and follow the age-appropriate approaches for establishing and maintaining positive feeding relationships I have described earlier in this book. The sick child needs love *and limits* just as much as a well child. You simply have to do all you can to parent well with food, then let go of it. If you do that, in the long run your child will eat better and you will save yourself, and your child, a lot of distress.

270

Breast-Feeding

More and more we see babies who don't grow well when they are breast-fed. They don't get enough to eat, they aren't demanding or assertive enough to let their parents know when they are going hungry, and they end up eating too little to grow well[5].

There are a lot of factors that contribute to the problem. Even with optimum support, while it's true that almost everybody *can* breast-feed, some people *can't*, and some people *don't want to*. Breast-feeding *is* better nutritionally, especially early on, but it's not enough better to make up for a feeding relationship that is going poorly. If you are breast-feeding and hating it, you won't enjoy the time with your baby, and you'll both know it. If you are worrying all the time that your breast-feeding isn't going well, and getting it to go better seems like a very steep and very uphill battle, it can again decrease your pleasure in feeding and spending time with your baby.

Some people try to breast-feed when they really shouldn't. They don't really *want* to. With the current emphasis on breast-feeding, almost everyone feels obligated, and some mothers comment that both professional and personal associates make them feel guilty if they decide not to. It's really all right to bottle feed. You and your baby can have an excellent feeding relationship, and your baby will be well nourished on a good formula.

At the same time that they are being encouraged to breast-feed, however, mothers (and fathers—their understanding and involvement is vital) don't get the kind of personal support and instruction they need in order to breast-feed successfully. With shorter hospital stays for delivery, most women go home before their milk even comes in. Learning on your own, without anyone knowledgeable to support you, can increase your tension and chances of failure.

It is very important when you are breast-feeding that you have a follow-up consultation with a knowledgeable person within 48 hours after you leave the hospital, again at one week, and again at two weeks. If you truly can't manage a direct visit, a telephone call will help. That way you'll get the support you need, you'll catch the problems early and have a chance to resolve them in a positive way. One of those ways might be choosing not to breast-feed.

271

Every breast-feeding relationship takes two—a mother who can, and wants to, and a baby who will. Every breast-feeding relationship takes time—feedings every two or three hours that last twenty to thirty minutes—at first, even longer. If you can't put in that kind of time, breast-feeding may not be for you. (Although bottle feeding may not be any different—it is just that someone else can help out.) Every breast-feeding relationship has problems. Most problems can be solved with little pain on either side. But some problems are insoluble.

The problems that can't be overcome include severely inverted nipples (nipples that go back rather than sticking out when you squeeze them). Inverted nipples can prove a complete barrier to breast-feeding, especially if you happen to get a baby whose suck isn't strong enough to pull them out during nursing.

Breast surgery may have disrupted the nipple and the milk ducts. The type of breast reduction surgery where the nipple has been removed and re-implanted completely rules out breast-feeding. Breast augmentation usually doesn't interfere, but if nipple sensation changes as a result of the surgery, there may be some damage to the milk-delivery system.

A few women don't have enough tissue for making milk. Those women have minimal breast changes with pregnancy, and don't experience engorgement. Some women don't have enough prolactin to stimulate breast milk production. Prolactin can also decrease if the mother is under stress.

A baby can also fail to contribute to the success of the breast feeding. Babies can be poor nursers for a lot of reasons—they suck poorly because they are premature, or small for gestational age, or have neurological or structural problems with their mouths.

A major reason breast-feeding doesn't go well is because the baby is too easily pleased. She seems contented and comfortable after feeding and sleeps a long time until the next feeding. Perhaps her feeding cues are subtle, and easy to overlook. Perhaps the mother is under stress, and unable to be attentive enough to catch those subtle cues. For whatever reason, everything seems to be going well until her parents take her in to be checked when she is two weeks or a month old, and discover to their dismay that she isn't growing properly. The cycle has to be reversed to allow her to do better with her eating. Observing the feeding relationship will provide clues to how to do that. But the problem has to be caught early, or breast milk production might not recover.

Stress can interfere with breast-feeding by decreasing milk production or preventing let-down of the milk to the milk ducts. When you are breast-feeding, you need a supportive environment—for your mothering, as well as your breast-feeding. Actually, the optimum breast-feeding relationship takes *three*, not two—a mother who can, a baby who will, and a father who is involved and supportive.

It's best to work out problems in relationships before the baby is born. But you can't always anticipate how you're going to feel, so if having a new baby has a particularly upsetting effect on you, your partner, or your relationship, get in for some counseling. A few sessions at that critical time can make a big difference in the way things go.

A mother I know got to be a baby, herself, after their daughter was born. She became so demanding that her husband didn't want anything to do with her. He withdrew, and her demandingness got even worse.

One father became very competitive with his baby, and sat right next to his wife during breast-feedings and actually, physically pushed their baby away from her breast. Another father was more subtle about it, but not much. He left the room whenever his wife breast-fed, and he acted very embarrassed when she breast-fed in front of their friends, even though she did it so discreetly they didn't even know that she was nursing. They didn't know, that is, until he started acting weird.

Some grandparents make no bones about their opposition to breast-feeding. They act pained when they see their grandchild nursing, and whenever she cries, they wonder if she is hungry and needs a bottle. Fathers need to function here, in defending the decision to breast-feed, and letting them know about the impact of their behavior on mother and baby.

Because of the theme of this chapter, I have given you a negative picture of breast-feeding. Let me remind you: By far the greatest proportion of breast-feeding relationships go well. If you want to do it and have a supportive mate, and are willing to spend time at it, your chances are extremely good that you will be able to breast feed.

The Child Who Is Defiant About Eating

I talked about Brian in Pressure Doesn't Work (Chapter 3). His growth chart is here, in Figure 13-3.

Brian was a three-year-old whose mother thought she had to stand over him and force him to eat or he would starve. I mean that literally. He showed so much resistance to eating and his growth had fallen off so much that it really seemed that way. His mother was frantic—and angry. At the same time that she was worried that Brian wouldn't eat enough to live, she felt like he was deliberately defying her and she was furious at him.

His eating had been a problem since birth. He had been breast fed—his mother did it because she felt like she *should*, but she didn't really like it. It bothered her not to know how much he ate. The best she could do was to take him to the doctor frequently to check on his progress.

It was a relief to her when it was time to start solid foods, because she finally could feel some control over his food intake. Her relief didn't last long. He was very hard to get onto solids. He refused to eat them, and it was only with pressure and the utmost persistence that she finally got them down him.

Getting him on table food was the same battle. In his mother's view, that battle had continued unabated until age three, when she was standing over him for an hour to get him to eat a piece of french toast.

Brian's growth chart told another story. He grew well during the first five months, and stayed right around the fiftieth percentile. Over the next year, however, his growth gradually fell off, until by age 18 months his weight was down around the fifth percentile. Then suddenly, he started to gain, and continued his gain until he was about two. Then again, he started to lose, and by age three had fallen well below the fifth percentile.

What had happened during the eight months when Brian grew well provided a clue to the problem. Mother had been ill. She had had a difficult pregnancy and had taken to her bed. Brian's younger sister had been born prematurely, and had taken a lot of time. During that difficult time, mother didn't have time or energy to devote to Brian and his eating.

When it was left up to him, Brian ate and grew. When it was left up to his mother, Brian did not eat and his growth fell off. It was not that Brian had a defect in his willingness or

274

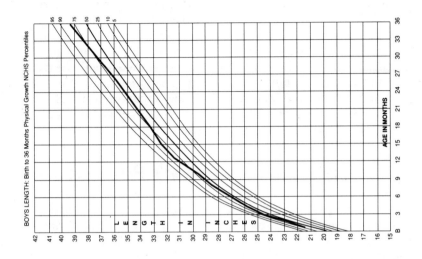

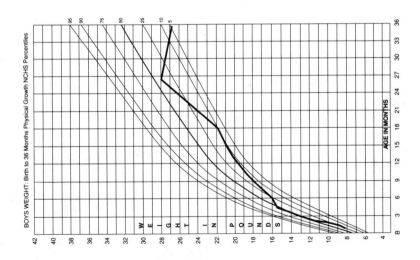

Figure 13-3   Brian's Growth Chart

ability to take in food. It was simply that, for whatever reason, he was not willing to go along with his mother's ideas about feeding. When she put pressure on him to eat, he fought back by eating very poorly.

It is all too easy to get in that sort of a self-perpetuating struggle with a child over eating. You get started seeing them as reluctant to eat and put on a little pressure, they react against it, you increase the pressure, and the whole situation escalates.

The next section will give some ideas about getting back OUT of some of these feeding struggles.

The Child Who Won't Progress

Some children eat enough and even get a nutritionally adequate diet, but get stuck at an early stage in feeding. Erik was a two-and-a-half-year-old who refused to progress to table foods—he ate only milk, juice, baby cereal, bananas and cookies. He was growing just fine. I'm not even going to show you his growth chart, because he had stayed right on the fiftieth percentile for height and weight throughout his growing-up. The problem was food acceptance: the variety in his diet was even less than when he had been younger. Erik had twin sisters, age fourteen months, and they were more grown up in their eating than he was.

The whole family came for a session—Erik, his parents, his grandmother, and his little sisters. The office was a real circus. It didn't take long to figure out that Erik's parents had too many responsibilities, too little money, and too much "help." Erik's mother had quit her job to take care of the children, and his father was making the minimum wage. The relatives lived entirely too close for Erik's sake, and every day a grandmother or a brother or sister called to find out how he was eating. And the answer was always the same: He was eating, but not what his audience wanted him to eat.

The neighbors thought the problem was that Erik was around younger children and he just didn't know how to eat like a grown-up boy. So one neighbor, who had older children, took him several days for lunch in hopes that he would eat what the other kids ate. They didn't take along any of Erik's special food, so he would either eat or go hungry. He went for lunch, but he didn't eat anything, nor did he ask for food when he got home.

Erik's uncle said they were just being soft on him and to bring Erik to his house and he'd get him straightened out. So they took him there and left him for three days and let his uncle work on him. After three days Erik emerged victorious—he still wasn't eating.

You no doubt have heard the standard advice, usually delivered in a belligerent tone of voice, "Let him go hungry. He'll eat when he gets hungry enough." Well, in some cases that might work, but probably not if you're so rude and crude about it.

It is a good idea to not let a child eat or drink whenever she wants to because she will spoil her appetite for nutritious meals and snacks. But when you have someone who is as turned off to eating as Brian or Erik, chances are if you try to starve them into submission you will get starvation but no submission. Eventually, you'll have to back down, and their reluctance to eat will be more entrenched than ever.

Erik's parents tried forcing him to eat, they tried depriving him of his favorite foods, they tried letting him help prepare it. None of the methods worked. Currently, they were enticing him. Before every meal, he and his mother were going through the cupboards, mother saying, "Do you want this?" and Erik saying, usually, "No." The babies had surpassed him in their ability to eat table food, but Erik was still eating his baby cereal.

There was nothing the matter with his chewing and swallowing. He could eat cookies like a whiz. There appeared to be nothing wrong with him mentally and developmentally. A child psychologist sat in on the case with me, and Erik seemed to be doing OK.

As Erik's uncle and most of the rest of the family saw it, the parents had to show Erik who was boss. As I saw it, they had to get the pressure off Erik, and off themselves to get Erik to eat. There were lots of things that they could get Erik to do, but eating wasn't one of them. They could get him, for instance, to come to the table and sit down and behave himself and not cause a big fuss about food. They could make it clear to him that they were the ones to choose what they were going to have for meals and snacks and that he would not be allowed to go through the cupboard with his mother, vetoing all her suggestions.

They could limit food availability to meal and snack time

277

and not allow him to have milk and juice between times or carry food around in hopes that he would eat it. Instead of trying to push eating onto him, they were to limit its availability and give the message that eating is a special thing that you can do at only certain times.

And they were to reassure him, once he got to the table, that he didn't have to eat if he didn't want to but that they wanted him to keep them company and behave himself. The reassurance was the most important part. With all the forcing and fussing about eating, Erik had gotten very touchy about being around food: He avoided it if at all possible. So the first step was to help him get over being so touchy.

They did allow him to have what he liked, but his mother was to choose from the short list of his preferred foods and present something to him. He was not to be given anything else he asked for. He was also not to get down from the table until they told him he could go.

When she was asked to be more firm with Erik, it emerged that the mother's feelings were part of the problem. She felt sad that, with all her responsibilities, she had missed out on much of his babyhood. She had mixed feelings about letting him grow up. It helped her when we told her that she needed to spend some alone time with him. At the same time they started being more matter-of-fact about feeding, it was going to be important for her to make up for some of that lost attention with some separate time for the two of them.

As the family left that first week, I told the grandmother the plan: They were not to force Erik to eat anything he didn't want to, but only to teach him to behave at the table. Her response was, "Do you mean you are going to let him get away with eating the way he does?" Cynical me, I wondered what she thought they *had* been doing. I also wondered how much help she would be.

During the first week, Erik made a lot of progress. His grandmother *was* some help: she bought him a high chair at a garage sale. She remembered that Erik had had to give his up when the babies got big enough to need high chairs. But he, unlike the babies, didn't have his tray on his high chair. He was a big boy, so he sat right up to the table with the adults.

And he behaved himself. He quietly ate his food, and didn't make a fuss about the other food that was on the table. His

278

adults had made some changes too: They expected Erik to do what he was capable of doing, and quit pressuring him about that of which he was incapable.

Each of his parents took some alone time with him every day. They liked that a lot, and seemed more comfortable about how they were providing for him.

Erik did as they asked him to at the table, and he also did some other things that were surprising: He paid more attention to what the rest of the family was eating, and asked his mother to leave the serving bowl of macaroni and cheese by his plate. He didn't eat it, he just left it there.

In that first week, Erik actually anticipated the next step in our treatment—getting him used to having other food around without having to eat it. The next step after that was to get him used to having the food on his *plate* without having to eat it.

As far as it went, the treatment plan was working. The rest of the plan was to continue that way for a while, keeping the pressure off him and letting his curiosity about food, and his desire to grow up with eating get him to try some new things. No doubt, it would have been slow. After a few weeks of relaxed, no pressure eating, we may have tried cutting back on his juice and milk a bit so he would be more hungry. Hungry kids are better at accepting new foods.

Erik's family had a good start, and then they moved away. It was disappointing for me not to see how it all turned out. I think, however, that they will continue their improvements in the way they managed his eating. They got the basic idea: Their job was the structure and limits and his was the eating. Once they shifted the way they looked at the problem, that freed them all up to operate more effectively with eating.

Failure To Thrive

Physical growth failure in the absence of a known medical cause has been called *nonorganic failure to thrive* (NOFTT). There are two types[1]. One, Type II NOFTT, is a fairly new diagnosis and resembles our earlier discussions in this chapter, and in this book, of children and their parents who are having struggles with feeding severe enough to have an impact on growth. This designation originated with the Georgetown Hospital feeding team. I heard about it from Thomas Linsheid, a psychologist who helped set up the team and has since moved to Cleveland Children's Hospital. (The Georgetown program is still active.)

The other, Type I NOFTT, is a diagnosis that is familiar to medical personnel. It is more severe, and management is really outside the scope of this book. I wouldn't expect any of my readers to be having this problem, because parents of Type I NOFTT babies aren't functioning well enough to read a book. You need to know about this condition, because you might recognize it in someone else.

Type I NOFTT begins in a baby's first few months of life. It is severe growth retardation secondary to underfeeding which, in turn, is the product of inadequate parenting. Babies with failure to thrive are severely limited in their physical and emotional growth. They don't like being around people. They tense or startle or withdraw when someone walks into the room, rather than showing the openness and curiosity of a normal baby. Parents of these babies are under a lot of stress, and have severe emotional limitations. They simply don't have the energy or capability to provide for themselves, let alone their child, or even to realize that they or their child have needs that are not being met.

When anyone expresses concern about their child's thinness, and wonders if she is getting enough to eat, parents of Type I NOFTT children will say she is. In fact, they will often protest that the child is getting enough even while they watch her child wolf down any food that may be offered. In most cases, the parent is not lying. She is functioning in such a limited way that she *simply doesn't know.*

Babies with Type I NOFTT often are distressed during feeding. Even though they are clearly starved, they fight the bottle—which is understandable in light of what goes on during feeding. In The Newborn (Chapter 7), I talked about Mary Ainsworth's observations of mothers and their babies. Among those cases were five which were typical of Type I NOFTT situations.

Feeding was absolutely arbitrary in timing, pacing or both. The mothers would put their babies away for long periods, and either tune out the crying or fail to realize the crying meant that the babies were hungry. Feeding times were erratic, as were feeding styles. Sometimes the mothers forced their babies to eat long past the point where they were full, and sometimes they interpreted any pause as satiety and stopped feeding. Feeding

was at the mother's whim, and showed little reflection of the
baby's wishes. As Ainsworth put it, a mother's determined stuffing of her baby "had to be seen to be believed." Little wonder
the babies were upset and confused when they had to deal with
feeding.

Treatment involves helping the parent, and helping the
interaction. Treatment teams work to reduce the stress on the
parent as much as they can, through social services like the vis-
iting nurse or financial assistance programs. They also teach and
support her in appropriate parenting.

Type II nonorganic failure to thrive is a term that means
poor or delayed growth in children usually over age eight
months who have previously experienced appropriate weight
gain. Problems include refusal to progress from liquid or pureed
foods, mealtime tantrums, exaggerated food dislikes and phobias
and delays in self-feeding. Type II NOFTT may be a disease of
over-concern, when children and parents have gotten into power
struggles over feeding that are so vehement that children simply
do not eat well. It may also be a disease of under-concern, when
parents are simply not involved enough with children to meet
their feeding needs or support age-appropriate behavior.

If you and your child have gotten into such a bind with
eating that it is impairing his social or physical growth, you will
need help getting out of it. You won't be able to see what you
are doing or, if you can see it, the pressures on you will be great
enough that it will be extremely difficult for you to resolve it.

Failure To Engage The Child

It takes a lot to draw some babies out. They are sleepy, not
terribly engaging, and easy to put down and leave down. They
don't demand much feeding and caring. If you combine them
with a parent who is over busy or over stressed or easily made
to feel unimportant, you can have a situation where the baby
doesn't get enough care and attention and might not even get
enough to eat.

Feeding babies requires time, and patience, and a willingness to check back at the end of the feeding and make sure the
baby has had enough to eat. It also requires that the parent be
engaging, and able to work out ways of helping the baby to

maintain a quiet alert state. She needs to be alert and organized enough to keep going with feeding, but not agitated or overwhelmed.

At times, putting the baby down and leaving her down is exactly what parents want. They are impatient with caring for her, and all too ready to stop feeding at the earliest sign of satiety. These same parents may or may not take their later responsibilities for feeding seriously. There may be a meal, or there may not. Children may be provided for, or they may be expected to forage for themselves. It's hard for children to get enough to eat under those circumstances, let alone getting the right *kind* of food.

Other kinds of neglect in feeding are more subtle. Parents might present inappropriate food to the child: Adult-type food that she has trouble eating, or food that is too low in calories. They might not give their child as much support as she needs to get served or get started eating. They might be emotionally remote, and ignore her at mealtime, and fail to give her the companionship and social support she needs to eat well. They might take advantage of mealtimes to vent gripes and impose discipline.

When mealtimes are tense and children don't have their emotional needs met, it has an impact on eating. They may be reluctant to experiment with new foods and have a hard time regulating their food intake: they may overeat or undereat. Eating becomes tense and anxious, and invested with all kinds of negative feelings that they are likely to carry with them into their adult life.

The Case Of The Pursuing Parent

A dietitian called me about a mother who was concerned about her 2½-year-old son's poor eating. The boy accepted only a very limited assortment of foods, despite the fact that she said she cooked well and presented them to him in pleasant fashion. She said they had meals, and snacks, and that he regularly turned down everything that was put in front of him. In our conversation, the dietitian and I couldn't figure out where there was any room for improvement, so she passed the case along to me.

I called the mother. I tried, I truly did, to be supportive and kind, but she was very edgy. I told her that, through no fault of their own, sometimes children and parents can get into unhelpful patterns with feeding. Those patterns are often subtle and difficult for parents to see because they are so closely involved with the situation. I went on to say that in view of the fact that she and the dietitian hadn't been able to come up with anything, and from hearing about it, I couldn't think of anything, it would most helpful if I could go to her home and observe the feeding process.

She didn't want that, she didn't see how it would help. And besides, if I were there, the child would just show off for me and I wouldn't be able to see anything anyway. But did I think it would turn out all right if she just kept doing what she was doing?

I said I couldn't possibly say, because I wasn't familiar with the situation. As an alternative suggestion, perhaps they could use their video camera and do some taping of them and the child in the feeding situation and then bring in the tape. They could just set it up on a tripod to show what eating was like at their house, and we would look at it together and see what we came up with.

She thought that was a pretty dumb idea. Why, in order for her to do that she would have to follow him all over the house and keep the camera going for six hours at a time, because he was always eating or drinking something and she was always trying to feed him. (She went on to say that the doctor said he needed meat, and she didn't think it was necessary. Did I think she should try to get him to eat his meat? I told her that until she was willing to establish a working relationship with me, I wasn't about to comment on anything her doctor had told her.)

I had my answer, but I wasn't going to tell her. I was afraid that any advice I gave her over the telephone would only be distorted.

In the first place, I now knew that she wanted to take the easy way out with the eating problem. It wasn't bothering her enough for her to really get serious about solving it. Until she was willing to take a look at the whole situation, her son's eating would continue to be poor.

In the second place, I was forming a picture of how she

283

handled eating. She provided no structure, no limits, and no expectations for him and his eating. She followed him around all day, feeding him little dibs and dabs, keeping food an issue all the time. She was grateful whenever he ate, for however much he ate. He never had the chance to get hungry, or to discover his own interest in eating. It was far too much his mother's affair.

I worked with lots of situations like that back in my medical clinic days. Poor growth is generally what the parent comes in complaining about, but poor food management emerges as the difficulty.

Having regular meals and snacks and limiting between-time eating is the beginning of the solution. It doesn't help children when they are allowed to simply run and eat. As one grandmother put it, it's like feeding a dog. Children who are fed that way don't learn how to behave well with food, and they don't eat well. It's not so bad when they are little, but when they are older they and their eating become a pain to their elders.

But the most negative aspect of all about that kind of feeding is the way children feel. It frightens them when feeding is irregular and unreliable. They worry that they won't be taken care of.

Establishing Normal Feeding

To solve a feeding problem with your child, work toward normal feeding. Read the age-appropriate chapter in the middle section of this book, have someone observe you and give you some suggestions about what you and your child are doing together that may be causing the problem. Chances are it started out with your child's doing something strange, and it pushed you into doing something counter-productive.

Chances are you either put on too much pressure or provided too little support—or both. Keep in mind that feeding demands a clear division of responsibility. Parents are responsible for picking food and providing meals and snacks. Children are responsible for deciding what and how much they eat. That charges you with providing appropriate food and establishing consistent meals and snacks. It lets you off the hook when you have done that.

Once you get past infancy, the first step in any feeding

284

intervention is to establish structure. This generalization applies whether a child eats too little or eats too much, whether parents push or withhold food. There have to be meals, there have to be snacks, and there has to be no food or drink (other than water) available in between times.

Once the structure is in place, the details of interacting with a child around feeding can be attended to. To do that, the division of responsibility can be interpreted in age-appropriate ways. Throughout this book, but particularly in the chronological chapters in the middle, I have discussed the specifics of dealing with children in eating.

No matter what the age of your child, Is the Toddler Jerking You Around At the Table?, (Chapter 9), will be helpful in establishing the basic routines. If your child hasn't yet learned to be a good toddler, you'll have to get that job taken care of.

Feeding problems are common. Everybody has some trouble with feeding, and in some situations, that trouble can disintegrate in major struggles. Once begun, feeding difficulties can become self perpetuating. The way *out* of the struggles is to share responsibility for eating. At every age, children eat best when parents provide appropriate meals and stacks, and children are left in charge of choosing from what is available and regulating the amounts they eat.

You may be able to get yourself out of your own difficulties about feeding, or you may require professional help. Whichever approach you use, the goal is to get back to doing your own job with feeding, and letting your child do hers. You must discharge your responsibilities as a parent, but you must free yourself from the impossible task of getting her to eat.

References

1. Linscheid, T.R.: Feeding disorders during infancy and early childhood. IN Feelings and Their Medical Significance. Columbus, OH: Ross Laboratories 241-C815, 1985.

2. Linscheid, T.R.: Disturbances of eating and feeding. IN Drotar, Dennis. New Directions in Failure to Thrive; Proceedings of a Conference. New York, Plenum, 1986.

285

3. Satter, E.M.: Childhood eating disorders. Journal of the American Dietetic Association 86:357-361, 1986.

4. Satter, E.M.: The feeding relationship. Journal of the American Dietetic Association 86:352-356, 1986.

5. Neifert, M.R. and Seacat, J.M.: A guide to successful breast feeding. Contemporary Pediatrics 3:1-14, 1986.

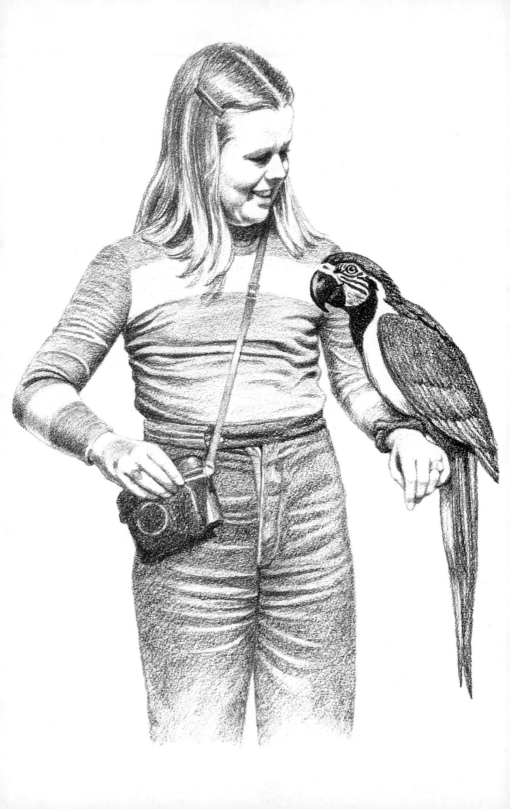

14

Helping All You Can To Keep Your Child From Being Fat

You can help your child to avoid becoming obese by maintaining a healthy feeding relationship. That relationship is the same as with any other child: You are primarily responsible for WHAT your child is offered to eat, he is responsible for HOW MUCH.

Your job with the obese child or the potentially-obese child is to do the same kind of good parenting with feeding, showing the same respect, sensitivity and self restraint, that we have been talking about throughout *How to Get Your Kid to Eat*. Once you have done that, your job is done, and you simply have to let go of it, let yourself off the hook, and let nature take its course.

I am absolutely opposed to putting children on diets. In my view, no person has the right to impose starvation on another, even if that other person is your child. Withholding food profoundly interferes with a child's autonomy, and you will both pay the price for that. He will grow up feeling angry with you, bad about himself, dependent on you to provide controls on his eating, and void of those controls within himself.

289

Resisting Pressure To Put Your Child On A Diet

You undoubtedly will get pressure to diet your child. The pressure may come from health professionals, school, media, family, friends, and your own feelings. The last is the most difficult to withstand. Parents feel watched, and they feel responsible. They can give in to the pressure—or not give in. Which they choose can have great consequences for the child.

A few years ago, my neighbor, Sandy, was telling me about her feelings about her then-adolescent son, Dan, who was quite fat. He had been a chubby little boy and at age 12 had developed a big spare tire. He was very active. In fact, his father coached one of the soccer teams and Dan played faithfully, year after year. But it didn't seem to help his weight much.

Sandy tried not to put pressure on him about it. But she said it was hard for her. Whenever she and Dan, for instance, went out for one of their very-rare ice cream cones, Sandy said she always felt like other people were watching them. And she just *knew* what they were thinking: "Why is she letting that fat boy have that ice cream cone? No wonder he's so fat!"

I was struck by the contrast between her attitude and that of another neighbor whose son, Jeff, was the same age as Dan and was equally fat. "You're getting too fat," she told him. "We are going to have to do something about it. No more ice cream." (I was shocked that she would talk like that in front of me. And no more ice cream? Who can live without ice cream?) So they put Jeff on diets, and tried to restrict him. It never worked very well, because they were always breaking their diets and then trying again.

A few days ago, I saw Dan on the bus. I had to look twice, and look up to him. He is 17, and well over six feet tall. He has slimmed down a lot from what he was at age 12. He is not thin, but he also is not fat. He is about normal weight and is pear-shaped and looks kind of soft, but that is a body type that a lot of men have. Dan looked good, he was dressed nicely, and he seemed to feel good about himself. Sandy tells me his eating and weight are not big concerns for him or the family.

Jeff is fatter than he was five years ago, even though he's a lot taller. He is embarrassed about his weight, and he won't eat with his parents. They generally prefer a low fat, low meat diet, and when they eat, Jeff goes out for hamburgers and french fries. With parents who are so intrusive, Jeff has to get completely away from them to declare his independence.

Using Indirect Methods

Dan's parents didn't apply a diet, but they *did* act on his behalf. They applied the indirect methods I will share with you in this chapter. These methods are intended to keep the child responsible for his own eating and help you control the availability of food and help prevent overeating.

They are not intended to promote under-eating. There is a big difference. You are out to help your child regulate the amount he eats as accurately as possible, and grow up with the body that is right for him. You are not out to try to get him to go hungry so he can achieve the body that you or your advisors *think* he should have or *wish* he would have.

The way it turns out might surprise you. A physician called and congratulated me about the Mills brothers (not the singers). I had seen them about their weight about five years previously, when they were ages 17 and 18. They were both pretty soft and round looking at that point, and each wanted to lose about 30 pounds. Neither had dieted before, and they came with their mother, who wanted to know how she should cook to help them. When they were little, she had done what I considered to be a very nice job of feeding her sons and maintaining a positive feeding relationship with them. She just *fed* them, and didn't try to get them slim.

I instructed them in some dietary modifications and behavior change techniques and they told me about their plans for increasing their exercise. I never saw them again. According to the doctor, they had lost all the weight they wanted and had maintained it. He told me what a good dietitian I had been, and I thanked him, even though I knew I didn't deserve all that much of the credit.

Weight reduction efforts worked for them because they were in a position to be successful. They had grown up with good attitudes about eating and themselves. When they tried to lose, it was because *they* were ready, not because someone else was pushing them. They had waited until they got their growth to make that one first effort that was most likely to be successful. Because their bodies hadn't adapted to previous under-eat-

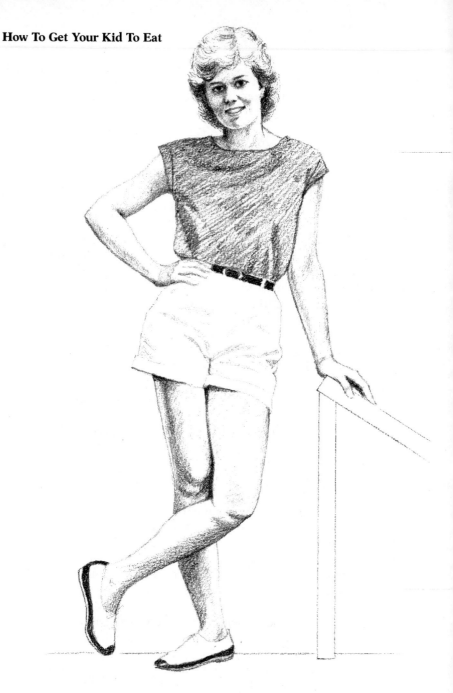

Figure 14-1 A girl who slimmed down. The 12-year-old from page 288 is now 21—and slim.

ing, they cooperated in letting go of the weight, and the brothers were able to do what they had to do to maintain.

I could tell you lots of stories about children I have known who were fat when they were little and slimmed down as they got older, all by themselves with no particular efforts. (See Figure 14-1.) The research bears me out[4]. Children often go through times when they are fat, and they lose that fatness. The idea is not to overreact and impose a diet, because that could promote the very problem you are trying to treat.

Eating Management

The methods I will describe are indirect and non-depriving, so you can apply them to everyone in the family—the skinny ones as well as the fat ones (or maybe the potentially-fat ones). If you apply them matter-of-factly, your children won't even know what you are doing. In fact, the methods are so doable and they can become so habitual that *you* won't remember what you are doing, either.

Don't underestimate, however, the amount of discipline it's going to take to institute them. Or the amount of discipline it will take to keep from putting pressure on your child about his eating and weight. You will be doing more than you realize. Over your child's growing-up years, your patience and persistence can make an enormous difference.

Maintain A Positive Feeding Relationship

Maintain a positive feeding relationship throughout the growing-up years. For instance, when you feed a baby with sensitivity and respect, you help to prevent obesity. When you do the same for a toddler and add on the kind of limits we talked about earlier, you help to prevent obesity. And so on. At all ages, the best plan for obesity prevention is the plan for *normal feeding* I laid out in the earlier chapters of this book.

When you maintain a positive feeding relationship, you allow your child to feel relaxed and comfortable about eating and in touch with his internal cues of hunger, appetite and

293

satiety. You help him hang on to these feelings as he grows up, so eventually he will get the body that is right for HIM.

If you maintain a positive feeding relationship, you will avoid overfeeding at one extreme, and withholding food at the other. Either extreme can make a child eat too much and gain too much weight.

Most people assume that fat children are the product of overfeeding. That does happen[1] but not always. At the other extreme, *under*feeding can make a child preoccupied with food and prone to overeat when he gets a chance[2]. For some people (probably the ones with a genetic predisposition to obesity), once gained, excess weight is extremely difficult to get off and keep off[3].

This is such a hard point to get across to people, that I will make it still again: *Even the fat child is entitled to regulate the amount of food he eats.* You don't have to do that, and you shouldn't try. Don't try to assume that responsibility even in sneaky ways, because your child will be on to you. Sneaky ways include saying, "Don't you think you have had enough?" Or, "Isn't that your second helping?" And we can't forget the reigning monarch of all sneaky ways, *the look.*

One of my young patients added her advice for parents: "Tell them, 'don't not offer food.' If they do that, it means that they don't trust their child. I would much rather have had it offered to me so I could have had the choice of eating it or turning it down."

Before you start berating yourself for any of your previously less-than-optimum feeding tactics, let's put this in perspective. Some people fail to make meals for their children, then yell at them about what and how much they eat. You can do better than that. Lots better.

Maintain The Structure Of Meals And Snacks

In a 14-year study of almost 200 children in the San Francisco Bay area[4], Dr. Leona Shapiro and her colleagues could find only one dietary factor that distinguished fat from thin children: The thinner children had more structure in their meals and snacks.

Structuring meals and snacks was the first and major intervention I made with Melissa, an obese five-year-old whose family came to me wanting help with her "compulsive eating." They were trying to cut Melissa back on her food intake, and she was constantly after them for food. She had tantrums when they refused her seconds and she sneaked to get food between meals. She was constantly hanging around, wanting something to eat.

Her parents felt very ambivalent about what was going on. They didn't like underfeeding her, but they were angry at her too for making such a nuisance of herself. It seemed like no matter what they tried, they just couldn't be successful with her.

As you can see by her growth chart, Figure 14-2, Melissa's weight had jumped from the fiftieth to the ninetieth percentile between ages 18 and 24 months, when her family was under a lot of stress. I don't know specifically why she got too fat then. Maybe she was upset and anxious, and they didn't have much tolerance for her fussing, and they used feeding to comfort her. But when things settled down in the family, her weight stabilized. She gained appropriately at the new, higher level for the next 18 months.

When Melissa was three and a half, they visited their pediatrician, who told them she was too fat and they should do something about it. They started cutting back on her food, and over the next eighteen months her rate of weight gain again increased. It appeared their attempts to withhold food, which I'll call restrained feeding, was currently at the heart of the problem. Her preoccupation with food that was resulting from the restrained feeding was making her eat more and actually making her gain more weight than when they had just been feeding her normally.

We set out to reestablish normal feeding and get rid of the restrained feeding. The first step was to reassure Melissa that she would get enough to eat. We let her know she could have snacks, and what times those snacks would be. We told her she could have as much as she wanted at meals and at snacks. And we told her she would not be allowed to eat between times.

Melissa's parents were ahead of the game, because they were doing a good job of having good meals. However, they were giving food handouts instead of having planned snacks, so they started to work on that. They set up regular snack times, and started choosing some food for snacks that she liked and was likely to be filling and satisfying.

The structure and reassurance worked. At first she ate

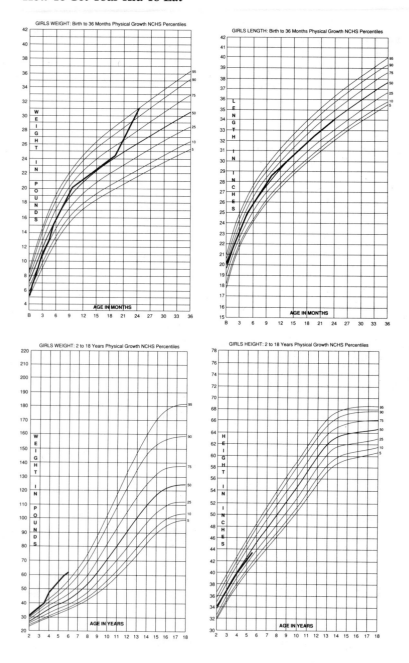

Figure 14-2   Melissa's Growth Chart

quite a bit, and she pestered them for food in between. But they held firm and kept their bargain about allowing her to eat as much as she wanted, and after a couple of weeks her pressure on food began to drop off. She still wanted a lot on her plate (it seemed she needed that to reassure herself she would get enough), but she often didn't finish it. She would go off and play, and occasionally she would even play through snack time.

Now Melissa's eating is more positive and relaxed, and her weight has leveled off. If her parents can continue to do a good job of parenting with feeding, we all have hopes that that trend will continue, and that she will even slim down over the next few years.

Teach Orderly And Positive Eating

Teach him to eat slowly and attentively. Have him sit down on his chair and get his backside planted and relax a little. Talk to him about eating slowly, and work on it with him. Make mealtimes pleasant with conversations and sharing and DON'T use that time for scolding or airing grievances.

Model slow and attentive eating, and let him know you expect the same from him. Put teeth into that expectation, if you must. If his eating style is disgusting, make him leave the table. About one trip should do it. If he eats fast, make him wait a couple of minutes before seconds. He'll particularly need good manners if he grows up to be fat. If he eats sloppy, he'll look like a glutton. If he eats in an orderly fashion, he'll feel and look like he is in charge of his food intake.

Eating slowly will give him time to enjoy his food and to find his internal stopping place. If you are not depriving him of food, he will be able to learn to tolerate his hunger and experience it as a positive, not a negative feeling. He will not fear his hunger because he'll know he can make it go away.

Paradoxically, as happened with Melissa, when you give people permission to eat and reassurance that they will get enough to eat, they can learn to become more controlled and orderly about their eating. I have used this method with lots of people who have eating disorders, and many others who are just chronic dieters who are eating chaotically. When they become more positive about their eating, they can settle down and eat in a more controlled fashion.

The slow eating technique, and the delay before seconds, are not tricks to get your child to eat less. They are methods to help him be sensitive in detecting his own hunger, appetite and satiety, and depending on those cues in regulating the amount he eats. The most delicious, wonderful and scrumptious food in the world won't be satisfying if he eats it too fast and doesn't pay attention to it.

To help your child regulate internally, you have to be able to do it yourself. If you are orderly and positive about eating, you can teach your child to eat in a way that is self-regulated and satisfying. I am not talking about the kind of "satisfying" that is promised by the weight loss organizations, where you smile cheesily and say, "It's so satisfying—I'm hardly hungry at all." Nor do I mean the kind of satisfying that leaves you feeling so full you wonder if you can get up from the table. I mean an eating-enough-but-not-too-much, hitting-the-spot, sticking-to-the-ribs type of satisfying that he can find within himself, again and again, and look forward to, and count on for his method of regulating his food intake.

Finally, turn off the TV. I am astonished that many families eat in front of the TV every single night. An occasional TV dinner for a special program that you all enjoy can feel good for the whole family. But having it there *all the time* destroys family interaction at the dinner table. It's simply not possible to gratify children's needs for attention, support, and limits when the TV set is on.

Cut Down On Feeding Cues (Reminders)

Some people are cue sensitive to food. That means that if there are food reminders to eat around, they are likely to eat. If there is a lot of food around, they are likely to eat more. Some people know when they are full, and then they don't eat another bite. Others groan, "Oh, I shouldn't, but it tastes so *good*." Some children will eat more when there is food around or it looks better, others will not. These appear to be innate differences.

Cue sensitivity, however, can be *caused* as well as inborn. While studies of obese people indicate that they are more cue sensitive than thin people, this can also be the product of restrained eating. Obese people who are *not* restrained eaters are no more cue sensitive than normal-weight people who are

298

not restrained eaters. Normal weight people who ARE restrained eaters are as cue sensitive as fat people[5].

A candy dish or a cookie jar is a booby trap for a cue sensitive eater. I am not saying we should give up candy or cookies. To me, this amounts to cruel and inhuman punishment. But what I AM suggesting is that we have candy or cookies when we WANT them and are hungry for them and can pay attention and really enjoy them. I think it's a waste of calories and pleasure just to grab a cookie and eat it without thinking because the cookie jar happens to be sitting there, calling.

If a child generally eats somewhere, say, on the floor in front of the TV, it can be a reminder to him to eat whenever he sits down there, whether he *really* wants to eat or not. Wouldn't it actually be nicer to spare him the necessity of thinking about food at all, except when he is hungry for it and really wants to eat it?

You can help by limiting his opportunities to eat. Maybe he should only eat at the eating tables (most houses have more than one). When he eats, you could have him eat *only*—no TV, no books. He'll have to choose between eating and doing something else. At times he'll choose one, at other times, the other.

Now, anybody who lives with children knows that if you impose that rule, everyone in the household will have to do it, too, including you. Otherwise, your at-risk child will say to you, "If it's such a hot idea and so good for me, how come the rest of you aren't doing it?" So do it. It's good for all of you. Compared with depriving and dieting, it's a piece of cake. Oh, excuse me. Unintentional eating cue.

Once again, these cue-limiting tactics are not intended as tricks to get him to undereat. They are intended as techniques to encourage deliberate and attentive eating that is likely to be satisfying.

Keep The Caloric Density Of Food Moderate

It will likely help your child to be thinner if you hold down on the caloric density of your usual food supply. Caloric density means the number of calories per bite in a food. Foods like french fries and candy pack quite a caloric wallop because they are so high in fat or high in sugar. That is also what makes those foods so very delicious. From birth, babies have a preference for

299

a sweet taste. Many of us learn a preference for fat because it carries the flavor in food and makes many foods taste better.

High-fat, high-sugar foods add pleasure and calories to the diet. Both are important. But if your child consumes too much fat or sugar it can impair the nutritional quality of his diet and contribute to excessive weight gain. Studies show, however, that fat children are no more likely to eat excessive amounts of high caloric density foods than thin children[4].

To me, this seemingly contradictory bit of information simply means that, unlike thin people, fat people pay a *price* for eating high-calorie foods, and that price is excessive weight gain. People who are genetically programmed to be fat are likely to have relatively low requirement for calories and relatively low metabolic ability to squander excess calories. For them, a high calorie diet could overwhelm their ability to regulate and make them get too fat.

(Exercise also comes into play here. If a person is too inactive, it is likely that their internal regulatory cues are easier to overwhelm[6]. I'll talk about that more in the *exercise* section of this chapter.)

As I'll explain in a minute, try to cook moderately in terms of fat and sugar, but not morbidly so. When your child is small and just developing his tastes, teach him to use modest amounts of sugar on his cereal and sour cream and cream cheese and spreads on his bread. That isn't intruding on his prerogative of food regulation, because you aren't trying to deprive him of food. Using modest amounts of fat and sugar are health concerns for *any* child, and when he gets a little older, you can teach him that.

Then it is his responsibility, your job is done, and you had better keep quiet. If you keep after him about the amount of sour cream or sugar he uses, it will be nagging and criticizing. He'll know better, but he may choose to eat more anyway, just because it tastes so good. Just like his elders.

But don't cut out the high-calorie foods. If you deprive, your child will want that, and so will everyone else in the family. I know a family that is *so* austere about eating: Everything is low sugar (the father is diabetic) or low fat (the mother has heart disease) or low calorie (the daughter has a weight problem). And everybody in the family has caches of food. The father's is the best: He keeps Godiva chocolate in a locked drawer in his study. He thinks it's his little secret.

Don't force your child to sneak to get "sinful" food, and don't go overboard on the low-calorie alternatives. I have had lots of patients, as adults, who couldn't *look* at a piece of broccoli because they had had so much of it foisted on them when they were children and had grown up to foist it on themselves when they were on diets. One of my patients who had been dieted by her mother said it best: "Don't push diet foods or withhold cupcakes. I got so I hated carrots and celery, and I was so envious of kids who had sweets in their lunch boxes."

Since you can't feed your (potentially) fat child one way and the rest of the family another, we have to shift the focus of our discussion to the *family* eating style. I have dealt with that topic in some detail in Nutritional Tactics for Preventing Food Fights (Chapter 6).

To summarize, you've got to find a balance between being depriving and being lavish. It is a personal balance, and only you and your family can decide where that balance will be. You might start by seeing a registered dietitian and getting a dietary evaluation. You might find you are already as austere as you should be. Or, if you are using excessive amounts of fat or sugar, you could start to cut down on some of those calorically concentrated and nutritionally dilute foods.

But make your changes SLOWLY. It is *hard* to change your eating. Since it is permanent change we are working on, you really have to be patient about it. If you *are* slow, and you *are* patient, you will get to the point where you all truly prefer and enjoy your new way of eating. If you try to do it too fast, it will always seem like a sacrifice and you'll all go on a family-style binge every chance you get. I see families who are too spartan all week and then cut loose at the drive-in on Friday nights or build in overeating as a part of their vacations. Don't try to do that. This whole regimen must be positive, not so negative that you have to take vacations from it.

The goal in all this is NOT to come up with a disguised weight reduction diet. It won't work to take all the fun out of eating, and caches of food all over the house you do not want. They draw bugs—and eaters. The goal is to come up with something that is tasty and satisfying for everyone and gives enough calories so everybody can get filled up on it—the big as well as the little eaters.

Do include high-calorie food, if you like it, and show your

301

child how to savor it. Eat it very slowly and really enjoy it. Moan, if you will. Teach the idea—and learn it yourself, that you don't have to eat a LOT of something to really enjoy it. Eat like a gourmet, tuning in on the exquisite pleasure of it all.

Don't Feed Unnecessarily

Comforting your child with a cookie when he skins his knee is feeding unnecessarily. So is giving soft drinks or juice for thirsty drinking between eating times, when water would do just as well. A child can take in a lot of extra calories in a day's time by drinking flavored beverages for thirst.

You will be going to extremes, however, if you try to avoid ever feeding for emotional reasons. Sharing food is a perfectly valid way of comforting or celebrating. The problem with most emotional eating is that it is done POORLY. People feel like they shouldn't *ever* use food for emotional reasons, but they go ahead and do it anyway and do it in a hurry and in a guilty, furtive fashion.

You can make good emotional use of food by being very orderly and positive about it. Go to some trouble to get something your child really likes, and take time eating and responding to it.

Think Of Your Child As "Normal" When Making Feeding Decisions

Don't treat your child differently because he is fat (or potentially fat). If you start making feeding decisions based on your desire to get him thinner, you soon will be into the area of depriving, and *that* will backfire. Try to think through feeding problems in the same way that you would for a normal-weight child.

Let me demonstrate how I used this principle with Christopher, a three-year-old obese patient whose parents I was helping with eating management. The first order of business was to establish structured meals and snacks. The second was for Christopher (and his parents) to learn that the parents were in charge of feeding, and after initially putting up quite a fuss to find out if they really meant it, he seemed relieved to have them take over.

They established a routine for meals and snacks, and stopped short-order-cooking and food handouts.

Feeding problems related to the obesity were more tricky, and the parents had a hard time figuring out how to deal with them. They were at a pot luck picnic, and everyone put their food out on the table and the adults were talking and the children playing while they waited to eat. Then SOMEBODY BROUGHT BROWNIES—wonderful, gooey chocolate brownies with lots of fudge frosting. And the kids made a bee line for them, Christopher right along with the rest. So what was Mother to do? She really didn't want him to eat them, but the only reason she could think to give was his weight.

I asked Mother what she would have done if she hadn't been concerned about Christopher's weight—if he had just been "any kid." And she said, "I would have made him stop, because those kids were eating up all the brownies and I wanted some for myself."

Perfect answer. He was also wrecking his dinner, but I liked her answer better, because it's pretty normal kid behavior for them to go for the sweets and wreck their dinners at parties like that. When they are little. When they get big they go for the sweets and the dinner too and you never let them go first in line.

Some eating situations are just going to be nutritionally hopeless. If it's an occasional thing, I wouldn't worry about it. If it happens a lot, you are going to have to deal with it. If, for instance, a neighbor is rolling out the goodie cart with the snack cakes and pop every afternoon, you are going to have to figure out a way of dealing with it.

I would suggest you go in by way of nutritional concerns rather than weight concerns. That will allow you to be much more matter-of-fact in telling your child, and your neighbor, that you don't want him having that food for his snack every day. Or maybe you don't mind, as long as it is *just* a snack, but you don't want him running over and eating that stuff all afternoon.

The point is, if your child is only behaving like the other kids, and the only reason you can think of for curbing his eating is your concern about his weight, you'd better let it pass. If you do anything, you'll end up putting pressure on his weight. He'll feel singled out, and embarrassed, and you may just make matters worse.

But normal-weight kids don't benefit from snacking all the

303

time and gobbling their meals and keeping after the cookie jar. You are not discriminating against your fat or potentially-fat child by preventing these behaviors, nor are you making your thin children suffer. You are only parenting well with food.

Use Your Own Good Judgment When Setting Feeding Limits

The major thing you have to avoid is ambivalence. Don't try to get yourself to do something you don't feel comfortable doing, and don't make feeble attempts. Either make a reasonable intervention and follow through with it, or forget it. Keep in mind that you are not punishing your child with this regimen as you would with a weight reduction diet. Setting limits is not the same thing as depriving. Your child will not go hungry unless he wants to.

You also have to agree with your partner on what you are going to do. If you want to limit eating to the table and your partner doesn't agree, you'll have to hammer that out, or your child will do exactly as he pleases. If he is allowed to eat in front of the TV one time and not another, it will still condition him to think of food when the TV goes on.

Encourage Exercise

Exercise can help. I have put exercise under the "eating management" section, because people have to get a certain minimum level of exercise to allow their hunger and appetite to accurately reflect their true calorie needs[6].

In the California study I talked about earlier[4], children who later became obese were shown to have exercised less when they were younger. To restate, when children were toddlers and preschoolers, they were still slender, but not as active. When they got into the school years, they remained less active, and became fatter.

What are we to make of this? We are probably justified in some modest optimism that exercise may help. We are probably NOT justified in saying that exercise is the *answer* to weight problems—for some people, perhaps, but not for everyone.

The best way to increase exercise for young children is to let them do what comes naturally. While activity levels vary,

304

even the least-active child is active by adult standards. Toddlers are constantly on the move. They prefer running to walking, and their running is so inefficient that they spend at least as much energy keeping themselves upright as they do moving forward. Parents, too, are on the run—fetching, bringing back.

Preschoolers are the same way. They are in a contest with the environment. They want to climb higher, run faster and play harder than they ever have before. They love rough and tumble play, and times together quickly disintegrate into a tangle of arms and legs and pummeling and riotous laughing.

Not all parents can take that. Not all parents have the judgment to know when normal activity disintegrates into destructiveness, nor do they have the nerve to let their child do things that have an element of danger. It's in this area that you should take a close look at exercise. Get some help adjusting your expectations of what children this age *do*. Observe in playgrounds, talk to day care workers. Think through your own history—were your parents very protective of you? As with eating, if you have real problems letting your child take the lead with exercise, you had better get some help for it.

But be *very* careful with encouraging add-on exercise. It's a good idea to pick out more active forms of recreation as a family (like biking and playing badminton rather than going out to eat or to the movies), and doing it because it's fun. It's not a good idea to take over your child's decision of whether or not he will exercise.

As with eating, exercise demands a division of responsibility: You need to make the opportunity available, your child has to choose whether or not he wants to do it.

Finding a middle-of-the-road approach to exercise is not a trivial issue. As with diet, parents of fat children are feeling pressure. The current trend in thinking among fitness and weight loss people is, "OK, apparently diet is not going to do it, but exercise will." That kind of thinking can entrap you into too-energetic efforts to get your child to exercise so he can be thin. If you put too much pressure on your child to exercise, he will be onto it in a flash. And he'll either plod along to please you, hating it every minute, or he will do the opposite.

I hope your child *will* be able to get interested in exercise. The advantages are many. Exercise *might* help him to be thinner. He can always hope, even if it is frustrating not to be able to

305

depend on it. But there are other advantages that he *can* depend on, like feeling strong and comfortable with his body.

Let Your Child Develop The Weight That's "Right"

If you consistently use these indirect methods throughout your child's growing-up years, you will give your child his very best chance of not getting fat. You will have controlled his eating environment in a very positive way, and prevented periods of overeating and excessive weight gain. You will have allowed him to go through periods of fatness and not scared him by putting him on a diet. Food will not be a major temptation to him because he will never have had to go without it.

At the most, the odds are with your child that he will be of normal weight—most children do slim down as they get older. At the least, I expect your child will turn out to be thinner than he otherwise might have been. Even if he turns out to be some-what fat, you will have to reassure yourself that you have done all you can, or perhaps, should. Anything beyond that would have involved imposing harm.

Help In Other Ways

Along with eating management techniques, there are many other ways you can help your fat, or potentially-fat child. You can help him grow up to be as emotionally healthy as possible, and you can help yourself to feel comfortable with what you are doing.

Help Your Child's Self-Esteem

Hilde Bruch, a specialist for many years in eating disorders, talked about emotional health and obesity in a way that so echos my patients' feelings that it is spooky[7]. Bruch says that she has come in contact with two kinds of obese people over the years: the emotionally healthy and the emotionally unhealthy. The unhealthy obese person sees his weight as being the single most salient feature about him. He hates it, and he is dedicated to getting rid of it. In his view, he *has* to do that, because until he gets thin he will not be able to do, be, or acquire anything he wants in life. He essentially has his life on hold until he can get thin.

The emotionally healthy obese person, in contrast, feels good about himself. He is well aware of his obesity and would probably prefer to be thinner and may even have tried at some point to be thinner. But it hasn't worked out, and he has decided that it isn't so centrally important anyway. He is living his life, and achieving things, and has friends and lovers and generally does just fine.

The difference between the two groups, says Bruch, is parental attitude. In the first case, parents have been vehemently preoccupied with their child's weight and have gone to extreme lengths to get rid of it. And, comments Bruch with some embarrassment, the greater the number of helpers the more negative the outcome. The helpers are people like me and other health workers and teachers and commercial weight loss businesses and YMCA workers and coaches and neighbors who are trying to get the child to eat less and lose weight. As one of my patients said: "All the help didn't really help, and just made me feel worse and worse about myself."

Redefining The Problem

I think I help people, and the way I help them is to define the problem in a way that it can be solved. I teach them to parent well with food, to enable and encourage exercise, to let their child's weight do what it will in response to their consistent and moderate efforts, and to reassure themselves that they are doing all they reasonably can. It is when people become adamant that they *must* achieve a certain weight level that they intensify their efforts and end up doing harm.

I also help by working with parents, and encouraging them to allow their child to grow up as emotionally healthy as possible. That starts out with good parenting, which depends on a good relationship between parents, or, at least making sure the child is not getting caught in battles between them. One divorcing couple I worked with had a son who became very obese at age six, just before they separated. The mother was overprotective, the father was overly demanding. Each criticized, and tried to compensate, for the excesses of the other. As a result, their son got no clear and reasonable guidelines from either.

307

When parents are able to work productively with each other, we work on the kinds of things we would with any child, such as respecting infants as individuals, by being sensitive and patient and curbing our responses so we don't overwhelm them. When they get older, we work on listening to and respecting their feelings and setting appropriate limits. And we work on dealing with the special problems of the fat child. One of the big ones is that other kids tease them about their weight.

Kids can be tough, and they can be hard on each other. They'll even tease somebody in a wheel chair. The popular kids of all descriptions learn to handle it; if you shelter him, you'll give him the message he can't take it. You'll have to listen to his hurt, and acknowledge that it must bother him, but then ask him how he intends to deal with the situation. His ideas might surprise you. The important thing is to give him some support, then turn him around and send him right back out there. You won't help him by being over protective.

It would also help if schools would do some consciousness-raising with the children. Special school programs can teach kids that "everybody's different," and everyone has feelings. They can help kids learn not to be so prejudiced and cruel with fat children.

Enhance His Appearance

Help him to look nice. Some clothing styles will look great on him, others will not. There are subtle differences in the cut of clothes that can make an enormous difference in the way kids feel and look. Teach him that, and encourage him (and yourself) to keep on shopping until he finds the styles and the cuts of pants and shirts that look and feel good.

Because he's a kid, he'll probably want to wear a style that looks ugly on him, and great on someone else. He's the one who has to make that choice. Lay it out to him: "Because of the way you're built, some styles will look better on you than others. You can make a difference in your appearance, depending on the way you dress. But I know that some of the things that don't look as good are the things that are stylish right now, and I can understand why you want them. So, you decide. All I ask is that you wear what we buy—I don't want to waste my money on clothes that hang in the closet."

Don't try to soften this for him. It's his body, and the sooner he reconciles himself to doing what he can to enhance himself, the better off he will be.

Keep Your Fingers Crossed

When Yogi Berra said "It ain't over 'til it's over," he could have been talking about raising children as easily as about playing baseball. You won't be able to tell whether your child will grow up thin until he grows up. Growth does some surprising things. Most babies are chubby during the first year or two, and they get thinner when they get older. Some children gain weight during times of family crisis, like when their parents divorce, but they lose it later[8].

We don't know why some children slim down and others don't. Some children are chubby throughout the school years, then slim down when they go through their pubertal growth spurt. Some children seem to get fat in *preparation* for their growth spurt, as if their body is storing up energy for all the demands of growing[9].

If you intervene by restricting food intake while your child is still growing and going through natural fluctuations in fatness, you could really mess things up. Adults who undereat decrease their metabolic rate, so they simply get along on less calories than they did before they dieted[10]. There is evidence that children who undereat do the same thing. They certainly can decrease their growth and their rate of maturation and will not have as much energy to enjoy life and physical activity.

Don't Be Tempted To Impose A Diet

Now is a critical time in the treatment of childhood obesity. The pressure on parents to diet their children is already high, and I am afraid it is going to get even worse. Statistics have recently been released that point to an alarming rise in the incidence of childhood obesity[11]. Obesity has increased by 54% among children age 6 to 11 and by 39% among children age 12 to 17. Most health workers and researchers attribute this increase to overeating and under-exercise, and recommend more exercise and less food.

While I can't quarrel with the essential truth of these impressions and advice, the notions are simplistic because they don't reflect any understanding about what is *causing* children to under-eat and over-exercise. Furthermore, the intervention, if applied in an insensitive fashion, can do more harm than good. Most health professionals don't think in terms of the feeding relationship. They don't realize how much potential there is for helping by enhancing the feeding relationship, from birth on. And they don't consider the impact of imposing diets on family interaction and on a child's self esteem.

It would be nice to put a child on a certain number of calories and have him lose weight, and then he could go back to eating normally and from then on be thin. But it doesn't work that way. In reality, you try to impose a diet and the child may go along with it at first. But then he will get hungry and want more to eat and pester you. And you will disagree with your spouse about how much he should have, and while you are arguing and angry with each other about it, your child will help himself to whatever he wants.

You will break your neck cooking low-fat, low-sugar everything and your child will go next door to the neighbors and eat eight cookies or go out with the gang for french fries, and you will feel like killing him. And you will rant and rave and, to your shame, you might even say, "If you are fat it is your own fault."

And the brothers and sisters will say, "Why do we have to eat this stuff just because Jeremy is fat? We haven't had chocolate chip cookies since he started this diet six weeks ago and it doesn't look like he is even losing!" And beastliest of all beastly behaviors, they will tattle, "Why, I saw him at the shopping center the other day eating an ice cream cone!"

I can think of no better way to get a family to fight, or to make a child a scapegoat, than by imposing a weight reduction diet on a child. And, as we observed with Melissa, our little girl who was labeled a compulsive eater, parents are always ambivalent about imposing a diet. It just doesn't feel right not to feed a hungry child.

(To get a feeling from a child's point of view for what it is like to be the subject of a family's weight reduction efforts, read *Dinah and the Green Fat Kingdom*[12].)

The formula doesn't work. Not only does it cause a lot of pain, in most cases it does not allow the kind of significant, permanent, life-changing weight loss people hope for. In adults, only about 5% of people who diet lose and maintain weight loss[13]. People lose over the short haul, but maintaining it is another story. Most regain.

Studies done on obese children and adolescents are more optimistic, but still definitely mixed. They lose about 10 to 30% of total body weight, on average[14]. For the 200-pound adolescent, that can mean becoming less obese, or it can mean resolving a weight problem.

Kids can't choose. They may do all the right things to lose weight, but fail to lose if their bodies won't cooperate. The limits on success hold true even for programs that are energetic: Lots of work on diet and exercise and, in the best ones, work on self esteem. If you talk personally to the professionals running the groups[15 16], they say that amounts the kids lose are secondary in importance to their improvements in other areas: Overall physical capability, nutritional status, and in feeling better about themselves.

They say that at some point the kids have to reconcile themselves to the idea that all their dreams about their weight may not come true. But that isn't so hard, once they have gotten far enough in the program to discover that they have other options. That reconciliation is extremely important. Out of a lack of resolution grows heightened anxiety about eating and weight, extreme methods to lose weight, and reactive overeating and further weight gain.

We, too, have to reconcile ourselves to the fact that our dreams about our children and their weight might not come true. I am talking about helpers as well as parents. We have to stop making kids feel like they will lose all their excess weight if they will only try hard enough. Being so unrealistic with them about their chances of being thinner is not motivating—it is just setting them up again and again for failure.

Some people *can* lose weight and keep it off because their body metabolism cooperates[3]. But the popular perception that anyone can get thinner if they only want it bad enough and are willing to work on it hard enough is simply not true. It is not true in a realistic sense, that is, in terms of the totality of their lives. Sure, if someone is willing to starve cruelly and exercise obsessively, and be so hungry all the time that all they think about is food, then they could be thin. But they would be thin,

311

lonely people who would have poor odds of success in work and in play, people hard to know and hard to deal with, who are so starved that they don't have the energy to devote to other things.

Don't Blame Yourself

It's not all your fault if your child is obese. The most significant influence on a child's weight appears to genetics. The particulars can vary, but generally the scientists say that if both parents are obese, a child has about an 80% risk of being obese. If one parent is obese, a child's risk drops to 40%, and if neither is obese, to 10%. (This was recently confirmed by a big Danish adoption study[17]. The weights of adoptive children reflected their birth parents' weights more closely than their adoptive parents' weights.)

However, while genetic factors exert a powerful influence, the fact that childhood obesity has increased so much in the last few years[11] indicates that there are environmental factors as well. On the other hand, it's hard to know what those environmental factors really *are*.

Some people say that obese people get that way because they overeat. Some do. But in most cases, obese people eat no more, and perhaps eat less than normal-weight people. OK, say the experts, obese people might not eat so much, but they exercise too little. Wrong again. Probably. By the time you realize that the obese person has to carry that much more around, walking a shorter distance or making less trips uses up just as many calories as more apparent activity does for the thinner person.

Well, then people get fat because their parents cook too rich or because they bottle fed them or started them on solids too soon. Wrong still again. No consistent evidence to support it. If you cook rich and you have two children and one is genetically programmed to be fat and one to be thin, one is likely to grow up fat and one likely to remain thin. Life is profoundly unfair.

So what is going on? It's probably not that eating and exercise management don't make any difference. It probably *is* that obese people pay the price for the same kinds of indiscretions that thin people get away with.

That view is at the same time both frustrating and hopeful.

312

If you can manage throughout your child's growing-up years to enhance his exercise and eating (but not so energetically in either area that he reacts and overeats or under-exercises), there is a chance that he will grow up to be of normal weight. Or he may be thinner than he would have been otherwise. It's not the ideal, but does offer some hope.

Attitudes Must Change

Sadly, some people are just going to be fat. Your child might be fat. I hope he can grow up feeling good about himself, and I hope societal attitudes continue to change so people recognize that if someone is fat it *isn't* necessarily his own fault, that he *isn't* necessarily unhealthy (or even unhappy) and that he *shouldn't* be willing (and able) to do whatever is necessary to get thinner.

The least we can do as a society is not blame fat people for their condition. The most we can do is loosen up on our ideas of attractiveness. Our society currently has ridiculously unrealistic attitudes about body weight and beauty. The standards of slimness are so stringent right now that even slender people do unhealthy things to themselves to get thinner.

I must remind you, however, that society's attitudes and standards have to be passed along by parents in order to do any real harm to the child. So the impact is on YOU—and it's not easy, because these standards make it hard for you to remain moderate and unobtrusive.

You have a challenge. Parents of any child who does not fit the norm have to come to grips with their special challenge. Part of doing that is letting go of the dream of what your child *could* have been like, part is learning not to overprotect.

Obesity in many ways is a handicapping condition. (However, unlike other handicapping conditions, it is blamed on the sufferer.) It is hard to raise an emotionally healthy, obese child in today's weight-prejudiced society. It can be done. To achieve it, you will need help, and support.

The best supports are going to come from other parents, from parenting groups, and from professionals who specialize in family dynamics. You'll have to keep the weight problem in proper perspective. Your child *can* be emotionally healthy at his present weight. But almost everyone, even professionals, has the

313

idea that a child has to get thinner before things can get any better.

Look For Underlying Causes

By the time an obese child or a child who is gaining too much weight comes to me for help, the doctor has seen him, and any medical basis for the problem has been ruled out. At that point, I assume the problem is being caused by one or more of four main factors: genetics, overfeeding, restrained feeding or emotional or physical stress. I TREAT them all the same. I use the same principles of management that I have talked about in this chapter. However, figuring out cause helps me decide if the family needs additional help beyond eating management.

I get clues to the source of a weight problem from the *pattern* of weight and the type of interactions around food that are going on in the family. If a child's weight has been consistently high throughout his growing-up years, and if family interactions are healthy, I suspect that the problem is genetic.

I go over the interventions with the parents, and see if instituting them makes any difference in the child's weight. If it does, it appears something in the environment was causing the child to overeat. If it doesn't, we assume the environment is pretty good to begin with, the cause is genetic, and the parents are doing all that they can to help him grow up slim.

If, however, a child suddenly puts on a lot of weight for no apparent reason, I suspect there is something going on in the family that could bear correcting. Children generally grow in a consistent fashion, and it takes a major stress to cause big variations in their growth. Family interactions can provide that kind of stress.

I ask the family what was different at the time the child gained too much weight. Usually, there was something happening in the family that encouraged the child to overeat or underexercise.

Melissa (the "compulsive eater" I talked about earlier in this chapter) gained a lot of weight when she was a baby and her parents were having a difficult time. After we got into treatment, it became apparent that her eating continued to be connected with her family's emotional functioning. We got rid of the restrained feeding and her eating stabilized. But from time to

314

time, the father would begin to complain that her eating was terrible and she was getting too fat.

In every instance, when we tracked down what was really happening, it emerged that he was upset and anxious about something that was going on with his wife—Melissa's mother. It was hard for him to deal directly with his wife, so he turned his upset and anxiety on to Melissa. Eating behaviors that he had overlooked before or that he had dealt with matter-of-factly began to look alarming to him. He started to criticize her eating and to withhold food from her and worry about her weight. Melissa then got scared she'd have to go hungry and went back to all her old food-seeking behaviors. If allowed to continue, that kind of pattern could have made Melissa overeat and gain too much weight.

Another example is Daniel, who started to gain too much weight when he was a baby. It was during the time his grandfather was dying, and his grandmother was staying with their family. His grandmother would go the hospital to visit, and get very upset. She would come home and get Daniel and get his bottle and they would rock and Daniel would eat. She found it so comforting; and Daniel loved eating, and would keep it up as long as grandmother wanted to.

Daniel's mother recognized what was happening, and chose not to intervene. She knew her mother-in-law was going through a difficult time, she didn't think Daniel was getting hurt that much, and she gambled that things would turn out. She was right. The grandfather died, the grandmother went back home, and when things settled down in the family they went back to feeding Daniel normally again. And his weight went back down to its previous level.

It is important to find and change the family interactions that promote the problem. If we just deal with the child's eating and weight, we'd be making the child pay for all the family's difficulties. The situations would likely not get resolved, and the weight problem would be perpetuated. Family problems have to be dealt with more directly, in counseling that gets the whole family involved.

Whatever You Do, Make It Permanent

The methods I have shared with you are pleasant and tolerable enough so you can live with them. Forever. They require

315

you to get organized and be firm about your organization and develop modest expectations of your child. They don't require you to deprive your child of enough food or good food.

If your ideas of what you should be doing to help your child made you feel depressed when I said you should apply the method *forever*, you are being too negative. You had better develop some more modest tactics. Figure out a realistic system that you *feel* comfortable with and that you can sustain. To feel good about yourselves, you and your child must feel successful in accomplishing your goals.

What If Your Child Wants To Diet?

Some time your child may choose to go on a diet to find out if he can lose weight. That might be a positive thing, under certain conditions. First, he should be through growing. The methods I have described here are surprisingly powerful ones, and, if carefully followed, can have a significant impact on your child's eating and weight. Until he gets his growth, he really isn't going to be able to tell what his body will be like, and nature just might take care of the problem. Plus, dieting could impair his growing[18], and that is too great a price to pay for thinness.

However, as I pointed out in the The Individualistic Teen-ager (Chapter 12), he will be governing much of his own eating and exercise, and he may benefit from some guidance. I wouldn't try to do it, if I were you. Encourage him to see a professional, a registered dietitian, to get some ideas of changes he can make in that area, changes that are modest enough so he won't do anything destructive to his growth.

When he *does* get through growing, and *does* want to make that first major effort (IF he does—it has to be his idea, and he has to be truly ready), he should follow all the guidelines for healthy dieting. It will be a matter of degree: a well-balanced diet with only a modest decrease in calories, moderate increase in exercise, allowing time to get it off.

Again, this is a good time for professional consultation. It will help him get started with methods that are truly helpful, and healthful, and may prevent a lot of damage along the way. A good book for him is *Winning Weight Loss for Teens* by Joanne Ikeda[19]. The author is a University of California teacher who knows her topic and knows kids, and she has written a realistic and helpful book.

316

Make sure you, and he, keep it his thing. Sure, you can help him by keeping certain foods around, and giving him encouragement. But don't get yourself in the role of supervisor or enforcer. He'll end up fighting with you rather than adhering to his diet.

You will have already done a great deal to help out. By not putting him on a diet while he was growing up, you have done him the favor of keeping him a virgin dieter. In my years of helping people lose weight, I have seen just a few who have lost weight and kept it off. They were all people who had never dieted before. Statistics show that the first diet is the one that is likely to be successful. All subsequent diets don't work as well. You have saved that one first try for him.

I wish I could reassure you that your child will turn out to be of normal weight if you do all that I recommend. The odds are with you, but there are no guarantees. I *can* reassure you that using these methods will help your child to be as thin as possible and will allow him to feel better about himself.

Self esteem is the bottom line. We are building feelings and behaviors for a lifetime. If all goes well, your child will grow up with good attitudes about himself and about food and with a habit of positive and deliberate eating.

If you need more convincing about the advisability of the moderate approach, read the next chapter, Eating Disorders. It will give you examples of what has happened with children and their weight when parents have tried too hard to help.

Parents feel an enormous amount of pressure to *do something* to keep their child thin. There are some things you can and should do, to help prevent obesity, and I have outlined them.

Beyond that, there is nothing you should do because there is nothing you *can* do. You can't withhold food from your child or force exercise on to your child, you shouldn't try, and if you *do* try, it will probably make matters worse.

It is as important to be careful about what you *don't* do as what you *do* do. It is so easy to move in and put pressure on a child's eating. I could write *another* chapter on all the ways. It is so hard not to. Like other issues in parenting, dealing with the whole issue of obesity requires restraint, and patience, and letting your child take the lead.

317

References

1. Klesges, R.C., Malott, J.M., Boschee, P.F. and Weber, J.M.: The effects of parental influences on children's food intake, physical activity, and relative weight. International Journal of Eating Disorders 5:335-346, 1986.

2. Costanzo, P.R. and Woody, E.Z.: Domain-specific parenting styles and their impact on the child's development of particular deviance: The example of obesity proneness. Journal of Social and Clinical Psychology 3: 425-445, 1985.

3. Garrow, J.S. and Warwick, P.M. Diet and obesity. IN T. Yudkin: The Diet of Man: Needs and Wants. Applied Science Publishing, Barking, 1978.

4. Shapiro, L.R., Crawford, P.B., Clark, M.J., Pearson, D.J., Raz, J. and Huenemann, R.L.: Obesity prognosis: A longitudinal study of children from the age of 6 months to 9 years. American Journal of Public Health 74:968-972, 1984.

5. Rodin, J.: Has the distinction between internal versus external control of feeding outlived its usefulness? IN Bray, G.A.: Recent Advances in Obesity Research. London: Newman, 1978.

6. Mayer, J.: Exercise and weight control. Postgraduate Medicine 3:25-37, 1959.

7. Bruch, H.: Eating Disorders: Obesity, Anorexia Nervosa and the Person Within. New York: Basic Books, 1973.

8. Shapiro, L.R.: Verbal communication. April, 1987.

9. Christian, J.L. and Greger, J.L. Nutrition for Living. Benjamin Cummings, Menlo Park, 1985.

10. Keys, A.J., Brozek, A, Henschel, O., Michelsen, O., and Taylor, H.S.: The Biology of Human Starvation. Vols. 1,2. Minneapolis: University of Minnesota Press, 1950.

11. Gortmaker, S. and Dietz, W. Increasing pediatric obesity in the United States. American Journal of Diseases of Children 141: 535-450. 1987.

12. Holland, I. Dinah and the Green Fat Kingdom. Philadelphia: Lippincott, 1978.

318

13. Stunkard, A. and McLaren-Hume, M.: The results of treatment for obesity: a review of the literature and report of a series. Archives of Internal Medicine 103:79-85, 1959.

14. Peck, E.B. and Ullrich, H.D.: Children and Weight: A Changing Perspective. Berkeley: Nutrition Communication Associates, 1985.

15. Mellin, L.: Verbal communication, April, 1987.

16. Ikeda, J.: Verbal communication, April, 1987.

17. Stunkard, A.J., et.al.: An Adoption study of human obesity. New England Journal of Mediciane 314:193-198, 1986.

18. Pugliese, M.T., Lifshitz, F., Grad, G., Fort, P., and Marks-Katz, M.: Fear of obesity: A cause of short stature and delayed puberty. The New England Journal of Medicine 309:513-518, 1983.

19. Ikeda, J.: Winning Weight Loss for Teens. Palo Alto, CA: Bull Publishing. 1987.

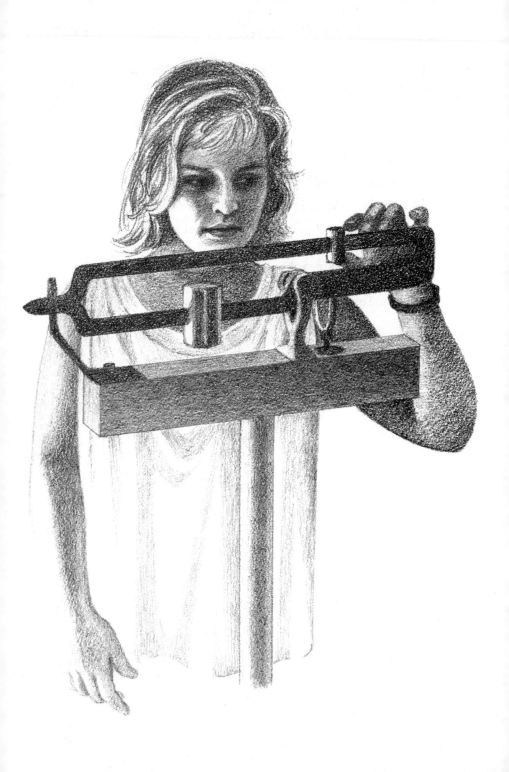

15

Eating Disorders

Disturbances in eating attitudes and behavior are on the increase. More and more people of all ages are confused about their eating, locked in a struggle to change their bodies, and limited in the time and energy they can devote to other activities. In some cases the struggle becomes so vehement and engrossing that we can call it an eating disorder.

People who struggle with their eating may be underweight, normal weight, or five, 50 or 150 pounds overweight. They may be starving, gorging, vomiting to get rid of excess food, or eating in a way that appears normal. What is common to all is the heightened anxiety about eating, vehement concern about maintaining a particular body weight, and eccentric thinking about what eating and weight control will do for them. They see thinness as being absolutely instrumental in being, accomplishing or acquiring what they think they want in life. Sometimes that longed-for thinness is a weight three or five pounds less than their present weight.

Eating disorders are extraordinarily complex. An eating disorder is a *biopsychosocial* illness, meaning it rises out of factors in a person's biological makeup, and from their psychological and social characteristics as well. An eating disorder, by definition, is a distortion in eating that is accompanied and supported by an emotional problem. The eating distortion is, in fact, considered to be a *symptom* of the underlying emotional difficulty.

People with eating disorders think that if they got thinner, they would be able to accomplish what they want, work things out with other people, and feel comfortable in the world. What they don't realize is that they basically don't feel good about themselves, they don't know how to work things out with other people, and that even becoming a beauty queen will not resolve those problems.

I say beauty "queen" because at this time, most people who are detected to have eating disorders are women and girls. There are a few men, and the issues are the same. The men, like the women, are having trouble making it in the world, or they are making it at extreme sacrifice. And they see achieving thinness as a way of helping themselves.

Let me emphasize that an eating disorder is *not* the same thing as an eating *problem*. I have talked in this book about many eating problems. Eating problems can exist in healthy families who are operating on the basis of misconceptions about feeding or who have been given bad advice. Many feeding problems grow out the idiosyncracies of children—they are sick or small or eat in a way that parents find upsetting. Families with eating problems *know* they are having problems because they are sensitive to their own feelings of upset and those of their children. They seek help, and, if they get good advice, are able to change the way they operate.

I have also talked in this book about many eating disorders (although I usually haven't labeled them as such): situations in which parents were having enough personal or relationship problems to interfere markedly with their ability to do an adequate job of managing feeding. Resolving the difficulty with the child's feeding has required working with both aspects of the problem: the eating and the emotions underlying it.

Until a problem becomes extreme, eating disordered families can't acknowledge their difficulties and deal with them. They persist in a given course of action, even if it isn't productive and even if it makes their child upset and unhappy. For them to realize there is something wrong, the child has to get *really* sick or upset (for instance, develop an eating disorder). That may finally force them to get help, and once they ask for help, it takes the utmost effort for them to change.

Making the distinction is important for choosing *treatment*. Families that have an eating problem will be able to read a book or to talk to a knowledgeable professional and get some advice and change the way they operate. Families that have an eating *disorder* will require psychotherapy that deals with the emotions and interactions in the family before they can resolve their struggles with eating.

To help orient you to what I will say in this chapter, I want to remind you that I am a mental health professional—a clinical social worker—as well as a registered dietitian. I treat eating disorders in my clinical practice. To do that, I have to draw on my skills as both a dietitian and a clinical social worker.

I want you to realize my dual roles, because I am going to explain both parts of the illness to you—the emotional part as well as the eating part. As we go through this chapter, I think you'll notice that sometimes we are talking about the eating aspect of the illness, sometimes the emotional aspect, and sometimes the two are intertwined.

Stories Of Eating Disorders

It will be easier for us all to understand this difficult topic if I tell you about the people involved. I will point out the issues as we go along.

Sharon

Sharon was a university sophomore at the time I met her. She had participated in an eating disorders emphasis week on the University of Wisconsin campus, and began to wonder how normal her eating was after one of the lectures. She had been hesitant to do so because she didn't fit the usual definition. But she thought she had an eating disorder, and I agreed with her. She had both emotional struggles and distorted eating. Her eating behavior most closely resembled the designation, "failed chronic reducer" in Figure 15-3, "Types of Eating Behaviors." (This table, which is on page 338, describes some variations in eating and distorted eating. I'll only refer you to it now, and say more about it later.)

Sharon had lost 50 pounds after a year of rigid dieting. At the time I met her, her control was starting to slip, and she was desperately afraid she would regain all of her weight. (She had, in fact, already regained 20 pounds.) She was totally sick of the rigorous means she was using to keep her weight down, and unsure of how much longer she would be able to sustain her efforts. She was resentful of the people she saw around her, because she saw them *eating* and having what they wanted and not having to go without the way she did.

But in spite of all her negative feelings, she tried to adhere to her 1400-calorie maintenance diet, eating the same monotonous foods that she had when she was dieting, because that was the only way she could keep her appetite under control. But even operating that way, periodically she would binge—she would eat prodigious amounts of all the foods she was trying to stay away from—chocolate bars, potato chips, chinese stir-fry on rice, bagels with cream cheese, and large quantities of cake (nibbling away at it a quarter-inch at a time).

Then she would feel TERRIBLE, and SO fat. She had tried vomiting and couldn't do it, so instead she would try to compensate by cutting back to her old weight reduction diet, and even below it. But that would last only so long, and then she would binge again. And try to cut back again.

She thought about food all the time. When she was depriving herself, she felt bad because she was missing out. But when she ate, she felt guilty and worried about getting fat. She was starting to wonder if thinness was worth the price she was paying for it.

Sharon had the psychosocial (emotional and social) characteristics of a person with an eating disorder. She was having a hard time personally. As a university student, she was around other kids all the time. But she was very lonely, and often felt depressed. She got good grades in school, but didn't really have much interest in what she was studying. She didn't know how to make friends, and had difficulty maintaining the friendships she had. She would often get angry at the way other people treated her, but she didn't know how to express her anger or work things out any better.

It was hard to tell, at first, how much of Sharon's negative feelings about herself and other people came from undernutrition. People who chronically underfeed themselves have no way of knowing how much of their tension, bad disposition, irritability and general lack of commitment is the direct result of undernutrition. The only way Sharon would find that out was to stop underfeeding herself, and see how she felt.

But her family history indicated that her problems went deeper than just suffering from an energy deficit. Sharon's struggles with eating and weight went back to her earliest childhood. As far back as she could remember, every time her mother took her to the doctor, the doctor would tell her mother she was too fat and that they had to do something about it.

Sharon's mother did express her ambivalence about Sharon's eating and weight. She told Sharon she looked OK—but then she took her around from one clinic to another, trying to find something that would solve the problem. On the one hand, Sharon's mother reassured her, but on the other hand, she tried to get her to go without second helpings and to skip snacks. Her messages, and methods, couldn't have been more contradictory —or unrealistic. She expected Sharon to eat apples, even when the other kids were having cookies.

Sharon wanted to cut down on her eating and lose weight, but she also wanted to *eat*. So sometimes she did what her mother said, and sometimes she defied her mother and ate. And sometimes she deliberately overate to irritate her mother, and they fought about it. "How can you eat like that?" Her mother would scream. "Look how fat you are!"

Sharon's eating became the focus of family fights. That was the *one* thing her family fought about. Other than that, they represented themselves as an "ideal" family. Her father was an MD, and her mother was a professional volunteer. Both were leaders in the community. The other kids thought Sharon's family was just great, and she couldn't imagine why she felt so miserable there.

The family worked hard to have no problems. Once Sharon had had a needle under the skin in her foot for six months. She kept telling her father it was there, and he kept saying there was nothing wrong. After they finally believed Sharon and got the needle out, her mother made excuses for him, saying, "He loves you so much he doesn't want there to be anything wrong with you."

325

Unlike Christine, whom I'll discuss next, when Sharon was in high school she didn't have anyone's help getting the family problems out in the open. As far as the parents were concerned, everything was just fine, even though Sharon's brother was doing very poorly in school and her older sister was wild and ran around and had sex with a lot of boys. Then one day, when Sharon was a senior in high school, her mother announced she was divorcing her father and went off to marry another man.

At the time, Sharon weighed 150 pounds. In that year, she gained thirty pounds. Her feelings were simply overwhelming, and she didn't know how to deal with them. She was furious at her mother, because her mother had always discounted Sharon's complaints about her father. Now here Mother was, putting in the ultimate complaint! She felt totally abandoned and left to a parent who had not been much help to her in the past. It was time for her to leave home, but she simply wasn't ready.

She felt so awful, and she took it out in eating. People do, and chronic dieting sets them up to do that. People who are chronic dieters are prone to *over*eat, not *under*eat in response to stress.

She tried to get support from her father. She told him, "I feel so frightened and overwhelmed about my eating." And her father responded, "Don't worry about it—just so long as it doesn't get out of control." The underlying message, of course, was, "Don't bother me with your struggles." The message under *that* was, "I can't handle this."

It wasn't that Sharon's parents were bad and awful people who didn't care about her. It *was* that they simply didn't know how to express or deal with their feelings. When they had a problem, or when they got into conflict with each other, it made them so anxious they did whatever they could to get the difficulty to go away. Many times when they were upset, they took their upset out on Sharon and her weight problem. They weren't doing it on purpose—it was all unconscious.

Christine

It's hard to reconstruct all the interworkings in Sharon's family, but we can get the flavor by looking at other families. Let's take a look at another, very similar family, and the way they dealt with each other and their high school age girl.

Christine sought help for her bingeing and vomiting. (In Figure 15-3, I describe her pattern of distorted eating as a "mid-range binge-purge cycler.") She was a skater, wanted to keep her weight low, and spent a lot of time working on it. Unlike Sharon, Christine had no glaring history of distorted eating management in her family. But she did have a history of distorted *achievement* management. It was very important to her parents that she do well in skating, and in school, and in everything else she put her hand to. Her eating got involved because her coach had told her she could skate better if she was thinner.

Christine was not at all open about letting me know what was going on with her, but she did respond when I observed that she seemed to be having some difficulty dealing with some of her feelings. She commented, briefly, that she was having trouble with friends at school. I listened, and encouraged her to say more. She did, a little, and on we went, with my doing lots of encouraging and her gradually doing more and more talking.

Eventually, when she began to trust me to pay attention to what she said, she told me of her difficulties with her family. But she didn't want her parents to come in to a counseling session. In fact, she was pretty put off by the idea.

Christine's feelings and experiences were almost identical to Sharon's—same experience with other kids, same pressure and lack of support at home, even though the pressure was on achievement instead of on eating.

During the first eight or ten weeks we talked together and worked on eating, and Christine told me more and more about what it was like for her at home and at school. She *had* friends, but she didn't have much fun with them. She thought they were kind of boring, but the kids she saw as not boring were doing things she said she didn't want to do, like partying. While she claimed she didn't care about that crowd anyway, she admitted her real concern was that she felt she wouldn't fit in.

She stayed home a lot, even though there wasn't anybody else at home. Her mother worked nights, and Christine was supposed to get dinner for her father when he came in from playing softball. Sometimes she did that, but other times she just stayed in her room, eating and throwing up. She couldn't express her anger and frustration directly, so she did it by stuffing herself and then purging.

Eventually she allowed her family to come in to a session,

327

and I found out why she was so reluctant to share what was on her mind. They simply wouldn't listen.

She began to tell them that she had been bingeing and vomiting, and that she was now realizing that her problem came largely from her sadness and loneliness. Her mother didn't say anything, just looked stony, and her father criticized her: "If you would try harder with your friends and be more sociable and do your work better you wouldn't be having all these problems. All you have to do is work harder and do better at your sport, and you would have all the friends you could ask for."

Not only was father discounting Christine's feelings, he was wrong. Being good at sports wasn't going to allow her to feel better about herself and feel comfortable approaching other people. What would help her was to share her feelings and have them accepted and find out different ways of dealing with people.

Christine's father simply didn't know any better. He had encouraged her to do what he had always done. He didn't know how to have friends and be comfortable with other people, so he used the structure of his work and play to provide social opportunities. But he never got close to anyone, because he didn't know how.

Christine's mother simply withdrew when Christine talked about her problems. The environment in which the mother had grown up was entirely different from the one she married into. She didn't know how to act, and she couldn't help her children. She was so anxious, she couldn't learn new ways of operating. Whenever she encountered a new situation, she blocked it out. To Christine, that felt like her mother didn't care.

Because the mother didn't feel comfortable making friends, she turned to her family for all of her companionship and support. Christine provided almost all the friendship her mother got, and was already starting to worry about what would happen to her mother when she left home.

Marion

It's easy, after the fact, to say Sharon's parents should never have gotten into that struggle with her about her eating. But it is hard for parents of overly-fat children to know how to be helpful to them. To get a feeling for what it is like for them, let's take a look at Marion and her parents. (I've talked about her before, if you remember—in What is Normal Eating (Chapter 5). Marion was the little girl who *loved* to eat, and mortified her mother by moaning audibly between bites.)

Marion was a chubby three-year-old who hadn't grown well on breast feeding, was regarded as overly enthusiastic about bottle feeding and eating solids, and had been pronounced "obese" by her physician at age 18 months. He had frightened Marion's mother by telling her that allowing Marion to remain fat at this age would condemn her to a lifetime of obesity. He encouraged her parents to cut back on the amounts they served her.

Marion *was* chubby, but I have my doubts whether she was really obese. Actually, that's beside the point. Once the doctor pronounced Marion obese, her parents started to worry about it, and it *became* a problem.

Marion's parents felt terrible. They felt like it was their fault that Marion was fat. When she was younger, they had fed her, even when she seemed like she wanted to eat a lot. But after the doctor's warning, they decided they had to start depriving her. They hated to do that, because eating gave her so much pleasure. But they did, because they felt so bad about "overfeeding" her, and were so worried about her weight. And Marion's habitual refrain became, "I'm hungry." Whenever she finished eating, she announced her hunger. All food had to be kept out of her reach, because it was certain to be raided, and she pestered everyone continually for food.

At age 2½, Marion's weight stabilized, but the doctor told her parents to cut back even further. And they tried. Mother tried to serve very small portions, and felt the father served too much. And they fought. It was constantly on their minds, and they felt guilty and ambivalent. They felt bad when she acted so hungry. But they also felt like Marion's fatness was their fault, and whenever they ate in public, it seemed like people were looking at them and saying, "Why are they letting that fat girl have that food—no wonder she is so fat!"

Marion's feeding got off on the wrong foot. With the bad advice they got from the doctor, the situation just got worse and worse. They made mistakes, felt bad, overcompensated, then over-reacted to their adjustments. Feeding was one distortion after another. If, at any point along the way, they could have

329

established *normal* feeding, the problems would not have escalated to the point they did.

I doubt if Marion will grow up to have an eating disorder. Even though her parents were very concerned about her, and about their situation, their over-all anxiety level was not as high as it was with Sharon and Christine's parents. They weren't as rigid. Marion's parents had the ability to look at what they were doing and to self-correct. It was a good sign that they were uneasy with their tactics and aware they were making Marion feel bad. They realized it was spoiling their relationship, always being engaged in that fruitless struggle about eating, and they wanted to change.

They didn't *need* to operate the way they were. They were simply being governed by some very bad advice. For some better advice, see The Newborn (Chapter 7), The Older Baby (Chapter 8), Is Your Toddler Jerking You Around at the Table? (Chapter 9) and Helping All You Can to Keep Your Child from Being Fat (Chapter 14).

Mary

Mary, a 19-year-old mid-range binge-purge cycler (see Figure 15-3) remembers being a Marion when she was little. Her parents did exactly the same thing with her eating that Marion's parents had. But, unlike Marion's parents, they couldn't, or didn't, evaluate themselves. They were determined to get Mary thin. They persisted in withholding food from her, year after year, even though it wasn't working and even though it made Mary miserable. Mary remained fat despite all their efforts. When I met her, she only ate when driven to it by extreme hunger. Then she overate, and vomited.

Mary felt profoundly hurt by her parents' actions, and singled out, and humiliated about her body. Her earliest memory of eating was of being dished up a very small portion of very carefully-chosen food. And she cried, because to her, not getting enough food seemed very much like not getting enough love. And their behavior *did* represent not giving enough love, in a way. They were so intent and single-minded about what *they* wanted that they didn't stop to think about what it was doing to Mary.

330

Even after Mary developed bulimia, her parents couldn't see the error of their ways. In their view, everything in their family was just fine, and if only Mary would clean up her act they wouldn't have anything to worry about. Their view was profoundly distorted. They showed absolutely no warmth for each other. The mother was depressed and anxious and apparently kept herself functioning at high speed with a steely self-will. The father was remote from the family, and only showed up to get his physical needs met and to tell them what to do. Mary had a depressed older brother who had no ideas or will of his own, and simply did whatever his father said.

In most families, I can see parents making mistakes, and I can be sympathetic with them because I sense where they're coming from. Usually I can see through their tough facade and get a feeling for their tender feelings and insecurities.

It was virtually impossible to do that with Mary's parents. They were *so* far removed from their feelings that they *seemed* to be exactly what they appeared to be: hard and self centered and uncaring. I have enough faith in people to believe that nobody is truly like that, through and through. But sometimes it is very hard to get to the point where people are willing to share enough so I can start to feel charitable toward them.

Other Stories

There are other disorders and other stories. I could tell you about the young, 180-pound woman who was so desperate to lose weight that she approached a surgeon about stomach stapling. Her weight, too, had been an issue with her parents throughout her growing-up years. When he told her he wouldn't consider doing the surgery for anyone under 200 pounds, she went home and gained another 20 pounds. She had the surgery, and lost sixty pounds, but she was still in enormous emotional pain.

I could tell you about a 300-pound woman who started out being dieted by her mother, and eventually dieting herself, just like Sharon did. In fact, the woman had weighed exactly what Sharon had—150 pounds—when she was a junior in high school. But, as is more typical than atypical, with each weight loss attempt she regained her weight, and more besides. Thus, in

331

stair-step fashion, she accumulated another 150 pounds over the next 20 years.

She wondered, as Sharon did as she looked back over her young life, whether it wouldn't have been better if her mother had simply let her grow up in the way she was going to grow up. Looking back from 300 pounds, she would have been glad to settle for Sharon's current 150 pounds.

When Sharon kept wanting to diet, I told her that story, and it made an impact. She was able to withstand the temptation of getting back into the depriving again and chasing that dream of making everything all better by getting thinner.

Even though, on the surface, all of the women I have described were very different, they all had eating disorders, and they all showed basic similarities in their behavior, feelings and family interactions.

They all had a history of early childhood distortions in feeding and weight management or, as with Christine, parents put an over-emphasis on achieving, especially physically. Parents were rigid and over-managing of the children's eating.

Family relationships were distorted in typical ways. There was a great deal of conflict in the families, but it was not resolved. In some cases, it was not even *acknowledged*. Children and parents were over-involved with each other, and unlikely to look to people outside the family for warmth and help. Parents, themselves, didn't understand how to make or keep friends, and tended to be over-protective or give unhelpful advice to their children about working things out with other people.

Christine's family was typical of those in the mid-range of eating disorders. They were aware of the emotional distress in the family[1]. In fact, each family member was willing to say that being in the family wasn't very comfortable for them, either. The interactions in the family were generally negative—there wasn't much warmth or emotional support.

Sharon and Mary's families were more typical of those in the crisis level or chronically severe range. Their manner of dealing with feelings was very similar to the way their daughters dealt with eating. They denied the feelings were there and they operated in a way that allowed them to ignore or discount any information that might make them uncomfortable. If you were to ask them, they would say their family was just fine—the only problems they were having were with their daughters' eating[2].

The Eating Behavior Continuum

Let's put these disorders in context with other eating disorders, and with normal eating. Eating behavior exists on a continuum, with normal balanced weight regulation on one end, and crisis level, or chronically severe disorders on the other. Figure 15-1, "Eating Behavior Continuum," illustrates this.

At one extreme, normal balanced weight regulation depends on *internal regulation*. It depends on your internal cues of hunger, appetite and satiety. You trust yourself to go to the table hungry and to eat until you get full. And then you can stop because you'll know there will be another meal or snack and then you can eat again until you are satisfied. When you eat in this automatic, self-regulated fashion, and exercise in a way that is comfortable to you, your weight will be more-or-less constitutionally determined. It will find its own level, depending on your genetic endowment.

The Consequences Of Dieting

The vertical line between "normal balanced weight regulation" and "voluntary food restriction" is a solid line, whereas the other vertical lines are dashed. The greatest single change on the continuum is made when you cross that first line. It is a profound change in eating, and has serious consequences; yet, in most cases, people make the shift very casually.

The shift is in the way you regulate your food intake. Rather than relying on internal processes, you have to start to depend on external processes, like a calorie level, a pattern of food selection, personalized lists of dos and don'ts, frequent weighing, etc. Ironically, however, as you attempt to shift your attention to the external processes, the *internal* processes become more insistent, and you have to invest more and more time and effort in overcoming them.

I am talking about the physical and emotional symptoms of energy deficit: Hunger, increased appetite, fatigue, lethargy, irritability and depression. You have to deprive yourself of eating enough and of eating some kinds of food you like. And you become preoccupied with food and with yourself.

In some cases, these negative feelings become very strong, perhaps because the person is depriving herself terribly, or

333

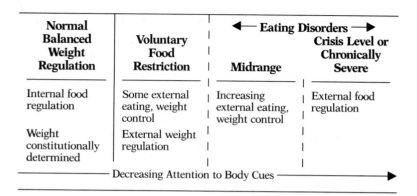

Normal Balanced Weight Regulation	Voluntary Food Restriction	◄— Eating Disorders —►	Crisis Level or Chronically Severe
		Midrange	
Internal food regulation	Some external eating, weight control	Increasing external eating, weight control	External food regulation
Weight constitutionally determined	External weight regulation		
	Decreasing Attention to Body Cues ————————————►		

Figure 15-1   Eating Behavior Continuum

because she is particularly sensitive to the feelings of deprivation, or because she doesn't lose weight very easily and she just
keeps trying harder and harder. When this happens, the person
has a choice: she can either decide the juice isn't worth the
squeeze, and go back to eating normally (or at least dieting less
harshly), or she can intensify her efforts.

Mid-range Eating Disorders

It is at this juncture that we have the potential of moving
to the next point along the continuum, the mid-range eating disorder. The person with an eating disorder does not, or cannot,
allow herself the option of giving up on the diet. A lowered body
weight, in her mind, is simply too important to allow for that
option. Besides, by this time other physiological and habit
responses may be kicking in that make it very difficult for her to
give up her diet.

She may be failing to lose weight on her weight reduction
diet. Many times, the first diet will work pretty well, and achieve
the desired results, but then people will gain their weight back,
and then each subsequent effort to diet gets harder.

When you starve, your body naturally shifts into metabolic
low gear to conserve itself. It is likely that each exposure to dieting makes that downshift more efficient. Your body has no way
of knowing whether you have voluntarily gone on a diet or have

334

been committed to a concentration camp, so it makes the same energy-conserving response.

You feel less energetic, and, whether you know it or not, will conserve energy in little ways as you go about your regular activities. You get cold more easily, because you start to conserve heat. You think about food all the time, and your appetite becomes keener, not because you are short on will power, but because this is your body's natural way of mobilizing you to seek food and save yourself from presumed starvation.

It is entirely possible to get crabby and irritable and depressed and hard to be around. People vary in their emotional sensitivity to undereating—some people feel only a modest effect, others suffer keenly. I don't know that that has anything to do with food seeking, but it does have an important point to make about emotional stability. You can't be as emotionally stable as possible as long as you are eating poorly. We are talking *calories* here. You might be getting all the protein and fatty acids and vitamins and minerals you need, but as long as you are low on *calories*, you will feel the effects. And so will the people around you.

Even with all these negative feelings and lack of success, the person with an eating disorder still cannot give up the diet. If she is maintaining on a *diet*, what will happen if she *stops* dieting? And, so she persists, and even redoubles her efforts. And the pressure on eating accumulates and, sooner or later, overwhelms her.

And she eats. At first, it feels like an enormous relief, and it is *so* reinforcing. Food never tastes so good and it never *feels* so good to eat as when you are starving. But, having no permission to eat, she can't just eat *enough*. At some point in the process, she says to herself, "Well, I've already blown it, I might as well really blow it." And she eats a lot, typically in a very chaotic fashion.

Then the remorse sets in, along with the nausea and lethargy and too-tight clothing from having eaten too much. And the only way, in the person's mind, to recover from the remorse is to diet again.

Starve-binge Cycle

People with eating disorders show a characteristic starve-binge cycle that is presented in Figure 15-2, "Starve-Binge Pattern."

335

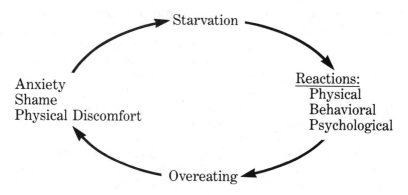

Figure 15-2   Starve-Binge Pattern

Almost everybody who deprives herself of food for any length of time gets into this pattern. It is common to all of the eating disordered people I talked about in this chapter.

People complain of the overeating, but it really all starts with deprivation. They undereat, the negatives build up until they can't stand it any more, and they eat.

It takes a lot of stamina to put up with the chronic pain of going hungry. People can at times diet successfully and get their weight down when things are going well, when stress is low or there is lots of encouragement coming in from the outside. But when outside stress builds up, or a person just plain feels tired or upset for whatever reason, that stamina just isn't there and they give in to the pressure to eat.

Again, at this point the person who is simply dieting can choose to give up the process and go back to eating normally. But the person with an eating disorder can't give it up. Besides, miserable as it is, being engrossed in the cycle has its compensation: It takes up a lot of time and physical and emotional energy and frees the person from having to deal with other, more distressing issues that seemingly have no resolution.

That's what Sharon and Christine and Mary were doing, and that's what their parents had done all the years they were growing up. They were all preoccupying themselves with the eating/weight problem, and not turning their attention to other, more important, more distressing underlying issues.

So we fit the emotional difficulty in with the distorted eating, and the picture of the eating disorder is complete.

Types Of Eating Behaviors

It will help our discussion if I am more specific about the eating behaviors that exist along the continuum. Eating behaviors in general appear in a variety of forms, including several varieties of eating disorders ranging from the mild to the severe. Figure 15-3, "Types of Eating Behaviors," describes some of the stops along the way of the eating continuum.

These are descriptive categories, for the purpose of detailing the type and range of eating behaviors involved, and to give you a feeling for when a behavior crosses from the "normal" to the "eating disordered." The descriptions' primary usefulness to you is in helping you to know when to be concerned. If you see an eating behavior in your child that I have placed in the eating disorder category, you had better get in for an evaluation with a mental health professional who is knowledgeable in the area. Only that person will be able to determine whether or not your child has an eating disorder.

There are other types of eating disorders as well. I have said in other places that at times the struggle between parent and child about eating really is the surface representation of a severe emotional problem in the family as a whole, and can be called an eating disorder[4]. Sharon and Mary's early history each fit that definition, and I think they (and their families) had an eating disorder when they were little, though according to the classical definitions of specific disorders it might be technically correct to insist on waiting until they got grown up to say that. It's really not important that we can't call it by the common labels of anorexia or bulimia. The eating distortion was there, the family emotional discord was there, and the kids were getting caught in it.

I have worked with other people in psychotherapy whose presenting problem was a struggle with eating that was so pronounced I recommended an eating disorder diagnosis. A person with diabetes comes to mind. Her feelings about eating were so conflicted she could no longer adhere to her diabetic regimen. She was doing many self-destructive things with her management, obsessing about it constantly and using her preoccupation

337

NORMAL EATING   Regulation of food intake by depending on internal cues of hunger, appetite and satiety. Body weight is likely to be pretty stable.

VOLUNTARY FOOD RESTRICTION   Intentional dieting with the goal of losing weight. It may be *occasional*, or *habitual*, but people can generally give it up when they want to or tolerate it and be successful with little distress.

EATING DISORDER   By definition, an eating disorder involves both significantly distorted eating attitudes and/or behavior and an emotional problem. People are no longer *voluntarily* dieting and, typically, can't discontinue it without help. Any of the patterns below can be precipitated by athletic training.

Mid-range eating disorders   People in this category are functioning, with difficulty, in their lives. They can get in touch with their feelings, and they can act on their own behalf in getting better.

Situational purger   Occasionally uses vomiting or laxatives or diuretics to get rid of extra calories; the behavior is voluntary and doesn't cause a lot of emotional distress, and may not even be an eating disorder[3]. This is categorized as an eating disorder because it's not a good idea and it could easily progress to something worse.

Failed Chronic reducer   Diets, and fails at dieting repeatedly, often regains weight to a higher level after each dieting attempt. Periodic starve-binge cycling.

Obligatory dieter   Successful at maintaining a lowered body weight, but must pay meticulous attention to eating and exercise to do so. The deprivation is severe enough to cause life-limiting symptoms: Fatigue, irritability, depression, and an inability to concentrate or to achieve social or emotional goals.

Binge-purge cycler—Mid-range   Repeated use of purging techniques to compensate for *perceived* overeating. Cycle is chaotic and causes shame and anxiety. Weight varies, except extreme underweight means a person is anorexic.

Crisis level or chronically severe eating disorders   Are in medical and/or emotional crisis and likely to require hospitalization or very intensive outpatient support. They are too anxious, depressed or disoriented to be able to detect that something is seriously wrong and act on their own behalf.

Binge-purge cycler—crisis May have disrupted body chemistry or have caused physical harm from the cycling, or may be in psychiatric crisis.

Bulimic anorexic Maintains an extremely low body weight by near starvation in conjunction with periodic binge-purge episodes.

Restrictor anorexic Consistently maintains very low food intake and body weight.

Figure 15-3 Types of Eating Behaviors

with her diabetic condition to distract her from her profound depression and anxiety.

I have seen people get as destructively preoccupied with a cholesterol-lowering diet, and with food allergies, as the most fanatic weight reducer. In all cases, I have asked the question: "Why do you need to be so obsessed about your eating?" Usually the answer, after a LOT of exploration is that they are having some emotional problem that they feel they can't deal with, so they (unconsciously) distract themselves from it by worrying about their eating.

Treatment

The eating disordered patient must first be medically stabilized. Some might have to be hospitalized, like a person with an alarmingly low body weight or someone who has been doing so much vomiting and laxative abuse that she has distorted her body chemistry.

Once the medical problems are resolved (and under the continued supervision of a medical doctor), treatment of eating disorders requires a two-pronged approach: symptom management to deal with the distorted eating attitudes and behaviors, and psychotherapy to deal with the disturbed feelings and social interactions. Since an eating disorder is primarily a mental disorder, treatment is under the supervision of a mental health professional. I generally do both parts of the treatment myself, because I am qualified in both areas. Other mental health

339

professionals collaborate with dietitians or clinical nurse specialists to give their patients symptom management.

I'm not going to tell you how to treat an eating disorder,
because it is not a do-it-yourself job. It is a problem that
requires professional help and demands participation of the
whole family.

To help your child with an eating disorder, you will first
have to help yourself, and change the way you operate. Do try to
forgive yourself for that. I know you care about your child and
have done what you thought was best for her. It could be that
you care so much that you try too hard to help. You are going to
have to resign yourself to the fact that, for whatever reason, if
your child has an eating disorder, your family interaction is
distorted and requires changing.

How Treatment Works

To give you a better idea of how treatment actually works,
let's go back to the people we started this chapter with. In all
cases, I did the symptom management as well as the psychotherapy. Sharon had individual therapy only, Christine and
Mary had family therapy as well as individual psychotherapy.

Sharon resolved her eating problem after two months of
symptom management. She had a total of about three months
of psychotherapy, and then she moved away. She developed
somewhat better feelings about herself, improved her ability to
work things out with other people, and grew to understand her
family better.

Because the therapy reduced the emotional pressure on
her, she was able to learn through symptom management to eat
normally. Her weight stabilized where it was when she started
therapy: at about 20 pounds higher than she would have liked.
She was lucky. There was no way of predicting where her weight
would go when she started controlling internally again, and
there was a risk it would have climbed back to her previous
high.

When Sharon left, I encouraged her to get more psychotherapy. She still doesn't like herself very much, she is unsure of
her ability to establish warm and close and lasting relationships
with other people. She has an enormous amount of anxiety
about doing well in school and at work.

340

I taught Christine, our vomiting high schooler, to eat normally, too. She, too, maintained her weight close to where she started. Getting her eating under control freed Christine to start to work in psychotherapy on the way she was feeling. After we worked individually for a few weeks, she was able to allow her family to come in to the therapy.

I worked with Christine's parents on paying more attention to what she was saying, and being more positively supportive of her. Then she and her family made the transfer from looking only at Christine's problems and began to look at the way the whole family operated. She was able let them know how concerned she was about her mother. Her father discounted that information, but she felt better anyway, because she had been able to share her concern.

The parents began to work on their relationship with each other, and the mother began to work on feeling better about herself. They started spending more time with each other, and became more open about their feelings. At present, they have taken a vacation from therapy, and may or may not be back. Often people will just get better to the point where the problem isn't such a crisis any more, and then they quit.

I didn't get to work things out with Mary—we did a little symptom management and we talked a little about her feelings. It was her parents' idea she come in for therapy, and when she needed help from them, they came in for two sessions. Their involvement ended the treatment. They made it clear to her that they considered her eating to be her problem, they refused to listen to her point of view on any issue, and it made her so angry she stopped seeing me. She wasn't going to change if they wouldn't change. Clearly, it was only hurting her, but she couldn't see that.

What Can We Do To Prevent Eating Disorders?

This whole book is about prevention. The way to really prevent eating disorders is to have a positive feeding relationship throughout the growing-up years. A healthy feeding relationship grows out of a healthy overall relationship. If things are going well with you and your child, you will be able to maintain the division of responsibility in feeding, be sensitive and accepting of your child's contribution to the feeding process, and be supportive of the way her body turns out.

Have A Healthy Family

Since parents are the architects of the family, that means you and your spouse need to have a good relationship with each other. If you can't swing a good relationship, at least fight directly, and don't get your kids involved in your fights.

The scary part is that you can be operating in an unhealthy fashion as a family and not recognize it—it might be the way every family you have been a part of has operated. To you, it is normal. But the big tip-off is if your children don't do well.

Children will show symptoms of some kind if things are going poorly in the family. Developing an eating disorder is only one of the patterns of symptoms they might show. They might become depressed, or very rebellious, or run away or drop out of school, or abuse alcohol and drugs.

Learn To Eat Normally Yourself

If you diet constantly, your child will grow up seeing that as normal eating. If your eating is fragile and chaotic and fraught with anxiety, her chances are increased of learning to eat in much the same way. It's hard to get weaned off of dieting, so if you know somebody who can help you learn normal, internally regulated eating, GO.

From reading this book and observing your children's eating, I think you will have a better idea of what normal eating is all about. But making the shift to internally regulated eating is hard and scary, and (if you fit my description) you could use some help.

Stop Putting Kids On Diets

Early obesity is NOT predictive of later obesity[5], and diets don't work very well, anyway[6]. Rather than imposing diets on kids, it is better to work on having a positive feeding relationship throughout the growing-up years. That way, your child will retain her inborn ability to regulate her food intake based on her internal cues of hunger, appetite and satiety.

If there is something about your child that indicates automatic food regulation processes might be easily overwhelmed, like a strong genetic tendency to obesity, then add on some indirect tactics like we talked about in Helping All You Can to Keep Your Child From Being Fat (Chapter 14).

Correct Society's Attitudes About Weight

We have to begin to moderate some of our societal terror about obesity. People are so afraid of becoming fat that they are willing to go to almost any lengths in order to avoid it. Even thin people do things to themselves that are unhealthy in order to prevent the fatness they dread.

We need to develop a, you should pardon the expression, broader definition of physical attractiveness. Some trends are changing—I see more and more articles about fashion shows for big people, and retailers and pattern manufacturers are starting to turn out stylish and flattering clothes in large sizes. More and more health professionals are speaking out about the dangers and futility of repeated dieting.

But other trends are going in the wrong direction. Playboy center folds are getting thinner, as are Miss America contest winners. One humorist calculated that if Miss America continues to get thinner at her present rate, in another twenty years, she will be dead! A study by a University of Minnesota psychologist indicated that the incidence of bulimia from 1980 to 1983 tripled, from 1% to 3% of incoming university freshmen women[7].

Despite these alarming statistics, and despite severe societal pressures to diet and be thin, you can help your child to be less vulnerable. You can be steady and accepting of her body the way it is turning out, and discourage her from dieting and trying to manipulate her weight. You can let her know that you think she is beautiful the way she is, and share what you know about the normal growth process. She will probably act like she doesn't believe you and like you don't know anything about it, but she will listen and be reassured by your steadiness.

If you think your child is having trouble with her eating and has some bad feelings about herself, get help as a family. It can make an enormous a difference for you all.

343

References

1.   Humphrey, L.L.: Family relations in bulimic-anorexic and nondistressed families. International Journal of Eating Disorders 5:223-232, 1986.

2.   Heilbrun, A.B. and Harris, A.: Psychological defenses in females at-risk for anorexia nervosa: An explanation for excessive stress found in anorexic patients. International Journal of Eating Disorders 5:503-516, 1986.

3.   Olmsted, M.P. and Garner, D.M.: The significance of self-induced vomiting as a weight control method among nonclinical samples. International Journal of Eating Disorders 5:683-700, 1986.

4.   Satter, E.M.: Childhood eating disorders. Journal of the American Dietetic Association 86:357-361, 1986.

5.   Shapiro, L.R., Crawford, P.B., Clark, M.J., Pearson, D.J., Raz, J. and Huenemann, R.L.: Obesity prognosis: A longitudinal study of children from the age of 6 months to 9 years. American Journal of Public Health 74:968-972, l984.

6.   Peck, E.B. and Ullrich, H.D.: Children and Weight: A Changing Perspective. Berkeley: Nutrition Communication Associates, 1985.

7.   Pyle, R.L., Halvorson, P.A., Neuman, P.A., and Mitchell, J.E.: The increasing prevalence of bulimia in freshman college students. International Journal of Eating Disorders 5:631-647, 1986.

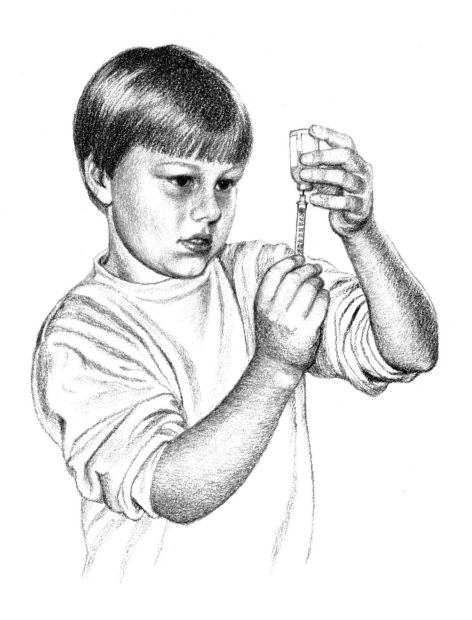

16

Feeding The Child With Special Needs

Some children have particular difficulty with eating. It may be hard for them to eat, period, as it is with the developmentally disabled child, and the one who has low-level nerve and muscle problems (that sometimes first show up with eating). Learning to eat is also hard for the child who gets a late start with eating, like the prematurely born child or the one who for some reason has been tube fed during his early months.

Some children have a hard time eating *enough*. For instance, the child with an unrepaired heart defect uses extra calories for breathing and circulating blood, but he doesn't have the energy to suck and take in those extra calories. The child with cystic fibrosis may have a hard time digesting and absorbing the calories from his food, in addition to needing more calories to fight infection and to breathe.

Some children face special challenges in *regulating* the amount they eat. Children with diabetes have to be more consistent in the amounts they eat to match their injected insulin.

Some children have special problems with food *selection*. Children with food allergies, for instance, have to become pretty sophisticated about what's IN food so they don't get in trouble.

347

Children with inborn errors of metabolism have to follow exquisitely regulated diets to function well, or even to survive.

Any of these problems can cause severe distortions in the feeding relationship, distortions that radiate outward to affect the whole parent-child interaction and the way a child feels about himself. It need not be so. It is possible to parent the child with special needs in such a way that he can hold on to his self esteem and grow up able to take as much responsibility for himself as he reasonably can. It is hard, but it *is* possible.

My intent in this chapter is to help you develop a positive feeding relationship with your special-needs child. I'm not going to try to tell you how to manage the condition or the nutritional problems that go along with it. You need to get that information from specialists. But specialists often don't tell you how to manage the feeding relationship. I know about that, and I'll give you some ideas about how you can do it.

In every case, it is vital for you to establish a good working relationship with your doctor, a registered dietitian, and the support people who specialize in your child's condition. The emphasis is on *good working relationship*. If they give you advice that precipitates feeding problems, they need to know that, and together you have to figure out something that works with your particular child.

You may find that you have to be your child's advocate in the area of feeding. When medical people are dealing with life-threatening conditions, paying attention to your child's eating may seem like a luxury. It's not. If your child is to grow up and fit into the world, he has to know how to eat.

Learning to eat is most easily accomplished early on. The eating function, and positive feeding relationships, are more easily maintained than restored. Be a pest, be a thorn under the saddle, if you must. But be persistent in seeing that feeding gets taken care of.

The Child Who Has A Hard Time Eating

In some cases, eating problems stem from neuromuscular (nerve and muscle) problems—severe ones like cerebral palsy or mental retardation. There are also not-so-severe but puzzling

348

nerve and muscle problems like slow development for no apparent reason with some babies whose mouths and throats just don't work right. Children with nerve and muscle problems are typically slow to develop, slow to show the signs that let us know they are ready to progress with their feeding, and slow to learn feeding skills once their capability does develop.

Sometimes children have a hard time learning to eat because they have had some medical problem and haven't been fed by mouth for a while. Many times children are tube fed, for whatever reason, and when it is time to get back on oral feedings again they have a terrible time making the transition.

The Child With Developmental Disabilities

Children with developmental disabilities have particular problems learning to eat. Children with cerebral palsy or Down's syndrome, for instance, have structural and neuromuscular problems that make it hard for them to work their mouths and deal with the mechanics of eating. Teaching them how to eat requires skilled and painstaking work by professionals, like occupational therapists, physical therapists and speech therapists who specialize in feeding.

Professionals who work with mentally and physically handicapped children give careful attention to engaging them in the process of feeding. They solicit their cooperation in opening their mouths, chewing and swallowing, rather than simply imposing feeding on them. In the same way, they recognize that even severely handicapped people have the ability to regulate the amounts they eat, and they depend on those regulatory cues to guide them in the amounts they feed.

Feeding handicapped children in this respectful fashion allows them the dignity of controlling that which they are able to control. As I will elaborate toward the end of this chapter, this and other subtle (and not so subtle) ways of protecting that child's self esteem will make all the difference in how successful he can be in life.

You might have to be a humane-feeding advocate for your child. To help you with that, and with other aspects of feeding, I highly recommend *Mealtimes for Persons with Severe Handicaps*[1]. In the introduction of the first release, in 1977, of this sensitive and uplifting book, authors observed the "excruciatingly

349

long. . .frustrating and unpleasant for everyone" mealtimes in the homes of handicapped children.

The situation they observed in some institutions and community service systems was even worse. The "quiet little murders" that went on at mealtimes in these places were long overdue for change. The authors saw mealtimes for handicapped people as a time of feeling comradeship and belonging, communicating, being accepted, making choices. In their book, they sounded "a gentle call to revolution. . .directed toward making mealtimes as important for persons who have a hard time speaking and doing for themselves as mealtimes are for the rest of us."

In the 9 years since its first publication, the authors see some signs of optimism: "We know better now, and we never want to go back to those terrible days again."

The Critically Ill Child

As more and more critically-ill children are being saved by modern medicine, we are seeing an increasing incidence of children who are getting through their first year, or their first several years, without learning to eat. They are fed through their veins or they are tube fed: given liquid feedings through tubes threaded through their nose and esophagus into the stomach, or surgically implanted into the stomach through the abdominal wall.

There are lots of medical problems that can end up requiring these special feeding procedures. One of the more common ones is bronchopulmonary dysplagia. This is a treatment-caused dysfunction of the lungs caused by respirators. Children with BPD have been subjected to the heroic procedures needed to preserve life in intensive care nurseries. Many of these impose a great deal of stress to the mouth and throat: respirators, suctioning, feeding tubes. In many cases, a child's mouth is monopolized by treatment apparatus, or if it is available for feeding, he gets so sensitive around his mouth that eating normally is revolting to him and entirely out of the question. The lung problem can go on for years, and children's feeding sensitivity can, too.

Children also may get tube fed because of some defect in their digestive system, like a girl who fractured her jaw in a

350

swing accident or a little boy who was born with no voice box and an abnormality in his throat and esophagus, or another who had a short gut so he couldn't digest his foods properly. Sometimes the child with a heart defect is fed by tube to promote growth so he can tolerate surgery. Tube feeding becomes even more of a necessity when a baby has multiple birth defects, such as nerve and muscle problems that go along with a heart defect, like many children born with cerebral palsy.

The best tube feeding situations are those in which the eating function can be maintained in a developmentally appropriate fashion. In many cases, tube fed children can still eat. Even if they can only eat tiny amounts, it is worth continuing oral feedings, and using the tube feeding as a supplement.

If the child absolutely *can't* eat, it may still be possible for him to mouth other things. He can, for instance, suck on a pacifier or be taught how to put his fingers or toys in his mouth. Putting things in his mouth will help tone down its sensitivity, and present one less hurdle to eating when the time comes.

Eventually, children get to the point where it is time for them to learn to eat. If a child has had no experience eating, he really has his work cut out for him. And so do we.

We are all learning together in the area of feeding problems. Many hospitals are setting up feeding teams to try to develop ways to help these handicapped children. Usually the team includes a speech therapist to deal with mouth and throat problems, an occupational therapist to deal with hand and arm movement, a physical therapist to deal with body positioning and control, a dietitian to help insure a nutritionally desirable food selection, and the physician who specializes in that particular child's condition.

Tom Tatum, a certified speech pathologist in Fresno, California, helped set up a feeding team in his area. He also has a private practice as a feeding therapist. He was gracious enough to share his information with me.

Tatum says, first off, that parents and professionals shouldn't automatically assume that if a child doesn't eat, he is just being stubborn. There may be things going on with him that are making it hard for him to eat. And don't assume that he will eat if he gets hungry enough. Whatever he has to overcome to be able to eat might be too pressing for that. For instance, the child who has been tube fed for a long time may find that

351

having anything in his mouth is extremely unpleasant, and if he tries to swallow he may gag a great deal and may even choke, which is very frightening.

Even the normal little baby has a very sensitive mouth and a very well-developed gag reflex. That sensitivity decreases as he has mouth experiences, such as learning to deal with the nipple. Before it is time to start eating solids, babies generally start sticking things in their mouths. At first they gag a lot, but eventually that gag reflex gets toned down, they learn to keep things off the back of their tongues, and the gagging and sensitivity decrease.

Kids who have poor muscle control can't put things in their mouths. If they were tube fed, they have had no experience with mouthing, so they stay very sensitive. To make matters worse, tube feeding allows the muscles at the back of the throat to get very tight. The area feels tense and irritated, and they feel like they are going to choke if they try to swallow anything. They gag and cough easily and the gagging puts them off. A dietitian on the pediatric intensive care unit at the University of Nebraska said they had one little boy who was so sensitive to eating that he would throw up when they brought food into the ROOM.

Tatum says that when you work with these little kids, first you have to make sure their medical issues have been taken care of. Then, he says, the most important thing is to insure TRUST. The child has to know that the therapist isn't going to try to get him to do anything he can't do. Then he makes it a clinical thing—they are very positive and orderly about what they work on and they just take it one step at a time.

At first Tatum only presents food for tasting. He doesn't ask the child to swallow. In fact, he tells him specifically that he is not to swallow and that he is to spit the food back out after he tastes it. They work quite a few sessions on that step, and Tatum keeps records on what the child does and doesn't like.

Then, he has the child come hungry, and they work on swallowing. He prepares something he knows the child likes in a very soft form so that it naturally flows around in the child's mouth, and part of it goes far enough back on his tongue to activate his swallow reflex. And he swallows. And discovers he can. That is the hardest step of all.

And so they go—ever so slowly. It takes an expert to know

how to gradually build up the child's abilities and how to challenge him without overwhelming him. Tatum says if you challenge too much and the child can't handle it, you have to start again, way back at the beginning. He says he can tell when a child will have trouble with a food, and he gets him to spit it out right away.

And so they progress. It is slow and painstaking, but eventually children *do* learn to eat.

Professionals who work with children have a variety of ways of getting the job done. Dr. Thomas Linscheid, a psychologist who works at Children's Hospital in Columbus, Ohio, has used behavioral modification techniques to resolve children's feeding problems ranging from teaching an autistic child to eat to stopping mealtime tantruming and food throwing[2].

When I visited with him in Cleveland, he told me about teaching a six-year-old boy to eat. This child had been fed by gastrostomy tube (a tube surgically inserted through the abdominal wall and into the stomach) since birth, and he had never eaten. He was going to regular school. He took his liquid feeding at school in the nurse's office, using his special syringe. As far as it went, he actually was taking pretty good care of himself. But he was missing out on the sociability of lunch hour, and the other kids were starting to think he was a little strange. He could, of course, have learned to live with that. But he didn't have to.

The original problem was that he had short gut syndrome. As a baby he had had to have a special formula, in quantity, one that had the protein, fat and carbohydrate in it predigested so with his limited intestine he could capture the nutrients as quickly as possible. As he had gotten older, the capacity of his bowel to digest and absorb food had improved, so he was able to make the transition to oral feedings.

When he was a baby, Dr. Linscheid's little patient had been through it all, and he had come out of it desperately afraid to eat. After they got acquainted, the first step in the eating treatment was for him to bring the spoon *to his mouth*. That's all. He didn't have to have anything on the spoon, and he didn't have to put it in his mouth. He just had to bring it *to* his mouth. And he was terrified.

Linscheid told him, once, what he wanted him to do, then simply sat there and waited. He did not remind him or try to

353

reassure or persuade or cajole him. Finally, after half an hour of crying, the little boy brought the spoon to his mouth.

They worked through the same careful progression that Tom Tatum does with his patients: something IN the spoon, to something mushy in the mouth, to swallowing, to chewing-and-swallowing. Throughout, the boy was afraid, and struggled to overcome his fear. And he complained about how sensitive his mouth was. To him, it was painful to eat bananas—because they had such "great big seeds." Spaghetti was too coarse. For a long time he couldn't manage turkey, because the fibers came apart in his mouth and he didn't have the skills with his tongue and jaws to chase the pieces.

Finally, they made it to the point where he could eat a variety of soft and cooked foods. The little boy was very proud, as he had every right to be. He had achieved something pretty great.

These children are so afraid of eating that they can be called *eating phobic*. Teaching an eating phobic child to eat is a task that is best taken on by a professional. If the child is in danger of choking, or if the treatment could temporarily make the child's condition worse, the task should be done under medical supervision, perhaps even in the hospital. Such precautions are needed for the kind of structure and follow-through that is necessary to teach such a child to eat.

As a parent, you can't do this. You are too worried and too emotionally involved. You don't have experience with a variety of children to fall back on, so you couldn't know that a child, who reacts so vehemently to the idea of eating, will eventually come around and do it. Behaviorists can do it because they are trained by experience to be less emotionally involved, and they have access to techniques like reinforcement, shaping, and fading to get new behaviors started. Even if they don't know much about treating eating, they can read about it in their professional literature[2,3], and apply the basic techniques, which are the same as for other problems, to eating treatment.

The feeding team at the University of Iowa uses forcing to get past the child's resistance and anxiety about eating. The feeder, in a matter-of-fact fashion, immobilizes the child, forces food into his mouth and physically keeps it there. After a few days of forcing, the child's resistance decreases, until eventually he gets to the point where he will eat.

354

The program works, because trainers are experienced and they don't chicken out. I object to the forcing, however, and Tatum and Linschied have demonstrated that it is unnecessary. The non-forcing programs may take longer, but they don't insult the child's dignity, and they don't increase his anxiety. Once you initiate a forcing program, you HAVE to see it through, or the child will end up more phobic about eating than he was before.

Prematurely-born Children

Children who have been born prematurely present their own particular set of problems with feeding. They may have the same mouth sensitivity problems as the other kids we talked about. On top of that, they have no concept of hunger, because in the premature nursery they have either been fed on a schedule or have been fed using a continuous-drip process of tube feeding around the clock. But most difficult of all, they are not sociable.

Preterm infants are less alert and responsive than full-term infants, and parents have more difficulty interacting with them. Parents of preterm infants, in comparison with those with full-term infants, do less talking, touching, smiling and mutual gazing with their infants during the period right after the baby is born. When the babies are somewhat older, parents are generally more active in stimulating preterm infants than they are with full-term ones, whereas the infants tend to remain relatively inattentive, and to be fussy, especially if they have been ill during the neonatal period. Parents are so active, in fact, during the first six months that babies may withdraw rather than engage During the second six months, some parents begin to tone down their approach and become more successful with their child. Others become *under*active, as if they have given up on the relationship[4].

I can understand why those babies would be hard to get through to. When I was in Akron, I toured the children's hospital. Their premature nursery is top-notch, and staffed by the most caring and dedicated people you can imagine. But it is still a heart rending place. The babies are in their little glass boxes and hooked up to all kinds of tubes and needles. They are working so hard just to stay alive. Some are on respirators—they are having their breathing done for them by machine—and their whole bodies seem to work *so* hard to help. It must be terribly hard to have your child go through that.

It is a tough world to be in, and those premature babies have their ways of coping. They devote all their energies to surviving, and they shut the rest out. They simply withdraw into themselves, and don't register what happens.

Once they get home, they continue to shut the world out. They have to be won over, and reassured that the world is not such an awful place after all. That is not easy for anyone, but it is especially difficult for a parent who has also been through so much and who is now being confronted with someone who seems so tiny and vulnerable.

Until they become more sociable, prematurely-born babies probably don't find it particularly gratifying to have someone feed them and take pleasure with them in the feeding situation. At first feeding may feel like just one more unpleasant procedure, of the sort that they have been exposed to all along.

Premature babies act like they are wired, and it takes them until about halfway through their second year before they really settle down. They have to be approached slowly and reassuringly, and demands made on them must be made in the most slow and painstaking way. Learning to nipple feed is a big accomplishment, and learning to eat semi-solid and then solid foods is another.

Generally, premature babies learn how to nipple feed before they go home from the hospital. While individual children vary, how well or poorly that transition goes seems to depend largely on the attitudes of the nursery personnel. I talked with professionals in one nursery who had a terrible time getting their babies on to nipple feeding. Babies were very resistant, and nursery workers were quite desperate. In another nursery, the attitude was very relaxed. "Oh, it takes a while," they said, "but eventually they all learn."

Even in the best of premature nurseries, babies are often sent home before they make one very important transition: shifting from external to internal control of their food intake. When they are first born they don't have the ability to regulate their food intake, or even to get food into themselves. By necessity, the professionals in the premature nursery decide what, when, and how much they will eat.

Once they learn how to suckle and gain enough strength to eat the amount they need, however, they can begin to go on their own and can start to be in charge of when and how much they eat. But a transition has to be made, and it's a big one for adults as well as for children. Adults are afraid they will starve.

To make the transition to internal regulation of food intake, it's necessary to back off on the feeding schedule and back off on amounts and begin to give the child a chance to get hungry. You need to realize that a premature infant's feeding cues may be entirely different from those of a baby who was not born prematurely. He may show only subtle signs of hunger—he may become tired, irritable or sleepy—rather than doing any crying or seeming distressed.

Eventually, he will start to make the association between his set of upset feelings and hunger, and he will develop ways of more clearly communicating that he wants to eat. You can help him begin to make that association. Before feeding, get him to wait a bit while he sits on your lap, and show him the breast or bottle and talk to him about being hungry. He needs a few moments to anticipate being fed.

It's very easy to get pushy with the bottle feeding, but so important not to. Forcing will just make him retreat all the more. When they feed their babies, many nursery people force nipples in or try to get babies to take a few more drops. Parents see that, and do the same thing. It doesn't help. Studies have shown that babies eat less, not more, when feeders get too active. Babies do better with eating when they have the feeling they are in control. The best feeding is as smooth and continuous as possible, with an absolute minimum of jiggling, burping and cleaning up[5].

The sensitive and observant infant-feeding techniques I talked about in The Newborn (Chapter 7) are especially important for the prematurely-born baby. If you have such a guarded little baby, it could be very helpful for you to get in an outside observer to help you pick up on what you are doing, and help you generate approaches to winning him over.

It's important not to rush. When you and your baby get bottle-feeding down pat, you need some time to enjoy your accomplishment—and each other. You and your baby truly need that pleasant and cozy time with each other. Starting solids can wait until you are ready.

Chances are you won't be ready until at least as much later as your baby was premature. Or later. Don't even *think* of starting solids for a preemie born at seven months gestation until he's eight months old—two months later than desirable for a baby born at term. With the preemie as with the child with no problems, wait to start solids until you see his signs of readiness: sitting up, following the spoon with his eyes, and opening up when he sees it approach his mouth.

Take it *real* easy in moving things along, and make as few demands as possible. Premature babies are sensitive, and they are likely to retreat like they did in the nursery when they are confronted with anything new. For instance, when you start cereal you should stick to one kind, only, always use the same spoon, and stir it up so it is smooth and thin. If you want to increase the thickness, you should do it very slowly. That might be enough for a month. Make sure feeding gets to the point where you both enjoy it, and take time to appreciate your accomplishments before you push on.

Then, when it is time to start fruits or vegetables, be very careful to start them one at a time, and offer the same food for three or four days until your baby gets really used to it. Use baby food or pureed food rather than anything that is lumpy. Flavor differences and subtle differences in consistency are probably all this cautious baby will be able to handle. Pureed bananas feel a lot different from baby cereal, which certainly feels a lot different from pureed pears. Once you have spent a lot of time with pureed food, then ever-so-gradually start with lumps. And so on.

Your baby may be 18 months old before he really gets on table food. That may cause problems for you—health workers and your friends may think you are being too slow. If there is any hazard to this approach, it is that your baby will get stuck on pureed foods and refuse to go any farther. I don't think you'll get stuck, however, if you gradually challenge your baby with eating all along the way, and if you are careful to engage him in the process and not force. The techniques I covered in The Older Baby (Chapter 8) are especially important for your careful little one.

This baby is also nutritionally fragile, so don't be in a hurry to switch from formula to regular milk. Make sure he is *well* established on table food before you make the switch, make it to WHOLE milk and do it gradually. You will probably just have to spike the formula with milk at first, and then gradually increase the proportion of whole milk until you have made the

358

switch. Remember, with these little kids, any change is a threat and can seem like something bad is about to happen to them.

A young mother came to see me about her fourteen month old son, who had been born two months prematurely. She wanted him to start eating table food, and he was being very cautious about it. He would sit and look at a new food for the longest time, and then he would knock it on the floor. Later, after it got a little more familiar, he had started to put some cooked carrot or potatoes or whatever in his mouth and chew it up, but he then he would spit it back out again. He had yet to swallow something. She thought she understood why he was doing that—it was a way of experimenting without having to over-commit himself. But she still worried about it. What should she do?

Before I tried to answer her question, we reviewed his feeding history. Sure enough, he had all the characteristics of the premature baby. He had a hard time getting the hang of nippling, solids and lumps. And unfortunately, the mother had been getting some bad advice from someone who was encouraging her to push her little boy along with feeding.

So she had tried to start him on solids at six months, and he didn't want anything to do with it. In fact, he rejected the whole idea very forcefully—he sealed over. So she had left him alone for a couple of months and tried him again, and then, even though he wasn't exactly enthusiastic he did go along with semi-solid foods.

Again, the unhelpful advisor had come along and wondered why she was feeding him all the purchased baby food. Why didn't she just mash and mill foods from the family table? She tried, but again he reacted. Even very smooth mashed banana was different enough from bottled baby-food banana to be a threat to him, and the graininess of the carrots she had milled with the baby food grinder turned him off completely.

So she backed off again and they went back to the baby foods. The experiment with the home-prepared foods had set them back a bit, but eventually he regained his confidence and began eating the commercial baby foods quite happily.

By now the mother was getting the hang of feeding this cautious little baby of hers. She was also getting the reputation for being an over-concerned mother, because her advisors didn't understand why she had to be so solicitous with this child. But

359

she had learned her lesson, so she persisted in her sensitive handling of him.

When they started with lumps she spiked a lot of baby food carrots with very little milled carrots. He was right on to it and kind of rared back in his high chair and glared at her. But she spoke to him very reassuringly and gave him time to open his mouth again before she went on with feeding. The carrots were close enough to what he was used to, and her attitude was reassuring enough, so that they got past the first exposure. And they continued to progress—ever so gradually and painstakingly.

Even though she was feeling her way and doing things just right, this mother was wondering in the back of her mind if she was being too concerned about her child. Maybe, she worried, she was remembering his rough start and being overprotective. Each time they got into difficulties with learning to eat solid foods, her doubts came up again. And *that* was the real reason she came in to see me. She knew how to do it—better than I did. She was just looking for reassurance and some recognition for what a fine job she was doing with her sensitive little son.

She got it. I was full of admiration. I thought she was doing just swell.

The Child Who Has A Hard Time Eating The Right Amounts

In one of my workshops, I commented that my general recommendations for feeding could be used with diabetic children. A dietitian who specialized in the treatment of children with diabetes challenged that, and insisted that a division of responsibility in feeding was out of the question with diabetic children. In her view, someone else *had* to control the amounts they ate because of the nature of the diabetic regimen.

Diabetic children get insulin by injection. A certain amount of insulin covers for a certain amount of food. If a child eats too much, blood sugar goes up too high. If he eats too little, blood sugar goes down too low. Going too high can cause problems over the long run. Going too low can cause an insulin reaction: A child can become shaky, have convulsions, or pass out.

If blood sugar starts to go too low, children *have* to eat to get their blood sugar back up again. The dietitian said that in her experience parents *had* to watch their diabetic children closely to see if they showed signs of low blood sugar (like weakness, dizziness, irritability or sleepiness). If those signs appeared, they had to try to get food into them. Quickly. And children learned early to manipulate their parent's desperation to get them to eat. The parents begged, they threatened, they argued, they cajoled. Some even paid their children to eat.

The philosophy of the local doctors was that blood sugars be kept as near normal as possible. To achieve that, children had to have two or more insulin injections a day, and their blood sugars were kept so low that they were always just across the line from having an insulin reaction. If they didn't eat, an insulin reaction was virtually a sure thing.

I was very concerned about this whole affair. It didn't make sense to me to promote distorted eating in the name of maintaining diabetic control. The tactic seemed counter-productive over the long run. Parents might be able to get their children through early childhood in tight control of their blood sugars, but their life-long eating habits would suffer. Eventually, those distortions would catch up with them, and their diabetic control would go haywire. Every pediatric practice has a number of diabetic children who stop adhering to their regimen when they become adolescents.

I shared my concern in a letter to Deb McMillon, a dietitian friend in Kansas who has a two-year-old son who is diabetic. She wrote me back, and I have asked her permission to quote from her letter. I think she has a very helpful perspective on the matter.

"I have had this on my mind since I received your letter because the attitudes of those practitioners really upset me. (That's putting it mildly for a lack of how to express how strongly it hit me wrong!!!)

"One of the statements that Dr. Guthrie and his staff made to us the first week Christopher was diagnosed as diabetic has always stuck with me and is the basis of any advice I would ever give: 'He is a child first and a diabetic second.' The principles and habits those parents are teaching those children by paying them to eat seem to point toward their having the opposite philosophy: First a diabetic and then a child. That attitude leads to the child and his disease state controlling him and his family.

This is a situation to be avoided at all costs—but that is difficult when their doctors are making or at least initiating the problem.

"Before I continue I would like to provide you some facts I have learned from Dr. Guthrie—who I might add is one of the leading authorities on juvenile diabetes in the world*.

1. Blood vessel damage (one of the major degenerative problems with diabetes) does not occur until puberty. He fully believes in tight control (keep the blood sugar as near normal as possible) but not so tight as to produce insulin reactions (loss of consciousness from low blood sugar), as convulsions in a person under the age of 5 can cause brain damage. He also believes control shouldn't be so tight as to be oppressive.

2. Multiple injections? How many? More than two? I cannot imagine subjecting a small child to more than two—occasionally three for traveling. Adults now sometimes use four or five but in most cases when control is that difficult an insulin pump is used.

Christopher gets two shots a day: Pre-breakfast and pre-supper. He is at the point of extreme needle aversion so we test his blood as little as we can to see how his sugars are doing. And his tests show that he is in excellent control—and we don't even have to pay him to eat.

3. We adjust Christopher's insulin dosage frequently and we have the ability to do that. During a period of low food consumption we decrease his insulin and vice versa."

"I was already practicing the majority of your child feeding principles with my kids. They work very well with diabetics, although of course some modification becomes necessary at times. Christopher cannot leave the table without eating anything as Kelly can—but he can eat a bare minimum. If he doesn't want to eat *anything* (which is rare), we then set out what he needs to eat to leave the table for his desired activity. And we tell him, 'If you would just like to sit in the chair and color you only need to drink this glass of milk' and so on. This then gives him choices and makes him feel in command.

---

*Dr. R.A. Guthrie is, indeed, an authority—he practices in Wichita, KS, and is the author of reference 6.

"Christopher's eating or not eating do not occupy my life or his 100% of the time—which surely it must in some of these other families. I think I could rave on for ages, but perhaps I have said enough. As you can tell, this is a subject near and dear to my heart."

Deb didn't say it, but I know from other experience that she gets cooperation from Christopher on his eating because she is firm and matter-of-fact in her expectations, at the same time that she gives him a proper sense of responsibility. There is a lot that goes into that. The family has to be operating pretty well to set appropriate limits for a child. Parents have to have their feelings resolved about the child's condition. If they feel sorry for their diabetic child (or the one with kidney disease or phenyketonuria or other chronic condition), they may waffle on their regimen. They are not able to be matter-of-fact and firm, and the child begins to manipulate the system.

Managing the diabetic regimen is harder than managing other diseases with dietary restrictions because with diabetes you have to worry about HOW MUCH. Overcoming someone's natural abilities to regulate the quantity they eat is considerably more difficult than limiting their food selection. It's better if you can avoid getting into the area of dictating quantities of food. Generally Deb was avoiding that—she offered balanced meals and snacks and let Christopher eat as much as he wanted. However, at times she did have to insist on quantity. When she did that she tried to make her demands as limited as possible and to leave as much control with Christopher as possible.

It is not my goal here to recommend a diabetic regimen for your child. Only your doctor can do that. But you need to know there are different ways of working the regimen, ways that might allow you to be more successful. You can be firm with a child and doing all the right things, but if what you are trying to do is unrealistic you don't have much chance of making things come out right.

For instance, I wrote to Dr. Guthrie, and sent him this section to check it for accuracy. He wrote back, concurring with what Deb had to say. He says they try to keep blood sugars below 150, and "...try for the most effective control we can without this becoming oppressive."

He went on to explain his approach to diabetic management. They teach parents to provide structured, nutritious meals

363

and snacks, they let the child eat in accordance with his hunger and appetite, and they teach parents to adjust his insulin to balance out his food intake. This is the opposite of most programs of diabetic management, which standardize the insulin and try to get the child to eat regulated amounts to balance it.

For parents (and later, children) to follow this regimen, they have to know enough about food composition and calories so they can do a good job of menu planning and can follow along with insulin dosages in a knowledgeable way. But they let the child's appetite, rather than the insulin dosage, take the lead. And that can make all the difference.

If you find you simply can't achieve the management goals that have been set for your child, you need to work with your doctor to set other goals. You can't be on your own with this. You and your doctor have to hang in there with each other, until you can come up with something that allows your child to be appropriately responsible for himself. Anything less will make your child's illness a condition that limits his emotional and social growth.

Being lax on the medical regimen is not an option. If you do that you will end up with a child who is a tyrant and sicker than he has to be. In the long run his disease will be more important to him, not less.

The Child Who Has A Hard Time With Food Selection

Even with dietary regimens that are absolutely essential to the child's well-being, some families do well and some do poorly. Phenyketonuria is only one of a number of a genetic diseases that will make a child mentally retarded unless he eats a very specially prepared diet.

Families of children with these inborn errors of metabolism often get lots of special attention: The kids are tested and followed, the families are instructed carefully on very special dietary procedures and get careful training. What happens after that is variable. In some families the kids and parents are creative and compliant with the regimen; they do it without a lot of fuss. Other families don't comply or fight about it.

There is a place to be firm about eating, and you can do it without stepping over the bounds we have talked about throughout this book—the division of responsibility. The parent is responsible for what the child is offered to eat, the child for eating it. The child with PKU has very narrow limits for what he can eat, and the parent need not feel apologetic about imposing those limits. The child with allergies has similar limits, and they are important ones.

My friend Rosie's son is allergic to a lot of things, from citrus to corn to seafood, and they have learned to avoid them. He can tell you all the unexpected places you find citrus and corn in foods—and there are a lot.

He's very responsible, but he doesn't think of everything. That's how he ended up in the emergency room in shock after he ate a lemon drop that a neighbor gave him. His mother didn't scold him. She just said, "That was a tricky one!" When you delegate responsibility, you also delegate the privilege of making mistakes.

The Child Who Has A Hard Time Eating Enough

Eating more than you want can be as bad as eating less than you want. Overeating can make you nauseated and uncomfortable and totally turned off to food. To do well, children with some medical problems have to eat more than they want.

Children with cystic fibrosis, unrepaired heart defects and malignancies have a particularly high energy requirement. It is hard for them to eat enough.

Cystic Fibrosis

Cystic fibrosis is a severe inherited disease of the pancreas that interferes with production of digestive enzymes and healthy functioning of the mucous membranes that line the intestine and lungs. Children with cystic fibrosis have a lot of lung congestion and breathing problems, and they aren't very efficient at digesting their food and getting the nutrients out of it. A lot of what they eat just goes right through the digestive tract.

365

As a consequence, they don't grow very well, and they always feel listless and tired.

Children with cystic fibrosis do much better when they get enough to eat. They grow better, they are more energetic, and they don't have as many problems with their lungs. It is worth going to considerable extra trouble to help them eat more.

There are a variety of ways to help children with cystic fibrosis get extra calories[7]. They can be offered meals and snacks of high fat content—fat carries a lot of calories in relatively little volume. Sugary foods also carry a lot of calories, but some children get tired of the sweet taste. There are some specially prepared foods that are helpful for getting in extra calories. Polycose® for instance, is a carbohydrate that is almost tasteless and can be added in larger quantities to foods without giving such an over-sweet taste as regular sugar. There are also some formulations (used particularly with younger children) that have special, more easily-digested fats in them, called medium chain triglycerides. Children might also have special high calorie drinks to supplement their meals and snacks, like milkshakes or Instant Breakfast®.

Sometimes children with cystic fibrosis have big appetites and eat enormous amounts, other times their appetites are poor. But whether they are eating a lot or eating a little, eventually they get full and have a hard time eating as much as they need. But when they are older and can understand their condition, they may be willing to overfeed themselves. When they are little, they won't overeat, and parents and children can get into the same pitched battles over eating that we saw earlier in this book.

Crista Dean, a dietitian at University of Wisconsin Hospitals Pediatric Special Clinics, often sees parents and children who have become entangled in struggles over eating. Parents become over anxious, and they try to force their children to eat. Children become resistant, and refuse to eat what and when their parents ask. Parents go to a lot of trouble to make special foods, and children refuse them, and parents feel hurt, angry and frustrated. Eating degenerates into a contest that nobody wins.

Dean says she can often help diffuse the struggle by asking the child directly to be responsible for his own eating. She tells him that he and she make a team, and together they will work out a way to manage his eating. And they do. She makes the child responsible for what and how much he eats, outlines the possible consequences of his behavior, and lets him make his decisions. She meets with parents periodically to advise them about what they can do to be supportive, but not managing, of the child's efforts.

When the pressure is taken off the situation, children with cystic fibrosis generally do better with their eating than they have before. The feeding relationship around home improves, and that is a relief to everyone.

However, even the best-intended and most motivated child may not be able to eat enough to keep himself as healthy as he can be. That is when treatment teams resort to tube feedings.

Some children with cystic fibrosis use supplemental tube feedings at night. Many of them find it a great relief to have this way of getting in the extra calories they need without having to put so much pressure on their eating.

Some children use nasogastric tubes to give those tube feedings, and even thread the tubes and swallow them by themselves. Other children have a gastrostomy tube surgically implanted, and use that for their night feedings. The tube may be "capped" with a gastric button. That works on the same principle, except instead of a tube sticking out of their stomach, they have a little valve that looks like the air valve on a beach ball. The button is less conspicuous, and that is important to children, who are concerned about the way they look.

Parents and children get pretty matter-of-fact about tube feedings. It is important, though, that once a child is old enough, he be involved in making the decision about tube feeding. If he truly doesn't want the tube feeding, going ahead with it anyway is force feeding just as surely as packing food in with a spoon.

Congenital Heart Defects

Children who have heart defects have to eat enough to be strong enough for surgery. It is hard for them to do that, because they breathe fast and that interferes with their nursing. They're tired because their hearts don't work very well—often too tired to eat.

Such babies look small and fragile, and it is hard for parents to contain their anxiety about feeding. The babies' eating goes up, and their eating goes down, and along with it, parents' spirits. When it goes up, parents are hopeful that the situation is finally improving. When it goes down they are devastated and fear that it is the beginning of the end.

With these children, as well, it is important not to get into struggles over feeding. It won't help. As one sensitive young mother commented, it just made them unhappy with each other, and her son didn't eat any better, anyway. He was growing ever so slowly, and she was beginning to despair that he ever would be ready for surgery. It helped her when she looked at the food intake chart of little baby J that I talked about in How Much Should Your Child Eat? (Chapter 4). When his eating fell off, she was able to reassure herself that this was just normal variation.

Sometimes babies with heart defects are given more concentrated formula so they can get more calories in with less work. This is tricky, however, because of their rapid breathing. They can lose a lot of body fluid that way, and if the formula has less total water in it, they can end up dehydrated. Sometimes babies with heart defects are given supplemental tube feedings. That is a very reasonable option, and really better than getting into feeding struggles.

Tube Feeding As A Supplement To Oral Feeding

The management of tube feeding requires careful nutritional supervision. The composition of the formula has to be right, and the amounts the baby takes have to be adjusted to his needs. That doesn't always happen.

A dietitian from Illinois called me, seeking help with her small patient. She was working with a one-year-old who had been on gastrostomy feedings since he was four months old. He was scheduled for heart surgery some time in the next half year. Until the mother sought out the dietitian on her own, there had been no clear plan for his feeding. He had four doctors, each with different advice on feeding: "Give him more protein—he doesn't have much muscle tone—cut down on his amounts—his stomach is getting too fat—feed him by mouth—don't bother." On her own, the mother began using formula with solids in it for a tube feeding, and also giving him solids from a spoon— which he vomited up.

Clearly, the mother needed a lot of help with feeding. The situation was so foreign and so overwhelming to her, the only question she could think to ask was whether they should persist with oral feedings.

The answer was, "Yes." He was getting bolus feedings (a set amount at set times, rather than "continuous drip" feedings where he would be fed all the time), and that was good. She could arrange to have the tube feeding at a different time from his oral feedings. Or she could only give part of a tube feeding and then let him eat. He might not be willing to stand for oral feeding when he was acutely hungry, but might go along with it part way through the feeding.

It was important that she not react to his vomiting. If she got excited about it, she could inadvertently reinforce it: He might continue do it just to get her reaction. The goal was to preserve his oral feeding skills and acceptance of oral feedings so when he got over his operation he would be willing to go back to eating. Otherwise, he could have an enormous barrier to overcome.

From responding to her immediate concerns, the dietitian was able to move with the mother to the more pressing nutritional concern of choosing an appropriate tube feeding and getting the quantities adjusted to the baby's needs.

From this example emerges some general principles you should observe if your child has to have tube feedings.

Take feeding seriously. With all his other problems, feeding might seem like the least of his concerns. But if you take the long view, your child will get past this crisis and will get to the point where he is going to be more like any other kid. Eating is an important part of that. You can't get birthday cake or school lunch through a gastrostomy tube. Well you can, but you'd have to blend it first, and that isn't really the point, is it?

Take nutrition seriously. It is astonishing to me that a child with this many feeding limitations could have gotten to be a year old without having any expert nutritional supervision. Ask for a referral to a registered dietitian. That person is the nutrition expert. Find out what to put in the tube, and how much, and how to go about oral feedings.

It is best to continue oral feedings, using developmentally appropriate food. It doesn't have to be a lot—even one or two teaspoons at regular feeding times will do it. Get your child up to the table with the rest of the family and teach him normal feeding behaviors, just like you would a child who wasn't being fed by tube. You might feed part of a meal, let him eat what he will from the table, then finish off afterwards with the right volume of food. It is even better to give the tube feeding as a snack, so it doesn't interfere with meal acceptance.

Be careful you don't associate over-fullness with oral feeding. If your child's appetite is poor, chances are you will be feeding past his feelings of fullness in order to get enough calories into him to grow appropriately. Getting too full feels bad. Make sure that you feed in such a way that he gets too full on the tube feeding, not on what he eats. Or, perhaps more to the point, don't try to entice him to eat after he has already had a full gastrostomy feeding.

Kids With Life-Threatening Disease

Children with leukemia or other forms of cancer present a special and heart-rending problem in feeding. Parents feel if they could only get them to eat, maybe they would get better. But they don't eat very well, because their appetites are poor and many times the treatments make their mouths sore and even make food revolting to them.

Dietitians who work with cancer patients know how to entice them to eat with specially-prepared foods. Children have their own motivations to eat, even when they are very sick or maybe because they are very sick. You just have to do what you can by way of enticement and encouragement, and then let go of it.

Even when he is very sick, your child deserves the dignity of choosing how much and whether he will eat. It is so important to remember the quality of life, to preserve the relationship, and not let your precious times together be used up with struggles over eating.

General Thoughts On Childhood Handicaps

It's tough enough to raise an emotionally and socially healthy child, and if your child is sick or handicapped, it is even harder. As I struggled to straighten out my thinking in this area,

370

I found it helpful to talk with Dr. Lynn McDonald, a specialist in parenting and family dynamics of the handicapped child. I'd like to share what she said with you, because I think you'll find it helpful, too.

Dr. McDonald has done studies about the stresses that families experience as they take on the challenge of raising a special-needs child. These stresses wax and wane over the life span, and sometimes families feel taxed in their abilities. However, most families report actually being strengthened by meeting this challenge[8].

A powerful predictor of how well a child will do in spite of a handicapping condition is that child's level of self esteem. If you can help your child feel better about himself, he will do better in life. He, like you, will be appreciative of his total potential, rather than simply focussing on his limitations.

Your attitude toward your child's disability will have an impact on how he feels about himself. If you are able to say, "That's the way you are, now let's get on with it," it will help his self esteem. It is important at every age, says Dr. McDonald, to tune in on what the child *does* do and be attentive and affirmative about that. It is important *not* to focus on what other children that age are doing, or on expectations for that particular child.

Parenting is probably the hardest job we'll ever do. It is particularly so with the child with special needs. I wish you well with your enormously difficult task. I hope *How to Get Your Kid to Eat* has helped.

References

1. Perske, R., Clifton, A., McLean, B.M. and Ishler Stein, J.: Mealtimes for Persons with Severe Handicaps. Baltimore: Paul H. Brookes. 1986.

2. Linscheid, T.R.: Eating problems in children. IN: Walker, C.E., and Roberts, M.: Handbook of Clinical Child Psychology, John Wiley and Sons, 1983.

3. Linscheid, T.R.: Disturbances of eating and feeding. IN Drotar, Dennis. New Directions in Failure to Thrive; Proceedings of a Conference. New York, Plenum, 1986.

371

4. Magyary, D.: Early social interactions: Preterm infant-parent dyads. Issues in Comprehensive Pediatric Nursing 7:233-254, 1984.

5. Satter, E.M.: The feeding relationship. Journal of the American Dietetic Association 86:352-356, 1986.

6. Guthrie, R.A. and Jackson, R.L.: Complications. IN Jackson, R.L. and Guthrie, R.A. The Physiological Management of Diabetes in Children. New York, Elsevier, 1986.

7. Sondel, S. and Tluczek, A.: Cystic fibrosis: Nutritional support. Unpublished paper, University of Wisconsin Hospitals Specialty Clinics, 1986.

8. McDonald, L, Hanusa, D., and Stoycheff, J. Home-based respite care, the child with developmental disabilities and family stress. IN Salisbury, C.L. Respite Care: Support for Persons with Developmental Disabilities and their Families. Baltimore: Paul R. Brookes, 1986.

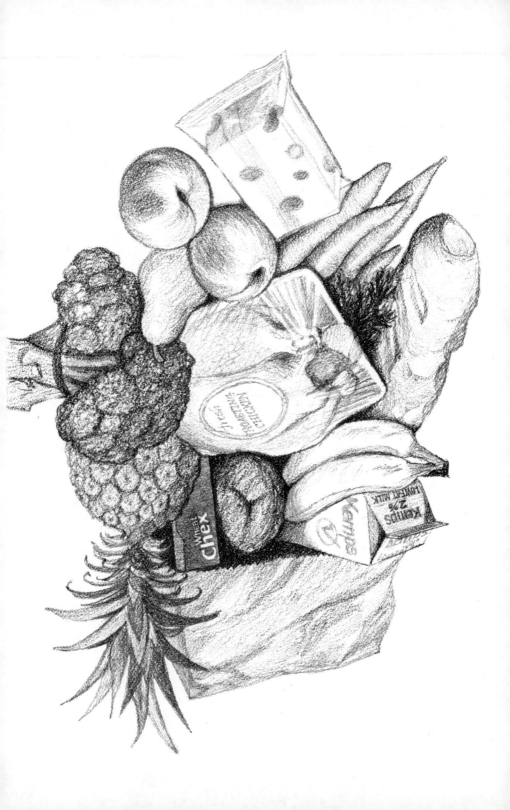

Tools & Strategies

Recommended Daily Pattern Of Food Selection

	Child 2-10	Adolescent Teenager	Adult
Milk	2 cups	4 cups	2 cups
Meat, fish, poultry, cooked dried beans, nuts	2-3 oz	4-5 oz	4-5 oz
Breads and cereals	4 serv.	4 serv.	4 serv.
Fruits and vegetables	4 serv.	4 serv.	4 serv.

Milk Group Portion Sizes

The following foods each give the calcium and at least the protein of an eight-ounce glass of milk. Fat and sugar content varies.

1 cup buttermilk or skim milk
1 cup chocolate milk or malted milk
1 cup yogurt
1½ ounces cheddar-type cheese
1 cup custard or milk pudding
1½ cup ice cream
1½ cup cottage cheese
¼ cheese pizza

Meat Group Portion Sizes

Foods from the meat group are good sources of protein, iron, B vitamins and trace elements. To help estimate portion sizes and think of alternatives, here are some examples of one- and three-ounce portions of meat and meat substitutes. Don't give nuts or seeds to small children as they might choke. Children like hot dogs and luncheon meats because they are soft and easy to chew. Don't overuse them, however. Once or twice a week is enough.

One ounce
1 egg
1 slice (1 oz) cheddar-type cheese
½ cup cooked dried beans, dried peas, lentils
2-3 tablespoons nuts or seeds
¼ cup cottage cheese
2 tablespoons peanut butter
2 slices bologna
1 hot dog
⅛ cheese pizza

Three ounces
One-fourth chicken (½ breast, or leg and thigh)
1 medium pork chop, ¾ inch thick
1 lean ground beef patty, made up four per pound
A piece of meat or fish the size and thickness of the palm of your hand

Breads and Cereals

Breads and cereals are good sources of B vitamins and iron and, if they are whole grain, fiber and trace elements. They are filling and satisfying and provide relatively few calories.

Use whole grain about half the time to get trace elements and fiber. Don't feel you have to use whole grain *all* the time. Too *much* fiber from whole grain can interfere with trace element absorption.

On the following list are one-serving equivalents of breads and cereals.

Bread: white, whole wheat, rye, raisin   1 slice

Bagel	½
Biscuit, dinner roll, muffin	1
Buns, hamburger, hot dog	½
Cereal, cooked	½ cup
Cereal, dry	¾ cup
Crackers	5-7 average
English muffin	½
Macaroni, spaghetti, noodles	½ cup cooked
Pancake, waffle	1 average
Rice, grits	½ cup
Taco shell, tortilla	1 average

Fruits And Vegetables

Fruits and vegetables are the primary sources of vitamins A and C in the diet. They contain other nutrients as well, such as calcium, B Vitamins, iron and trace elements. However, in selecting fruits and vegetables we look particularly for the ones that are good in vitamins A and C. If you get these two nutrients from natural foods and in adequate amounts, you can generally assume that you will get enough of the other nutrients you need.

Vitamin A in fruits and vegetables

Choose one excellent source every other day, or a combination of two good sources, or at least one good plus one fair source. If a child won't eat his vegetables, it is really vitamin A we are concerned about. Notice that there are fruits that are good "A" sources.

Excellent Sources	Good Sources	Fair Sources
Apricots, dried	Apricot nectar	Apricots
Cantaloupe	Asparagus	Brussel sprouts
Carrots	Broccoli	Peaches
Mixed vegetables	Nectarine	Peach nectar
Mango	Purple plums	Prunes
Pumpkin		Prune juice
Spinach, other greens		Tomatoes
Squash		Tomato juice
Sweet potatoes		Watermelon

U.S.D.A. Home and Garden Bulletin Number 72

Vitamin C in fruits and vegetables

Choose one excellent or two good sources per day. Almost all fruits and vegetables have some vitamin C, so eating a variety will assure good vitamin C nutrition.

Excellent Sources	Good Sources
Broccoli	Asparagus
Brussel sprouts	Bean sprouts, raw
Cabbage	Chard
Cauliflower	Honeydew melon
Cantaloupe	Potato
Grapefruit; grapefruit juice	Tangerine
Kohlrabi	Tomatoes, tomato juice
Mango	Pureed baby fruits
Oranges, orange juice	
Papaya	
Peppers	
Spinach	
Strawberries	
Vitamin-C fortified infant juices	

U.S.D.A. Home and Garden Bulletin number 72.

Fun Foods That Make Nutritional Sense

You don't have to be a puritan about good nutrition. "Snack" food, franchise food, convenience food can all be nutritious. Use it in moderation, like you should everything else in your diet. Here is a list of foods that can "perk up" your food selection. The list also tells you what the foods give you. Once you get the idea, you will have more ideas of your own.

Food	Meat	Milk	Fruit & veg	Bread
Chili	•		•	•
Tacos, burritos	•	•	•	•
Pizza	•	•	•	•
Spaghetti & meat balls or meat sauce	•		•	•
Lasagna	•	•	•	•
Beans: Bean soup, bean salads, refried beans, pork and beans	•		•	
Sandwiches: Hamburgers, hot dogs, peanut butter	•			•
With cheese	•	•		•
With lettuce, tomato, etc.	•	•	•	•

378

Choosing Nutritious Snacks

A snack that is filling and also that will keep your child satisfied should include some starch, some protein and some fat. The starch provides the bulk, the protein and fat the staying power. If your child is really hungry or if he has to wait quite a while until the next meal, an apple or some carrots just won't do the trick.

Here are some suggestions for nutritious snacks that will tide you over from one meal to the next.

Vegetable Snacks
Cut up fresh, raw vegetables. Serve with peanut butter, cheese, cottage cheese or milk* to get protein and fat. Add crackers or fruit juice to get carbohydrate.

Broccoli	Green beans
Carrots	Green peas
Cauliflower	Turnip sticks
Celery	Zucchini
Cucumber	

Use either 2% or whole milk to give fat.

Fresh Fruit Snacks
Slice or serve whole. Serve with peanut butter, cottage cheese, yogurt, ricotta cheese or milk to give protein and fat.

Apples	Berries	Peaches
Apricots	Grapefruit	Pears
Bananas	Grapes	Pineapple
	Melons	

Dried Fruit Snacks
Serve with nuts, almonds, cashews, peanuts, or with seeds (pumpkin, squash, sunflower) to give protein and fat. *Be very cautious about giving seeds and nuts to young children.*

Apples	Figs	Prunes
Apricots	Peaches	Raisins
Dates	Pears	

Nuts and Seeds
Peanuts, Pumpkin and squash kernels, Sunflower seeds.

Grain Products
A. *Bread products.* Use whole wheat about half the time. Read the label to make sure the flour is enriched or whole grain. (The first listed ingredient should be *whole* wheat.) Try a variety of yeast breads and quick breads—whole wheat, rye, oatmeal, mixed grains, bran—plain or with

379

dried fruit. Try rye crisps, whole grain flat bread, and whole grain crackers. Serve bread and crackers with cheese, peanut butter or a glass of milk to give protein and fat.

B. *Dry cereals:* Choose varieties with less than three grams of "sucrose or other sugar," *read the label,* per serving. Serve with milk to give protein and fat. Add dried fruits, nuts and seeds for variety and increased nutrients.

C. *Popcorn:* Try using grated cheese instead of salt and butter. Serve with milk or cocoa to give protein and fat.

D. *Cookies:* Bake your own, substituting ½ whole wheat flour for white flour. Try oatmeal, peanut butter or molasses cookies. Experiment with cutting down on sugar in recipes, often you can decrease sugar by ⅓ to ½. Serve cookies with milk to give protein (cookies already have fat).

Beverages

A. Use fruit juices and vegetable juices rather than powdered or canned fruit drinks which are high in sugar and lower in vitamins.

B. Milk: Serve plain with bread, crackers, cereal, etc. Mix in blender with banana, other fruit or orange juice for a healthy milkshake. Try adding vanilla extract, honey, molasses, even a little sugar. Use chocolate and strawberry flavorings for an occasional treat.

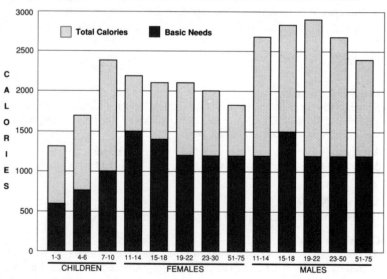

CALORIE REQUIREMENTS COMPARED WITH BASIC NEEDS

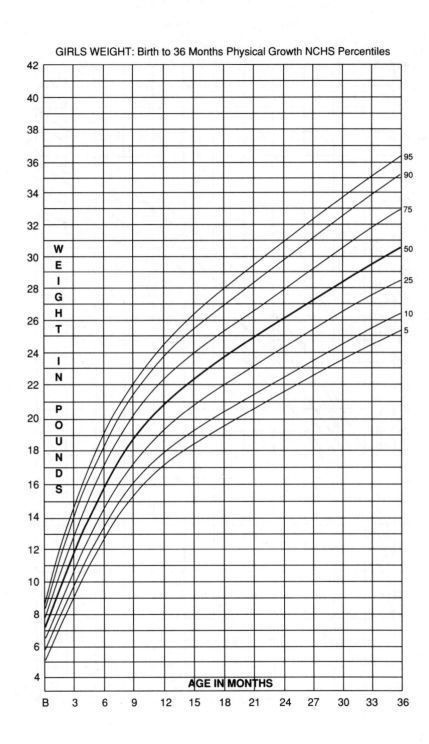

GIRLS WEIGHT: Birth to 36 Months Physical Growth NCHS Percentiles

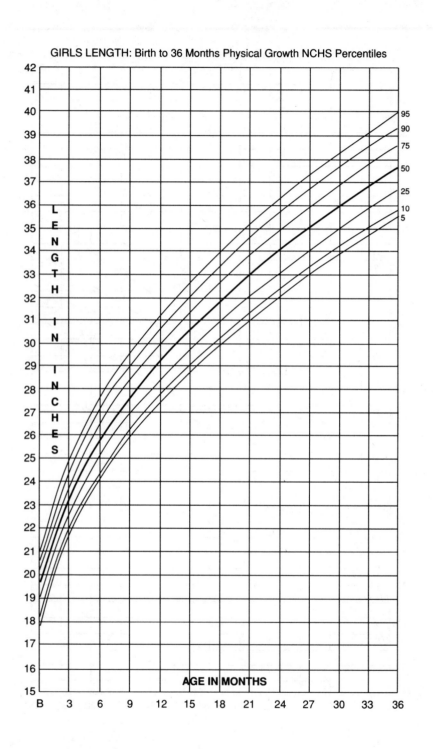

GIRLS LENGTH: Birth to 36 Months Physical Growth NCHS Percentiles

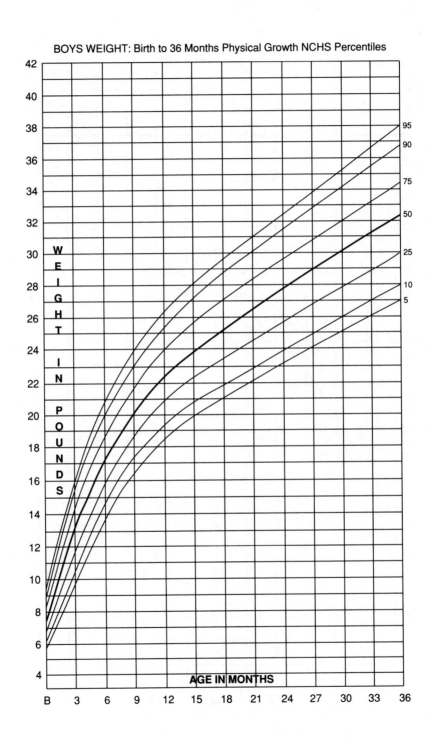

BOYS WEIGHT: Birth to 36 Months Physical Growth NCHS Percentiles

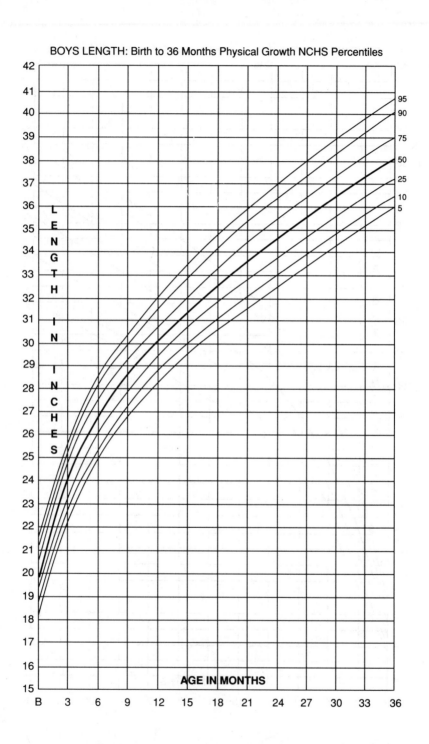

BOYS LENGTH: Birth to 36 Months Physical Growth NCHS Percentiles

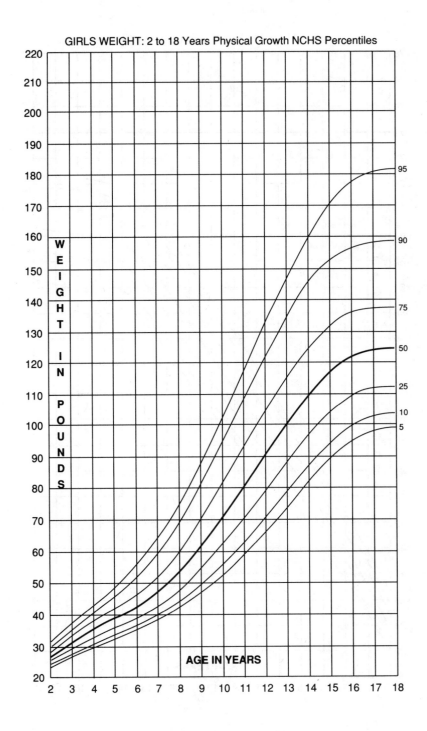

GIRLS WEIGHT: 2 to 18 Years Physical Growth NCHS Percentiles

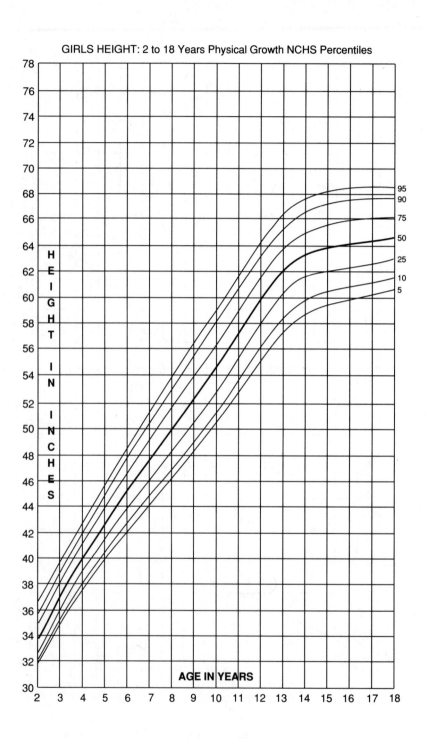

GIRLS HEIGHT: 2 to 18 Years Physical Growth NCHS Percentiles

BOYS WEIGHT: 2 to 18 Years Physical Growth NCHS Percentiles

BOYS HEIGHT: 2 to 18 Years Physical Growth NCHS Percentiles

Index

Titles of Related Interest

Child of Mine: Feeding with Love and Good Sense, by Ellyn Satter, RD, ACSW, 560 pages, $16.95

This book covers all the basics of child nutrition, including: nutrition for pregnancy; breastfeeding versus bottle feeding; calories and normal growth; introduction of solid foods to the infant diet; feeding the toddler; overweight children and childhood eating disorders.

Childhood Emergencies—What To Do, by Marin Child Care Council, 8$^1/_2$" x 11" flip-up format, $14.95

This is an easy-to-use quick reference guide that explains exactly what steps to take while waiting for medical assistance.

Topics covered include: CPR, choking, abdominal pain, abrasions, cuts, splinters, bites, bleeding, burns, broken bones, eye and ear injuries, poisons, toothaches, broken teeth. This booklet also includes information about childhood immunization, communicable diseases, diapering recommendations, proper handwashing techniques and a suggested list of contents for a first aid kit.